Oxford Medical Publications
Opioids in Cancer Pain

Opioids in Cancer Pain

Edited by

Mellar Davis
Director Research,
The Harry R. Horovitz Center for Palliative Medicine,
Cleveland, Ohio, USA

Paul Glare
Head, Dept of Palliative Care,
Royal Prince Alfred Hospital,
Sydney, Australia

and

Janet Hardy
Director of Palliative Care,
Mater Health Services, South Brisbane
Queensland, Australia

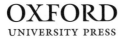

OXFORD
UNIVERSITY PRESS

OXFORD
UNIVERSITY PRESS

Great Clarendon Street, Oxford OX2 6DP

Oxford University Press is a department of the University of Oxford.
It furthers the University's objective of excellence in research, scholarship,
and education by publishing worldwide in

Oxford New York

Auckland Cape Town Dar es Salaam Hong Kong Karachi
Kuala Lumpur Madrid Melbourne Mexico City Nairobi
New Delhi Shanghai Taipei Toronto

With offices in

Argentina Austria Brazil Chile Czech Republic France Greece
Guatemala Hungary Italy Japan Poland Portugal Singapore
South Korea Switzerland Thailand Turkey Ukraine Vietnam

Oxford is a registered trade mark of Oxford University Press
in the UK and in certain other countries

Published in the United States
by Oxford University Press Inc., New York

A catalogue record for this title is available from the British Library

Library of Congress Cataloging in Publication Data

(Data available)

Typeset by Newgen Imaging Systems (P) Ltd., Chennai, India
Printed in Great Britain
on acid-free paper by Biddles Ltd, King's Lynn

ISBN 0–19–852943–0 978–0–19–852943–9

10 9 8 7 6 5 4 3 2 1

Acknowledgements

I would like to recognize my two co-editors, who without hesitation agreed to become partners in authoring this book. Both Janet Hardy and Paul Glare are well known to the Palliative community, and I am flattered by being associated with them. Gavril Pasternak took time out from his exhausting research schedule to orchestrate his chapter. Kenneth Jackson was wonderful to efficiently add the chapter on pharmacokinetics.

I want to recognize my mentor Declan Walsh who has encouraged me in this project. I am indebted to Robert Twycross for the time and effort he put into my education in 1996 and 1997.

Michele Wells has worked tirelessly on the manuscripts, without her skills this book would have been impossible to complete. Many thanks to Becky Phillips who contributed her skills in revising various chapters.

This book is dedicated to Deborah Doan Davis who edited many of the chapters. Her sacrifice of time and effort made *Opioids in Cancer Pain* possible. Thanks are also due to Ross Pinkerton and Monica Glare.

Contents

Contributors

Mellar Davis
MD, FCCP,
Director,
Harry R Horvitz Center for
Palliative Medicine,
Cleveland Clinic Taussig Cancer Center,
Cleveland, USA

Paul Glare
MBBS, FRACP,
Clinical Associate Professor
Director of Central Sydney
Palliative Care Service,
Royal Prince Alfred Hospital, Sydney,
New South Wales, Australia

Tony Hall
Assistant Director of Pharmacy
(Clinical),
Mater Health Services, South Brisbane,
Queensland, Australia

J. R. Hardy
Associate Professor,
Director of Palliative Care,
Mater Health Services, South Brisbane,
Queensland, Australia

Kenneth C. Jackson
Pharm D,
Assistant Professor of Pharmacy Practice,
Pain and Palliative Care,
Texas Technical University Health
Sciences Center School of Pharmacy;
Clinical Specialist,
International Pain Institute,
Texas Tech Medical Center;
Clinical Consultant,
Hospice of Lubbock,
Texas, USA

Gavril Pasternak
MD, PhD
Member and Attending Neurologist,
Head,
Laboratory of Molecular
Neuropharmacology,
Memorial Sloan-Kettering Cancer
Center,
New York, USA

List of Abbreviations

6-AM	6-monoacetylmorphine		CXB	a breed of mice
AAG	Alpha$_1$ acid glycoprotein		CYP	cytochrome P450
AC	adenylyl cyclase		DAMGO	[D-Ala^2, MePhe^4, Gly(ol)^5] enkephalin
ACTH	adrenocorticotrophic hormone		DM	diamorphine
AHCPR	Agency for Health Care Policy and Research		DOR	delta opioid receptor
AMP	adenosine 5'-phosphate		DPP	dextropropoxyphene
AMPA	alpha-amino-3-hydroxy-5-methyl-4-isoxazolepropionate		EAA	excitatory amino acids
			EAPC	European Association for Palliative Care
ASA	Aspirin		ECG	electrocardiogram
ATC	around-the-clock		EDDP	2-ethylidene 1–5-dimethyl-3–3-dephenyl pyrrolidine
AUC	area under curve			
AWP	average wholesale price		EM	extensive metabolizers
BA	bioavailability		FDA	Federal Drug Administration
BBB	blood brain barrier		FNCLCC	French National Federation of Cancer Centers
BI	basal opioid infusion			
BPOMS	Brief Profile of Mood States		FSH	follicle stimulating hormone
C6G	codeine-6-glucuronide		GABA	γ–aminobutyric acid
CADD	computer-activated drug dose		GBC	guideline-based care
CADD-PCA	computer assisted delivery device-patient controlled analgesia		GDP	guanosine 5'-diphosphate
			GFR	glomerular filtration rate
CBZ	carbamazapine		GI	gastrointestinal
CCK	cholecystokinin		GIT	gastrointestinal tract
CCK$_B$	CCK type B receptors		GTP	guanine triphosphate
CGRP	calcitonin gene-related protein		GTP	guanosine 5'-triphosphate
CI	continuous infusion		HAART	highly active anti-retroviral therapy
CIVI	continuous intravenous infusion		HM	hydromorphine
Clcr	creatinine clearance		HM3G	HM-3-glucuronide
C_{max}	Mean maximal plasma concentrations		HMOR	human mu opioid receptor
			i.m.	intramuscular
CNS	central nervous system		i.v.	intravenous
CPS	Cancer Pain Prognostic Scale		ICV	intracerebroventricular
Cp_{ss}	steady state plasma concentrations		IDDS	implantable drug delivery system
CR	controlled release		K_i	enzyme affinity of the competing drug
CSCI	continuous subcutaneous infusion			
CSF	cerebrospinal fluid		KOR	kappa opioid receptor
CSI	continuous subcutaneous infusion		KOR$_{1+3}$	kappa opioid receptor

LA	local anesthetic	PR	per rectum
LH	luteinizing hormone	PRN	pro re nata
M3G	morphine-3-glucuronide	QOL	quality of life
M6G	morphine-6-glucuronide	QTc	time interval between Q wave and end of T wave on ECG
MAPK	mitogen-activated protein kinase or	R(L) methadone	dextro and levo enantiomers of methadone
MDR-1	multi-drug resistance		
MEC	minimum effective concentration	RCT	randomized controlled trial
MOPP	multiagent chemotherapy	RDI	relative dose indicator
MOR	mu opioid receptor	RGS	regulators of G-protein signaling
MR	modified-release	RVM	rostroventromedial medulla
MRM	modified-release morphine	S(D) methadone	levo and dextro enantiomers of methadone
MS	morphine sulfate		
NK1	neurokinin I	s.c.	subcutaneous
NMDA	N-methyl-D-aspartate	SCI	subcutaneous continuous infusion
NMDA	N-methyl-D-aspirate receptors	SL	sublingual
NNT	number-needed-to-treat	SQ	subcutaneous
NOS	nitric oxide synthase	SR	slow release
NPP	norpropoxyphene	SR	sustained-release
NR	normal-release	SSRIs	selective serotonin re-uptake inhibitors
NRM	normal-release morphine		
NRS	numerical rating score	$t^{1/2}\alpha$	distribution half-life
NSAIDs	non-steroidal anti-inflammatory drugs	$t^{1/2}\beta$	elimination half-life
		TM	transmucosal
OBC	oncology-based care	TTS	transdermal fentanyl
OM	oral morphine	TTS	transdermal therapeutic system
OTFC	oral transmucosal fentanyl citrate	UC	usual care
PAG	periaqueductal gray	UDP	uridine diphosphate
PCA	patient controlled analgesia	UGT	UDP glucuronyl transferase
PCA	parenteral analgesia	VAS	visual analog scale
PKA	protein kinase-A	Vd	volume of distribution
PKC	protein kinase-C,	VRS	verbal rating scale
PK-PCA	pharmacokinetic modulated PCA pump	WDR	wide dynamic range
		WHO	World Health Organization
PM	poor metabolizers		

Chapter 1

Introduction

Mellar P. Davis

In Dennis Turk's insightful editorial entitled 'Remember the Distinction Between Malignant and Benign Pain? Well Forget It'[1] list 12 points that question the separation of cancer pain from non-malignant pain:

- The difference between nociception and pain is the same for cancer patients and non-cancer patients.
- No pain is benign (particularly when I experience it).
- Anatomically, physiologically and biochemically, malignant and non-malignant pain does not differ.
- Cancer patients do experience more symptoms (cachexia, anorexia, dyspnea), but patients with chronic non-malignant pain will experience symptoms that can overlap with cancer patients.
- Although cancer pain patients experience anxiety and depression with their life-limiting illness, chronic pain patients face the same emotions when they have no reprieve from their pain.
- Pain interferes with function, and is related to severity and not cause (cancer, non-cancer).
- Health care professionals can learn from the cancer pain literature and vice versa. Psychological factors, behavioral and social factors contribute to the pain experience and are scrutinized to a greater extent in the chronic non-malignant pain.
- Acute and chronic pain can be conceptualized upon two domains time and physical pathology, rather than etiology (cancer versus non-cancer pain).
- Acute pain is nociceptive and chronic pain is largely altered pain processing from neuroplasticity (and not malignant versus non-malignant).
- The balance between physical pathology and psychosocial contributions to pain may differ between cancer and non-cancer pain; nevertheless, both play a role in the experience of pain.
- The disadvantages of separating malignant from non-malignant pain are that this classification of pain is not based upon relevant mechanisms[1].

Perhaps the differences are in nuances and focus. The psychosocial factors that contribute to the pain experience approximate to a normal curve within the chronic pain population to which persons with cancer and persons with non-cancer pain are distributed differently[2]. The context within which patients experience pain and the meaning of pain contributes to the disability of pain. Cancer patients who experience pain as a life-limiting illness experience greater degrees of disability from their pain[2].

Rehabilitation and restoration of function are the primary goals of therapy for non-cancer chronic pain, whereas relief balanced by side effects is the primary purpose of cancer pain management. This may seem artificial, but we in palliative medicine may have neglected rehabilitation and restoration to the detriment of patient care.

Perhaps other differences are the risk of drug interactions, frequency of polypharmacy (greater in the cancer population) and organ dysfunction (again, greater in the cancer population), which influences the pharmacokinetics of analgesics to a greater extent in cancer patients. As a generalization, the therapeutic index of most analgesics will narrow near the end of life and the risk of adverse effects (particularly delirium) becomes greater than in non-cancer patients.

Cancer patients experience greater pain and distress, but they also experience greater social support[2]. The hospice movement is the 'poster child' of this support structure. Finally, addiction is not a major an issue in cancer pain management, but a major barrier to the use of opioids in chronic 'benign' pain. On the other hand, sedation is an acceptable practice for severe cancer pain, but not so for severe non-malignant pain.

Hence, the separation of chronic non-malignant cancer pain is by degree and not absolute. A text that focuses on the opioids in cancer pain may therefore appear rather one-sided or lop-sided. Yet it is our belief that these differences justify a text that focuses on cancer and opioids.

This book has a narrower focus than a general approach to cancer pain management. There are no chapters devoted to cancer pain classification, epidemiology or assessment. The subject is only approached tangentially in various chapters involving equianalgesia, opioid choices and dosing strategies. This does not mean that it is not important nor is it our intent to minimize the complexity of pain assessment. Poor pain assessment is a major reason for lack of pain control in developed countries[3]. The influence of mood on pain severity, the patient's functional activity, as well as pain pattern, location and severity, should be evaluated routinely[4]. 'Timely, appropriate and thorough assessment in treatment of cancer patients experiencing pain should reduce their suffering and improve the quality of their lives'[4].

Non-pharmacological modalities and pain rehabilitation are of equal importance to the treatment of cancer pain. Surgery, radiation and orthotics are critical to improving functional outcome and reducing pain for some patients[1]. Increased social support, physical activities and a well-developed adaptive coping strategy should minimize 'catastrophizing', which is strongly associated with intense pain[5]. Cognitive behavioral therapies and psychosupportive measures may do far more to reduce pain severity than opioid dose escalation[6]. Finally, religious beliefs may be either a boon or a bane to the success of cancer pain management[7].

Economic analysis of cancer pain management (and pharmacology) will become increasingly important as the healthcare dollar becomes limited and newly released, highly expensive opioids come onto the market. This is particularly true for American hospices, which have a capped reimbursement. Economic analysis of guidelines are now published, which may influence clinicians, patients and healthcare policy-makers in selecting various strategies for cancer pain management[8].

The text is divided into three parts:

♦ a section on opioid pharmacokinetics and pharmacodynamics;

♦ a section on individual opioids;

♦ a section on opioid choices, opioid rotation, equianalgesia and dosing strategies, which is subdivided into dosing strategies, patient controlled analgesia, spinal opioids and opioid-resistant pain.

The initial chapter on opioid receptors was orchestrated by Gavril Pasternak, an internationally known researcher on opioid receptor molecular genetics. I was fortunate to assist him with this chapter. This chapter contains a great deal of detail, which may be a 'reach' for some, but sets the stage the rest of the text. This will become evident when reading the chapter on opioid-resistant pain. The unique molecular pharmacology of opioid receptors and counter-opioid responses provides an understanding of analgesic non-cross tolerance, the benefits of opioid rotation, analgesic tolerance with chronic opioid exposure, opioid-resistant pain and opioid-facilitated pain.

An understanding of differences in opioid ligand receptor interactions has recently lead to trials of combination opioids[9]. Receptor genotype differences centered upon single nucleotide polymorphisms may help to explain differences in opioid responses between individuals[10]. An understanding of counter-opioid responses, particularly activation of the N-methyl-D-aspartate receptors has lead to explorations in the use of dextomethorphan and ketamine in the prevention of opioid analgesic tolerance, and facilitate pain and the management of opioid-resistant pain[11,12]. Available evidence is not enough to make any of the above-mentioned practices routine. However, in the future, as pain management moves into the era of molecular medicine and receptor proteonomics, as well as micro-array techniques may provide a means to rational opioid choices that will move beyond empiric trials[13].

The chapter on pharmacokinetics was kindly provided by Kenneth Jackson. This chapter provides the foundation for discussions on the kinetics of the particular opioids within the next section.

Morphine kinetics and analgesia remain a mystery. Despite previous suggestions that there are therapeutic (serum) levels of morphine and morphine metabolites[14], a study published this last year again suggested that there were both large inter-individual differences in levels, and no association between peak or trough morphine or metabolite levels, and pain relief or toxicity[15]. This confirms the previous findings by other investigators[16–18]. The overwhelming evidence is that opioid pharmacodynamics, rather than pharmacokinetics are the major determinants to effective doses.

The UDP-glucuronosyl transferases, UGT-2B7 and UGT-1A1, are responsible for metabolizing morphine[19,20]. Studies published within the last year or two do not suggest that structural polymorphisms of either gene play a major role in clinical variations of glucuronide to morphine ratios, although one study has suggested some association[21–23]. There are also differences in glucuronide to morphine ratios depending upon the route of administration[24]. It has been suggested that the UGT2B7 activity within the gastrointestinal tract is a major factor in the large individual variations in morphine metabolites[25]. Perhaps the answer to the glucuronide to morphine ratio question lies not with the structural gene or location, but to single nucleotide polymorphisms involving the reporter-promoter gene sequence[26]. I am certain that this will become more evident in the future.

Technical advancements, using high performance liquid chromatography, have identified new morphine metabolites that could potentially be active and may explain individual differences in opioid responses[27]. Similarly, gas chromatography has recently identified new oxycodone metabolites, which may do the same[28].

Another mystery (at least to myself) that I have not seen formally addressed in the literature is why methadone can be given orally with good bioavailability and fentanyl cannot. Both are metabolized by CPY3A4, which is located within enterocytes[29–31]. Perhaps it has to do with differences in enzyme interactions and affinity, but this remains speculative.

I have had the good fortune to coax both Paul Glare and Janet Hardy to join me as co-editors in this endeavor. Both have published extensively and are gifted clinicians. Both willingly took on the task of gathering materials for the sections on individual opioids, opioid rotation and opioid selection. We have included the most commonly used 'Step II' (weak) and 'Step III' (potent) opioids. Selections were personal and admittedly biased. Some would have preferred adding or subtracting to our list. Buprenorphine is not included, although in some circles this particular opioid is gaining popularity[32,33].

'Weak' opioids are a major question in the management of cancer pain, where potent opioids are readily available. A recent review has minimized the benefits of weak opioids (codeine, tramadol and dextroproxyphene)[34]. Admittedly, our use of weak opioids at the Harry R. Horvitz Center for Palliative Medicine, Cleveland Clinic, is negligible. However, several trials compared either tramadol or dextroproxyphene with morphine for moderate cancer pain and found the two weak opioids better tolerated by patients than morphine[35] (see chapters on respective opioids). It may be a little hasty for us to abandon this group of opioids altogether for low doses of potent opioids.

The second major question is whether morphine should remain the potent analgesic of choice. Recent publications have found fentanyl better tolerated[36]. Yet pain relief is not better with fentanyl. A recently completed randomized trial found methadone no better or worse than morphine[37]. Oxycodone is no better than morphine[38]. The choice of fentanyl must therefore be on the basis of side effect profile and ease of administration, which is weighed against cost and lack of versatility. The choice of methadone as a first line agent is not justified based upon efficacy, but may be so based upon cost and patient characteristics. Methadone is the least expensive of the short- and long-acting potent opioids. Oxycodone has no particular advantage and is a financial burden if the sustained release preparation is used (either to the patient or to the health care system). Hydromorphone is the American 'diamorphine', since it is highly soluble and can be given in large doses by subcutaneous infusion[35]. So, as of mid-2004, morphine remains the opioid of choice for managing moderate to severe cancer pain, since there is nothing better available. Since morphine responses range between 60 and 80%, it would take a study involving hundreds of patients to detect a difference (depending upon what would be considered reasonably expected and relevant).

Guidelines for treating cancer pain have surprisingly weak evidence to justify their status as guidelines. The World Health Organization Analgesic Step Ladder has been validated prospectively, but strategies for treating pain based upon pain pattern, opioid selection, rotation and adjuvant analgesics are weak at best, but are recommended based upon expert opinion from the few available studies[39–43]. This was evident to this author when researching material for opioid dosing strategies and patient-controlled analgesia. In fact, to my surprise, there are no prospective trials of hydrocodone in the management of cancer pain.

We live in an era of evidence-based medicine, systematic reviews and meta-analysis. Evidence-based graded studies provide the basis for recommendations to guidelines. The strength of recommendations can then be graded by levels of evidence. Such 'disciplines' help physicians make decisions with regard to diagnosis and treatment of disease, and may provide the impetus for research trials to further validate recommendations and guidelines. Yet there are drawbacks to evidence-based guidelines (Table 1.1)[44].

A good balance between guidelines, pragmatism and clinical experience should guide the practice of medicine. One of the problems with entering the evidence-based medicine era is the tendency to neglect case reports. Single patient reports can be both instructive and introduce new paradigms to the understanding of disease or treatment[45]. The introduction of the World Health Organization Analgesic Ladder guidelines (nearly 18 years ago) was done without having prospective controlled trials to validate the adequacy of analgesia using this guideline[46]. Subsequent studies have demonstrated a high degree of pain relief using the World Health Organization (WHO) analgesic ladder. A major criticism to the published WHO ladder was that it was difficult to prove that cancer pain management actually improved with the institution of the WHO analgesic ladder as there were no prospective studies prior to the WHO guidelines[46]. However, the purpose of publishing the guidelines was to facilitate

Table 1.1 Risk of evidence-based guidelines

- There are many guidelines that are heterogenous (different).

- Guidelines appear to make physician involvement and the art of medicine dispensable.

- Evidence-based medicine excludes outliers and those who do not fit the study criteria (unfortunately many of the palliative medicine population fit this category).

- Guidelines are workable in simple clinical situations, but are hard to apply to polysymptomatic patients on polypharmacy with multiple co-morbidities, and a relative high frequency of organ dysfunction or failure.

- Clinical trials to generate guidelines may involve patient populations, which do not represent the population for whom the guidelines are to be applied.

- The study aims may diverge from the treatment goals for the particular patient for whom the guidelines are to be applied.

- Guidelines are not followed or involve patients who are not compliant to guidelines.

- Individual patient choice (autonomy) is neglected by rigid application of evidence-based guidelines.

- Guidelines are not law and are not a means of limiting therapy (for those in managed care).

- The practice of guidelines will not relieve physicians of their moral obligation to care for their patients as individuals nor provide medicolegal protection.

---

the acceptance of opioids to treat cancer pain, since historically this was discouraged by medical authorities[47]. In the same vein, I doubt that there will ever be a randomized trials comparing multiagent chemotherapy (MOPP) with single agent chemotherapy in Hodgkins disease to prove the point of improved survival.

Guidelines (including the grade of evidence for recommendations) for opioid choices, dosing strategies, breakthrough and rescue dosing, alternative opioids, opioid rotation, conversion and management of opioid toxicity have been published by the French National Federation of Cancer Centers (FNCLCC) and the Expert Working Group of the Research Network of the European Association for Palliative Care (EAPC)[42,48–50]. These publications should be read by all caring for cancer patients. The last section in the book deals with opioid rotation, equianalgesia, opioid dosing strategies, patient controlled analgesia, spinal opioids and opioid refractory pain. These chapters are a detailed supplement to these guidelines. Dosing strategies are a bit biased towards my experience at the Cleveland Clinic. Both the EAPC recommendations and publications by Declan Walsh play a large role in the final chapters of the book[48,51]. Other publications that are important were written by Dr Paul Glare, Dr Sebastiano Mercandate, Dr Geoffrey Hanks and Dr Carla Ripamonti (among others)[52–59].

Opioid tolerance, the opioid withdrawal syndrome, neuropathic pain and opioid-facilitated pain have overlapping mechanisms as discussed in the opioid receptor chapter. Case reports of opioid-induced hyperalgesia continue to be published[60]. Two excellent reviews on the pathophysiology of opioid tolerance, physical dependence and opioid-facilitated pain have been published within the last year[61,62], and provide the background to the chapter on opioid-resistant pain. Initial management of opioid-resistant pain requires assessment for idiopathic (somatized) pain. Opioid-resistant pain may be relieved by adjuvant analgesics, opioid rotation or conversion, and non-pharmacological supportive therapies (radiation, surgery, neurolytic blocks, orthotics and psychosocial support).

Pain that arises from the soul or spirit is idiopathic only when we do not recognize the source of pain. Psychological and spiritual pain can be described by patients in physical terms, and thus can be frequently missed by physicians. This type of pain is ill served by opioids, which will only produce toxicity without relief. Even those with physical reasons for pain (cancer treatment or co-morbidities) may suffer largely from 'idiopathic' pain, resulting in a poor or incomplete response to analgesics. Perhaps we should consider expanding our classification of pain from nociceptive and neuropathic to nociceptive, neuropathic, psychosocial, spiritual, mixed and move away from a bio-medical concept of pain[63].

A good book should not be like bronzed shoes that once finished are placed on the shelf to be admired as something past, never to be worn again. My hope and prayer is that this book will be well-thumbed and worn out from use. I hope that those who read *Opioids in Cancer Pain* find something new and useful. If one patient benefits from our work, the endeavor will have been well worth the effort.

References

1 Turk DC. Remember the distinction between malignant and benign pain? Well, forget it. *Clin J Pain* 2002; **18**(2): 75–6.

2 Fordyce W. Pain in cancer and chronic non-cancer conditions: similarities and differences. *Acta Anaesthesiol Scand* 2001; **45**: 1086–9.

3 Davis MP, Walsh D. Epidemiology of cancer pain and factors influencing poor pain control. *Am J Hosp Palliat Care* 2004; **21**(2): 137–42.

4 Turk DC. Clinical effectiveness and cost-effectiveness of treatments for patients with chronic pain. *Clin J Pain* 2002; **18**(6): 355–65.

5 Zaza C, Baine N. Cancer pain and psychosocial factors: a critical review of the literature. *J Pain Sympt Manag* 2002; **24**(5): 526–42.

6 O'Leary U. Psychosocial influences on pain perceptions in cancer. *Nurs Times* 2002; **98**(43): 36–8.

7 Bosch F, Banos JE. Religious beliefs of patients and caregivers as a barrier to the pharmacologic control of cancer pain. *Clin Pharmacol Ther* 2002; **72**(2): 107–11.

8 Abernethy AP, Samsa GP, Matchar DB. A clinical decision and economic analysis model of cancer pain management. *Am J Managed Care* 2003; **9**(10): 651–64.

9 Lauretti GR, Oliveria GM, Pereira NL. Comparison of sustained-release oxycodone in advanced cancer patients. *Br J Cancer* 2003; **89**(11): 2027–30.

10 Hirota T, Ieiri I, Takane H, *et al.* Sequence variability and candidate gene analysis in two cancer patients with complex clinical outcomes during morphine therapy. Drug Metab Disposit 2003; **31**(5): 677–80.

11 Weinbroum AA, Bender B, Nirkin A, *et al.* Dextromethrophan-associated epidural patient-controlled analgesia provides better pain- and analgesics-sparing effects than dextromethorphan-associated

intravenous patient-controlled analgesia after bone-malignancy resection: a randomized, placebo-controlled, double-blinded study. *Anesth Analg* 2004; **98**(3): 714–22.

12 Bell RF, Eccleston C, Kalso E, *et al.* Ketamine as adjuvant to opioids for cancer pain. A qualitative systematic review. *J Pain Symptom Manag* 2003; **26**(3): 867–75.

13 Futterman LG, Lemberg L. The mysteries of the human genome uncovered—medicine is changed forever. *Am J Crit Care* 2001; **10**(2): 125–32.

14 Faura CC, Moore RA, Horga JF, *et al.* Morphine and morphine-6-glucuronide plasma concentrations and effect in cancer pain. *J Pain Symptom Manag* 1996; **11**(2): 95–102.

15 Quigley C, Joel S, Patel N, *et al.* Plasma concentrations of morphine, morphine-6-glucuronide and morphine-3-glucuronide and their relationship with analgesia and side effects in patients with cancer-related pain. *Palliat Med* 2003; **17**: 185–90.

16 Wolff T, Samuelsson H, Hedner T. Morphine and morphine metabolite concentrations in cerebrospinal fluid and plasma in cancer pain patients after slow-release oral morphine administration. *Pain* 1995; **62**(2): 147–54.

17 Goucke CR, Hackett LP, Ilett JF. Concentrations of morphine, morphine-6-glucuronide and morphine-3-glucuronide in serum and cerebrospinal fluid following morphine administration to patients with morphine-resistant pain. *Pain* 1994; **56**(2): 145–9.

18 van Dongen RT, Crul BJ, Koopman-Kimenai PM, *et al.* Morphine and morphine-glucuronide concentrations in plasma ratios are unaffected by the UGT2B7 H268Y and UGT1A1*28 polymorphisms in cancer patients on chronic morphine therapy. *Eur J Clin Pharmacol* 2002; **58**(5): 353–6.

19 Stone AN, Mackenzie PI, Galetin A, *et al.* Isoform selectivity and kinetics of morphine 3- and 6-glucuronidation by human udpglucuronosyltransferases: evidence for atypical glucuronidation kinetics by UGT2B7. *Drug Metab Dispos* 2003; **31**(9): 1086–9.

20 Radominska-Pandya A, Little JM, Czernik PJ. Human UDP-glucuronosyltransferase 2B7. *Curr Drug Metab* 2001; **2**(3): 283–98.

21 Holthe M, Klepsted P, Zahlsen K, *et al.* Morphine glucuronide-to-morphine plasma ratios are unaffected by the UGT2B7 H268Y and UGT1A1*28 polymorphisms in cancer patients on chronic morphine therapy. *Eur J Clin Pharmacol* 2002; **58**(5): 353–6.

22 Holthe M, Rakvag TN, Klepstad P, *et al.* Sequence variations in the UDP-glucurononosyltransferase 2B7 (UGT2B7) gene: identification of 10 novel single nucleotide polymorphisms (SNPs) and analysis of their relevance to morphine glucuronidation in cancer patients. *Pharmacogenomics J* 2003; **3**(1): 17–26.

23 Sawyer MB, Innocenti F, Das S, *et al.* A pharmacogenetic study of uridine diphosphate-glucuronosyltransferase 2B7 in patients receiving morphine. *Clin Pharmacol Ther* 2003; **73**(6): 566–74.

24 Takahashi M, Ohara T, Yamanaka H, *et al.* The oral-to-intravenous equianalgesic ratio of morphine based plasma concentrations of morphine and metabolites in advanced cancer patients receiving chronic morphine treatment. *Palliat Med* 2003; **17**(8): 673–8.

25 Tateishi M, Ohashi K, Kobayashi K, *et al.* Interindividual variation in the ratio between plasma morphine and its metabolites in cancer patients. *Int J Clin Pharmacol Res* 2003; **23**(2/3): 75–82.

26 Duguay Y, Baar C, Skorpen F, *et al.* A novel functional polymorphism in the uridine diphosphate-glucuroniosyltransferase 2B7 promotor with significant impact on promoter activity. *Clin Pharmacol Ther* 2004; **75**: 223–33.

27 Chen XY, Zhao LM, Zhong DF. A novel metabolic pathway of morphine: formation of morphine glucosides in cancer patients. *Br J Clin Pharmacol* 2003; **55**: 570–8.

28 Moore KA, Ramcharitar V, Levine B, *et al*. Tentative identification of novel oxycodone metabolites in human urine. *J Anal Toxicol* 2003; **27(6):** 346–52.

29 von Richter O, Burk O, Fromm MF, *et al*. Cytochrome P450 3A4 and P-glycoprotein expression in human small intestinal enterocytes and hepatocytes: a comparative analysis in paired tissue specimens. *Clin Pharmacol Therapeut* 2004; **55(3):** 172–83.

30 Labroo RB, Paine MF, Thummel KE, *et al*. Fentanyl metabolism by human hepatic and intestinal cytochrome P450 3A4: implications for interindividual variability in disposition, efficacy, and drug interactions. *Drug Metab Dispos* 1997; **25(9):** 1072–80.

31 Shinderman M, Maxwell S, Brawand-Amey M, *et al*. Cytochrome P4503A4 metabolic activity, methadone blood concentrations, and methadone doses. *Drug Alcohol Depend* 2003; **69(2):** 205–11.

32 Radbruch L. Buprenorphine TDS: use in daily practice, benefits for patients. *Internat J Clin Pract Suppl* 2003; **133:** 19–22.

33 Budd K. Buprenorphine and the transdermal system: the ideal match in pain management. *Internat J Clin Pract Suppl* 2003; **133:** 9–14.

34 Anon. Weak opiate analgesics: modest practical merits. *Prescrire Int* 2004; **13(69):** 22–5.

35 Mercadante S. Is morphine the drug of choice in cancer pain? *Progr Palliat Care* 2001; **9(5):** 190–3.

36 van Seventer R, Smit JM, Schipper RM, *et al*. Comparison of TTS-fentanyl with sustained-release oral morphine in the treatment of patients not using opioids for mild-to-moderate pain. *Curr Med Res Opin* 2003; **19(6):** 457–69.

37 Bruera E, Palmer L, Bodnjak S, *et al*. Methadone versus morphine as a first-line strong opioid for cancer pain: a randomized, double-blind study. *J Clin Oncol* 2004; **22(1):** 185–92.

38 Anon. Oral oxycodone: new preparation. No better than oral morphine. *Prescrire Internat* 2003; **12(65):** 83–4.

39 Lewis CR. Adjuvant analgesic therapy for cancer-related pain: does the evidence support the practice? *ASCO Ann Meet Proc* 2004; **23:** 733.

40 Curatolo M, Sveticic G. Drug combinations in pain treatment: a review of the published evidence and a method for finding the optimal combination. *Best Pract Res Clin Anaesthesiol* 2002; **16(4):** 507–9.

41 Wootton M. Morphine is not the only analgesic in palliative care: literature review. *J Adv Nurs* 2004; **45(5):** 527–32.

42 Krakowski ST, Balp K, Bonnefoi MP, *et al*. Summary version of the standards, options and recommendations for the use of analgesia for the treatment of nociceptive pain in adults with cancer pain (update 2002). *Br J Cancer* 2003; **89(1):** 567–72.

43 McNicol E, Strassels S, Goudas L, *et al*. Nonsteroidal anti-inflammatory drugs, alone or combined with opioids, for cancer pain: a systematic review. *J Clin Oncol* 2004; **22(10):** 1975–92.

44 Lubbe AS. Risks and misconceptions of guidelines in medicine and palliative medicine in particular. *Progr Palliat Care* 2002; **10(6):** 275–9.

45 Mercandate S, Serretta R, Sapio M, *et al*. When all else fails: stepwise multiple solutions for a complex cancer pain syndrome. *Support Care Cancer* 1999; **7:** 47–50.

46 Jadad AR, Browman GP. The WHO analgesic ladder for cancer pain management stepping up the quality of its evaluation. *J Am Med Ass* 1995; **274(23):** 1870–2.

47 Reidenberg MM. Pain control and the World Health Organization analgesic ladder. *J Am Med Ass* 1996; **275(11):** 835.

48 Hanks GW, de Conno F, Cherny N, *et al*. Morphine and alternative opioids in cancer pain: the EAPC recommendations. *Br J Cancer* 2001; **84(5):** 587–93.

49 Mercadante S, Radbruch L, Caraceni A, *et al*. Episodic (breakthrough) pain. *Cancer* 2002; **94:** 832–9.

50 Cherny N, Ripamonti C, Pereira J, *et al.* Strategies to manage the adverse effects of oral morphine: an evidence-based report. *J Clin Oncol* 2001; **19(9)**: 2542–54.

51 Walsh D. Pharmacological management of cancer. *Semin Oncol* 2000; **27(1)**: 45–63.

52 Glare P, Walsh D, Groh E, *et al.* The efficacy and side effects of continuous infusion intravenous morphine (CIVM) for pain and symptoms due to advanced cancer. *Am J Hosp Palliat Care* 2002; **19(5)**: 343–50.

53 Glare P. Problems with opiates in cancer pain: parenteral opioids. *Support Care Cancer* 1997; **5(6)**: 445–50.

54 Glare P, Aggarwal G, Clark K. Ongoing controversies in the pharmacological management of cancer pain. *Intern Med J* 2004; **34(1/2)**: 45–9.

55 Mercadante S, Fulfaro F. Alternatives to oral opioids for cancer pain. *Oncology* 1999; **13(2)**: 215–20.

56 Mercadante S. Opioid rotation for cancer pain: rationale and clinical aspects. *Cancer* 1999; **86(9)**: 1856–66.

57 Mercadante S. Controversies over spinal treatment in advanced cancer. *Support Care Cancer* 1998; **6(6)**: 495–502.

58 Ripamonti C, Zecca E, De Conno F. Pharmacological treatment of cancer pain: alternative routes of opioid administration. *Tumori* 1998; **84(3)**: 289–300.

59 Hanks GW, Forbes K. Opioid responsiveness. *Acta Anesthesiol Scand* 1997; **41(1 Pt 2)**: 154–8.

60 Mercadante S, Ferrera P, Villari P, *et al.* Hyperalgesia: an emerging iatrogenic syndrome. *J Pain Symptom Manag* 2003; **26(2)**: 769–75.

61 Udea H, Inoue M, Mizuno K. New approaches to study the development of morphine tolerance and dependence. *Life Sci* 2003; **74(2/3)**: 313–20.

62 Ossipov MH, Lai J, Vanderah TW, *et al.* Induction of pain facilitation by sustained opioid exposure: relationship to opioid antinociceptive tolerance. *Life Sci* 2003; **73(6)**: 783–800.

63 Turk DC, Monarch ES, Williams AD. Cancer patients in pain: considerations for assessing the whole person. *Hematol Oncol Clin N Am* 2002; **16(3)**: 511–25.

Chapter 2

Opioid receptors and opioid pharmacodynamics

Mellar P. Davis and Gavril W. Pasternak

Introduction

Opioids have a long and rich pharmacology. They are widely used throughout medicine and have been invaluable. However, they come with problems, including side effects such as constipation, respiratory depression and sedation, as well as the potential of abuse. Investigators have long believed that more selective drugs lacking these drawbacks could be developed, leading to the synthesis of novel analgesics that have proven to be extraordinary tools for the early pharmacologists in the field (Fig. 2.1). The structure–activity relationships for the vast number of agents led to the conclusion that there must be specific recognition sites or receptors for these drugs[1–3], going so far as to suggest specific molecular interactions between the ligand and its binding pocket. However, the biochemical demonstration of these receptors had to wait until 1973[4–7]. These binding sites were highly selective for opioid analgesics and their antagonists, and demonstrated the same structure–activity relationships seen pharmacologically, including stereospecificity. Much of the work in the past 30 years has focused upon identifying, characterizing and, most recently, cloning these receptors, and correlating them with opioid action.

Opiates and opioid peptides

The original opiates, morphine and codeine, come from opium. Over the years, thousands of derivatives were synthesized in an effort to dissociate analgesia from problematic side effects, particularly respiratory depression, constipation and dependence liability. Morphine has a rigid structure (Fig. 2.1). Systematic studies showed that a number of modifications of the morphine structure could be tolerated without losing analgesic activity, including eliminating significant portions of the molecule. For example, elimination of the 'C' ring provided the framework for the benzomorphans, such as ketocyclazocine, ethylketocyclazocine and pentazocine. Although these ligands retained analgesic activity, their pharmacology was quite distinct from morphine and led to the identification of kappa receptors[8] long before the discovery of their endogenous ligand, dynorphin A[9,10]. However, further simplification of the structure led to other opioids with actions more similar to those of morphine, including methadone, meperidine and the fentanyl series of mu opioids[11] (Fig. 2.1).

The strict structure–activity relationships of the opioids followed by the demonstration of their receptors clearly indicated that there must be an endogenous ligand for these sites. The first physiological evidence for the presence of endogenous opioids

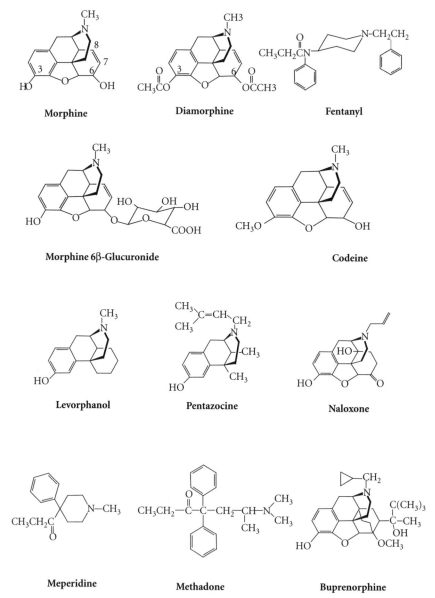

Fig. 2.1 Structure of common opioids.

Table 2.1 Structure of some common opioid peptides

Natural opioid peptides	
[Leu⁵]enkephalin	Tyr-Gly-Gly-Phe-Leu
[Met⁵]enkephalin	Tyr-Gly-Gly-Phe-Met
Dynorphin A	Tyr-Gly-Gly-Phe-Leu-Arg-Arg-Ile-Arg–Pro-Lys–Leu-Lys-Trp-Asp-Asn-Gln
Dynorphin B	Tyr-Gly-Gly-Phe-Leu-Arg-Arg-Gln-Phe-Lys-Val-Val-Thr
α-Neoendorphin	Tyr-Gly-Gly-Phe-Leu-Arg-Lys-Tyr-Pro-Lys
β-Neoendorphin	Tyr-Gly-Gly-Phe-Leu-Arg-Lys-Tyr-Pro
β-Endorphin	Tyr-Gly-Gly-Phe-Met-Thr-Ser-Glu-Lys-Ser-Gln-Thr-Pro-Leu-Val-Thr-Leu-Phe-Lys-Asn-Ala-Ile-Ile-Lys-Asn-Ala-Tyr-Lys-Lys-Gly-Glu
Endomorphin-1	Tyr-Pro-Trp-Phe-NH₂
Endomorphin-2	Tyr-Pro-Phe-Phe-NH₂
Orphanin FQ/Nociceptin	Phe-Gly-Gly-Phe-Thr-Gly-Ala-Arg-Lys-Ser-Ala-Arg-Lys-Leu-Ala-Asp-Glu
Synthetic opioid peptides	
DPDPE	[D-Pen²,D-Pen⁵]enkephalin
DADLE	[D-Ala²,D-Leu⁵]enkephalin
DALDA	Tyr-D-Arg-Phe-LysNH₂
DAMGO	[D-Ala²,MePhe⁴,Gly(ol)⁵]enkephalin
DSLET	[D-Ser²,Leu⁵]enkephalin-Thr⁶
Deltorphin II	Tyr-D-Ala-Phe-Glu-Val-Val-Gly-NH₂
CTOP	D-Phe-c[Cys-Tyr-D-Trp-Orn-Thr-Pen]-Thr-NH₂

came from the studies of Liebeskind and co-workers, who demonstrated analgesia following stimulation of the periaqueductal gray, an action that was reversed by the opioid receptor antagonist naloxone[7,12,13]. The isolation of opioid-like materials from the brain[14–17], led to the determination of the structure of the enkephalins, β-endorphin and the dynorphins (Table 2.1)[18,19]. The term endorphins was proposed by Eric Simon to encompass all the endogenous opioids, with the enkephalins referring to the two pentapeptides first identified by Kosterlitz[7] (Table 2.1).

Goldstein later described the dynorphins, a series of peptides that shared the same first five amino acids as the enkephalins and had high affinity for kappa receptors[7,9,10]. Although all these endogenous peptides display affinity for the three main opioid receptors, dynorphin A binds preferentially to kappa opioid receptors and the enkephalins to delta opioid receptors. The endogenous ligand for the mu receptors is still not entirely clear, although the endomorphins label this site with high affinity and specificity[20].

The endogenous opiates are derived from a family of three precursor proteins that are processed to generate the various peptides[21]. The dynorphins are produced from preprodynorphin, while the enkephalins are generated from a distinct precursor protein, preproenkephalin. β-Endorphin is a 31-amino acid peptide that also possesses potent opioid activity[22], but what makes it unique is its localization to the pituitary gland and the fact that it is produced from the same precursor protein (β-lipotropin) that generates adrenocorticotrophic hormone (ACTH) and other hormones. Furthermore, it is co-released into the blood with ACTH as part of the stress response, perhaps contributing to the role of stress to modulate pain perception[23]. Thus, the opioid peptides represent a family of highly related neurotransmitters.

Antagonists

Antagonists have been extremely valuable, both clinically and in studies of opioid mechanisms. Antagonists such as naloxone effectively reverse the actions of traditional opioids. However, their clinical use is complicated by their ability to precipitate withdrawal in dependent subjects. Thus, care must be taken when administering an antagonist to a subject who has been on opioids chronically, particularly since sensitivity towards an antagonist progressively increases as the subject becomes more physically dependent. Although naloxone is used clinically to reverse opioid actions, its duration of action is relatively brief with the actions of many agonists lasting longer. Thus, care must be taken to re-administer it when counteracting longer-acting agonists.

Although agonists and antagonists bind to the same receptor, they interact with different conformations of the protein that can be influenced biochemically in a variety of ways, including monovalent and divalent cations[24–26], enzymes and protein modifying treatments[27–29], and guanine nucleotides[30]. Our understanding of how these different conformations actually bind their ligands is now being explored at the molecular level with detailed modeling approaches.

Antagonists have proved valuable in studies of pharmacological mechanisms. They can verify the opioid nature of a response and the availability of highly selective antagonists has greatly facilitated our understanding of opioid receptor multiplicity. Selective mu antagonists, such as β-funaltrexamine[31,32], have proven valuable in defining mu actions both *in vivo* and *in vitro*, while other agents, such as naloxonazine, have demonstrated subpopulations of mu receptors[33–36]. Naltrindole is an excellent delta receptor antagonist, while nor-binaltorphimine selectively blocks kappa$_1$ receptors[37,38].

Partial agonists

Many opioid analgesics are partial agonists, which may impact their analgesic activity. Unlike full opioid agonists, partial agonists may display a ceiling effect. This reflects their limited intrinsic efficacy or their ability to activate the receptor. Depending upon the situation, drugs with limited intrinsic efficacy may not achieve a complete response at full receptor occupancy. This ability to produce a full response, termed efficacy, is dependent upon the situation in which it is measured. For example, opioids exhibiting full efficacy in low intensity pain models may be unable to provide a complete response with higher pain intensities. This can result in either a shift to the right of the dose–response curve, which leads to the appearance of dose-limited side effects and/or the appearance of a ceiling effect, as shown by a plateau in the response that cannot be overcome with further increases in dose.

It is possible to assess the intrinsic activity and efficacy of drugs at the molecular level. Earlier studies utilized receptor-binding approaches to assess the agonist/antagonist character of the drugs[24,25]. However, this approach has a number of limitations. Functional approaches are more direct. The most straightforward involves looking at the activation of G-proteins. Opioid receptors are coupled to G-proteins that generate the downstream processes following receptor activation. Agonists activate the receptor and initiate the dissociation of guanosine 5′-diphosphate (GDP) from the G_α subunit of the heterotrimeric G-protein complex, which is then replaced by guanosine 5′-triphosphate (GTP). The G_α subunit then dissociates, liberating the $G_{\beta\gamma}$ subunit, which can then interact with downstream transduction systems. The ability of a drug to activate the G-protein is dependent upon its intrinsic activity. Partial agonists, which have low intrinsic activities, activate G-proteins less efficiently, resulting in a lower overall activation at full receptor occupancy. Pure antagonists do not activate the G-protein and have no effect. The ability of drugs to activate the G-proteins can be assessed experimentally by measuring the dissociation of GDP and its replacement by a non-hydrolysable radiolabeled GTP analog, [^{35}S]GTPγS. Partial agonists are unable to activate as many G_α subunits as full agonists and thus have lower levels of [^{35}S]GTPγS binding than full agonists. Comparing the potency (EC_{50}) of an opioid to induce [^{35}S]GTPγS binding with the binding affinity of the ligand determined through receptor binding assays (K_i) can provide an indication of intrinsic activity. Antagonists do not induce binding of the GTP analog.

Inverse agonists are unusual and differ from both agonists or antagonists. Most receptors typically have low levels of constitutive activity, leading to a low level of G-protein activation in the absence of agonist. Antagonists are neutral, neither inducing G-protein activation nor reversing the constitutive receptor activity. In contrast, inverse agonists block the constitutive receptor activity.

Classification of opioid receptors

Opiates and the opioid peptides act through a family of receptors. Classical pharmacological studies indicated the presence of multiple classes of opioid receptors long before their identification biochemically. Based upon the interactions of nalorphine and morphine in clinical studies, Martin proposed distinct receptors for the two drugs over 35 years ago[39], which subsequently led to the current classification of mu and kappa receptors[8]. Delta receptors, selective for the enkephalins, were identified in bioassays and then biochemically[40]. Initially, opioids were classified by their actions in bioassays. The guinea pig ileum bioassay is relatively selective for mu opioids, while delta drugs are defined by their actions in the mouse vas deferens bioassays. However, drugs are currently classified by their affinities against mu, delta and kappa receptors in traditional receptor binding assays.

Mu receptors display high selectivity for morphine and related synthetic compounds. Identification of the endogenous ligand for the mu receptor has proven difficult. Many of the endogenous opioids, particularly β-endorphin, have reasonably high affinity for mu sites, but the most selective of the endogenous ligands are the endomorphins. The structural requirements of the synthetic compounds for affinity for mu receptors are met by a broad range of opiates, ranging from the rigid structure of morphine to flexible structures like methadone and fentanyl, and even synthetic enkephalin derivatives[11]. Kappa receptors were initially proposed, based upon the actions of keto-cyclazocine[8] before the discovery of their endogenous ligand, dynorphin A[9,10]. Delta receptors were then proposed, based upon their selectivity for the enkephalins[41,42]. The pharmacology of these receptor families has been facilitated by the synthesis of highly selective agonists for all of them.

Pharmacological evidence from a number of laboratories has suggested subtypes of these receptors. Within the mu opioid receptor family, the ability of the highly selective mu antagonist naloxonazine to dissociate supraspinal morphine analgesia from both respiratory depression and the inhibition of gastrointestinal transit, coupled with binding studies, led to the suggestion of mu_1 and mu_2 receptor subtypes[33,34,43–49]. The possibility of distinct mu receptors for morphine-6β-glucuronide then arose[50,51]. The concept of mu receptor multiplicity has now been confirmed at the molecular level through the cloning of a number of mu opioid receptor splice variants[52–57].

Multiple kappa receptors also have been proposed, starting with the initial suggestion of $kappa_2$ by Zukin and colleagues[58]. This was then extended to $kappa_3$ receptors, based upon the pharmacology of a novel opioid naloxone benzoylhydrazone[59–64]. Finally, computer modeling of binding data suggested the presence of subtypes, even with the $kappa_1$ receptor classification[64,65], with one being highly sensitive to the endogenous opioids dynorphin B and α-neoendorphin[64]. Finally, pharmacological studies also have led to the suggestion of delta receptor heterogeneity[66–69].

Anatomical localization of opioid receptors

Opioid receptors have been demonstrated throughout the nervous system, from peripheral nerves to the spinal cord to the brain. Peripheral opioid receptors are synthesized in the dorsal root ganglion, and transported to nerve endings and centrally to the dorsal horn of the spinal cord. Axonal opioid transport is enhanced by inflammation[70,71]. Many of the immune cells associated with an inflammatory response can synthesize endogenous opioids, including enkephalins[70] and they also contain opioid receptors. This may help explain the utility of peripheral opioids for inflammatory conditions and the clinical use of topical opioids in open wounds and within joints[72–74].

All three classes of opioid receptors are localized with high density within the superficial layers (lamina I and II) of the spinal cord, with lower levels in the deeper lamina. Within the dorsal horn, mu receptors are the most dense, accounting for 70% of the receptors, followed by delta receptors (24%) and kappa$_1$ (6%)[75–78]. These receptors are localized both pre- and post-synaptically[77].

Supraspinally, mu opioid receptors are found within the amygdale and nucleus accumbens, as well as the striatum. The nucleus acumens has been associated with the reinforcing behavior of opioids. Their functional significance within the motor systems is not clear, but they are presumed to be associated with analgesic responses within the limbic system, which is important in the emotional components of pain. Within the thalamus, mu opioid receptors are more prominent within the medial structures than the lateral ones. The medial thalamic nuclei relay spinothalamic input from the spinal cord to the cingulate gyrus and limbic structures[75]. Mu receptors also have a well established distribution within the brainstem, with high densities in a number of structures associated with analgesia, including the periaqueductal gray, the reticular formation, the locus coeruleus and rostral ventromedial medulla[70,79,80]. The periaqueductal gray, the locus coeruleus and rostral ventromedial medulla are responsible for a descending modulatory system, which dampens or facilitates dorsal horn pain processing. Opioid receptors are also found within the hypothalamus, where they are presumed to be involved with hormonal regulation, as well as medullary vagal complex, the nucleus tractus solitarius and area postrema. These locations mediate the endocrine and autonomic actions of opioid, as well as nausea[79–82].

The distributions of the delta and kappa receptors also have been described. Although they demonstrate similar distributions within the spinal cord, their supraspinal distributions differ[79,83,84].

Behavioral opioid actions

Analgesia

The utility of morphine and related drugs rests with their ability to modulate pain. They differ in many respects from other analgesics. First, pure opioid agonists do not display a ceiling effect. Thus, increasing the dosage will continue to increase pain relief, although side effects commonly interfere with dose escalation. Partial agonists may show ceiling effects in selected circumstances, depending upon the nature and intensity of the pain. In contrast, other analgesics, such as the non-steroidal anti-inflammatory drugs (NSAIDs), all display ceiling effects. More important, opioids act upon the subjective 'hurt' associated with pain without affecting primary sensory modalities. This distinguishes them from local anesthetics, which interfere with all sensory input and, at sufficiently high concentrations, motor function as well.

Opioid analgesia is mediated within both the central and peripheral nervous systems. Numerous sites of action of action have been mapped in the brainstem, including the periaqueductal gray, nucleus raphe magnus and locus coeruleus, as well as in the dorsal horn of the spinal cord[85], regions known to have high levels of opioid receptors. In the periphery, opioid receptors have been demonstrated on peripheral nerves and peripheral opioids have clear analgesic actions. Although each site is important and can elicit an analgesic response independent of the others, simultaneous activation of more than one site elicits synergistic responses. First demonstrated with spinal and supraspinal morphine[86], synergistic interactions also have been documented between the periphery and the central sites[87,88] and even among brainstem nuclei[89]. These regional interactions are important since systemic drugs activate all sites.

Epidural opioids present a unique clinical situation. The instillation of opioids epidurally leads to high levels at the spinal level due to diffusion into the subarachnoid space. However, epidural drugs also have an appreciable systemic absorption. Animal models demonstrate that even low doses of spinal morphine will dramatically potentiate the analgesic response of systemic morphine, shifting the systemic dose–response curve 10-fold or more to the left (Table 2.2). Thus, the synergy due to the combination of elevated opioid levels spinally, along with the systemically absorbed drug may help explain the utility of this approach. Since intrathecal opioids have reduced systemic absorption, their actions are mediated spinally. Synergy is observed with the co-administration of a systemic with an intrathecal opioid.

Kappa and delta drugs also display analgesia peripherally, spinally and supraspinally. However, their overall clinical utility is far less than mu systems due to the limited availability of selective opioids. There are some agents with kappa activity, including

Table 2.2 Systemic/spinal opioid synergy

Morphine route	Morphine ED$_{50}$		Systemic shift
Systemic alone	3.1 mg/kg	(1.6, 4.4)	
Intrathecal alone	305 ng	(153, 501)	
Systemic			
+25 ng, i.t.	0.5 mg/kg	(0.4, 0.8)	6.2
+50 ng, i.t.	0.3 mg/kg	(0.2, 0.5)	10.3
+100 ng, i.t.	0.2 mg/kg	(0.1, 0.3)	15.5
+200 ng, i.t.	0.037 mg/kg	(0.01,0.10)	83.8

Morphine analgesia was assessed in groups of mice and the ED$_{50}$ determined following systemic administration alone, intrathecal administration alone and for systemic administration with the indicated fixed dose of intrathecal morphine. Administration of low doses of morphine intrathecally that are insufficient to produce an analgesic action alone are still capable of potentiating the activity of systemic morphine. Results are from the literature[87].

Table 2.3 Sensitivity of mouse strains to morphine

Strain	Morphine Analgesia
BALB/c	90%
CD-1	76%
C57/bgʲ	62%
HS	62%
Swiss Webster	40%
C57/+	40%
CXBK	0%

Groups of mice ($n \geq 10$) from the indicated strain received a single dose of morphine (5 mg/kg, s.c.) and analgesia tested 30 min later using the radiant heat tailflick assay. Analgesia was defined as a doubling or greater of the baseline tailflick latency. Adapted from the literature[93].

pentazocine and nalbuphine, but they are not very selective. There are not yet any clinically useful delta opioids.

Pharmacogenomics and opioid analgesia

Although virtually all strains of mice respond to opioids, there are intriguing genetic differences in sensitivity. The genetics of opioid sensitivity has been extremely well studied by a number of laboratories[90–92]. However, these differences are illustrated by a simple study examining the responses of different strains of mice to a fixed dose of morphine (Table 2.3). The responses ranged from 80 to 0%[93].

However, these genetic differences are even more complex, as illustrated by comparisons of the CD-1 and CXBK strains (Fig. 2.2). Doses of a series of mu opioids were chosen that elicited similar analgesic actions in CD-1 mice and then were given to the CXBK mice. Although the CXBK mice were not very sensitive to morphine, they responded normally to several other mu opioids, including methadone and heroin[94,95]. These variable responses to mu opioids are similar to the clinical situation, where the responses of individual patients to different mu opioids can vary.

Analgesic tolerance

Chronic opioid use leads to a progressive decline in potency, a phenomenon termed tolerance. Put another way, with continued usage, the dose of opioids must be increased to maintain a fixed response. Tolerance is due to a wide range of responses ranging from biochemical changes at the receptor to more generalized changes within N-methyl-D-aspartate (NMDA) neuronal circuits. The roles of other neurotransmitter systems, including NMDA receptors and nitric oxide, are particularly interesting, since

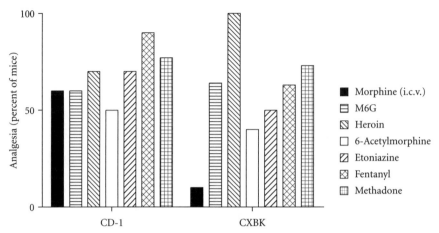

Fig. 2.2 Analgesic activity of opioids in CD-1 and CXBK mice. Doses of the indicated drugs were chosen to give similar analgesic actions in CD-1 mice and then were administered to the CD-1 mice. From the literature[94,95].

inhibitors of nitric oxide synthase and NMDA receptor antagonists can diminish or reverse tolerance in animal models[96–101].

Cross-tolerance implies that subjects tolerant to one opioid will be tolerant to another and is limited to drugs acting the same receptors. Thus, animals tolerant to mu opioids do not show cross-tolerance to kappa or delta drugs. Complete cross-tolerance implies identical receptor mechanisms of action while incomplete cross-tolerance suggests some differences. Within the mu opioid family, preclinical studies show both complete and incomplete cross-tolerance (Fig. 2.3). In mice made tolerant to morphine, codeine shows complete cross-tolerance, but a number of other mu opioids do not, including methadone and heroin[102]. These preclinical studies are similar to observations made with patients who often show incomplete cross-tolerance, helping to explain the utility of opioid rotation[103].

Opioid dependence

Dependence is a physiological response to chronic administration of opioids. It has been most closely studied with mu opioids. Withdrawal is associated with a number of standard signs and symptoms. However, it is important to distinguish dependence from addiction. Dependence is a physiological response seen in all subjects maintained on opioids, whereas addiction implies a psychological dependence and is uncommonly seen in patients with no prior history of drug abuse.

Clinically, dependence is not a concern so long as patients continue to take their opioid. However, if their analgesic is withheld, they will undergo withdrawal. Care must taken with dependent patients, since switching them to a partial agonist, such as pentazocine, will precipitate withdrawal in some situations. Antagonists can precipitate withdrawal within seconds. The clinician can titrate the antagonist in a dependent patient

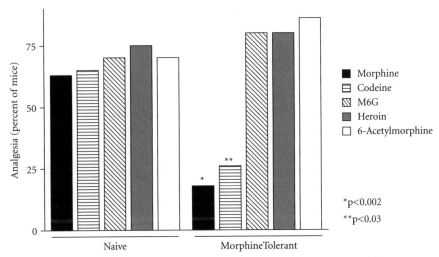

Fig. 2.3 Incomplete cross-tolerance among mu opioids. Doses of the indicated drugs were chosen to give similar analgesic actions in naïve animals. Groups of mice were given morphine daily for 4 days and then tested with the same doses of the indicated drugs on the fifth day. From the literature[95].

by diluting the antagonists, typically naloxone and administering it very slowly in order to reverse opioid induced sedation but not precipitate a withdrawal syndrome.

Other actions

Morphine and related drugs have a variety of other actions other than analgesia, including respiratory depression and the inhibition of gastrointestinal transit, which is associated with constipation[102,104,105]. Opioids also have a number of neuroendocrine actions. These actions, like analgesia, are reversed by opioid antagonists, such as naloxone, which confirms that they are opioid receptor-mediated. Respiratory depression and the inhibition of gastrointestinal transit are of greatest concern clinically. There is evidence raising the possibility of distinct populations of mu receptor subtypes for these side effects and morphine analgesia[102,104,105]. Thus, it may be possible to develop opioids lacking these undesirable actions. Alternatively, selective delta and kappa drugs might avoid some of these problems. Some highly selective kappa drugs have been examined in humans. Although they displayed analgesia, their clinical utility was impaired by the high incidence of psychotomimetic effects and a profound diuresis. Delta drugs have not been studied in detail clinically.

Molecular opioid actions

Opioid actions can be defined at the level of the receptor, the cell and in the modulation of circuitry within the nervous system. Much progress in these areas has been made over the past few decades, although it is still difficult to integrate all these various

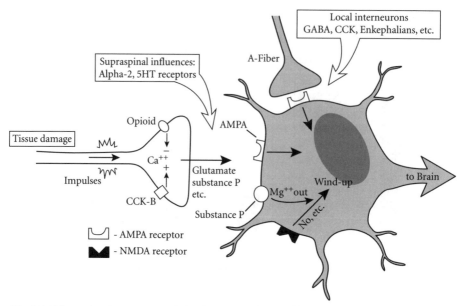

Fig. 2.4 Schematic of neurotransmission between primary afferents and wide dynamic range neurons (WDR).

foci of investigation. At the cellular level, the three opioid receptors are inhibitory, preventing the presynpatic release of a number of neurotransmitters. The ability to inhibit the release of acetylcholine was first demonstrated in the guinea pig ileum[106,107]. Of particular interest were the observations that opioids inhibited the release of glutamate, calcitonin gene-related protein (CGRP) and substance P in view of their established roles in pain circuitry and nociceptive transmission[75] (Fig. 2.4). The substance P within the dorsal horn of the spinal cord originates from dorsal root ganglia neurons, as well as neurons intrinsic to the cord. The receptor for substance P, termed the neurokinin I (NK1) receptor, is present on postsynaptic afferent terminals within lamina I, II, IX[108]. Calcitonin gene-related peptide (CGRP), another peptide associated with pain modulation, is released from primary afferents and facilitates the activity of substance P within the dorsal horn[76]. Glutamate is one of the most important transmitters, with actions throughout the nervous system. There are a number of glutamate receptors, including the ionotropic NMDA and alpha-amino-3-hydroxy-5-methyl-4-isoxazolepropionate (AMPA) receptors, as well as the metabotropic glutamate receptors that belong within the G-protein coupled receptor family. Nociceptive transmission is thought to involve all three transmitter systems. Glutamate has a unique place in nociception since activation of NMDA receptors has been associated with the production of centrally mediated chronic neuropathic pain and hyperalgesia. Indeed, spinal cord 'wind up' is induced by sustained depolarization of wide dynamic range (WDR) neurons found in deeper layers of the dorsal horn[76,109–112].

Opioids modulate both ion channels and transduction systems involved with G-protein coupled receptors.

Electrophysiology

Opioids have a variety of effects on channels and, thus, the ionic conductances in the cell. Cyclic adenosine $5'$-phosphate (cAMP) modulates the membrane 'pacemaker' current that influences the excitability of the cell. Opioids inhibit cyclic AMP formation and thereby reduce spontaneous neuronal depolarization by maintaining the membrane in a hyperpolarized state[113,114]. This, in turn, reduces neurotransmitter release, consistent with the results described above.

Opioids induce postsynaptic neuron membrane hyperpolarization through activation of G-protein-activating inwardly rectifying potassium channels (GIRK)[75,115]. Four GIRK channels have been identified (GIRK I, II, III, V). The GIRK-II is particularly important in opioid analgesia[116]. High efficacy opioids maintain GIRK in an active state and produce a longer duration of potassium influx. Overall, the coupling of opioids with GIRK appears to be less efficient than opioid-calcium channel interactions or cyclic AMP inhibition[113,114].

Opioids also block the voltage-gated calcium channels[75,117], presumably through their activation of pertussis toxin-sensitive G_i and/or G_o proteins. The $G_{\beta\gamma}$ subunits of the heterotrimeric G protein are thought to be primarily responsible for voltage gated calcium channel blockade[113]. Although calcium channels are blocked by opioids through activation of G_o and by $G_{\beta\gamma}$ subunits, intracellular calcium can be mobilized through opioid activation of phospholipase C, which is initiated by certain G-proteins such as G_{11}, G_{14} and G_{16}. Intracellular calcium activates several kinases, which blunt opioid responsiveness through opioid receptor phosphorylation and receptor desensitization[118].

Opioid receptors and G-proteins

Opioid receptors are coupled to pertussis toxin-sensitive inhibitory G-proteins, principally $G_{i/o}$, although there is some evidence for excitatory activity in selected situations[75,119–121] (Fig. 2.5). Opioid receptors reduce cyclic AMP through blocking adenylyl cyclase (AC) activity, which, in turn, is responsible for a multitude of actions, including modulation of sodium channel activity[118]. G-protein-mediated actions include blocking calcium and GIRK channels, as well as increasing intracellular calcium through membrane phospholipase C and the activation of a number of kinases (mitogen-activated protein kinase or MAPK), which act to balance opioid inhibitory responses[118,121]. Opioid receptors are 'promiscuous' in that they can interact with several different G-protein complexes[118]. The type of opioid G-protein coupling appears to be independent of type of opioid receptors, opioid affinity to the receptor, receptor density and availability of G-protein[118,121]. All three receptors can activate $G_{i/o}$ proteins with equal efficacy although there are specific preferences for certain G-protein subtypes[118,122,123]. Opioid receptor G-protein interactions are also tissue and cell

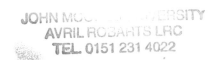

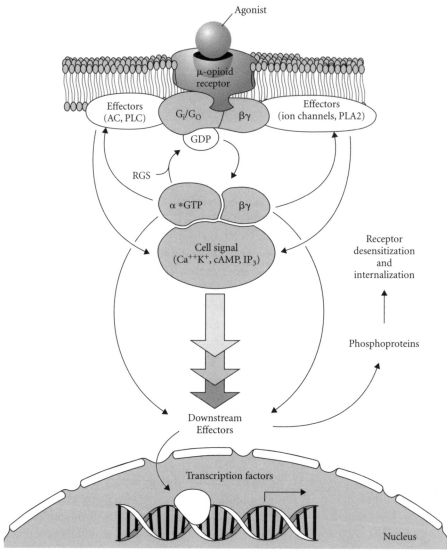

Fig. 2.5 Schematic of interactions between opioids receptors and G proteins.

specific[124]. Subtle differences in receptor structural conformation among the three major opioid receptors can influence the type of G protein coupling specificity[124]. Opioid receptors will also interact with certain pertussis toxin- insensitive G-proteins, such as G_z, G_{14} and G_{16}. Similar to pertussis toxin-sensitive G proteins, these G proteins also stimulate GIRK and inhibit AC[118].

One of the paradoxes of opioid pharmacology is the excitatory actions seen at very low concentrations that stimulate adenylyl cyclase activity[119,120]. At this point, it is not clear whether this effect involves unique receptor subtypes, unusual complements of G-proteins or adenylyl cyclase isoforms that are stimulated by $G_{\beta\gamma}$ subunits of Gi and/or Go[118]. The 'superactivation' of adenylyl cyclase produced by the opioids can mimic many of the observations seen with opioid withdrawal.

Regulators of G-protein signaling (RGS) are important modulators of G-protein responses, influencing the duration of G-protein signaling[124]. RGS proteins serve as GTPase activating proteins, which curtail receptor signaling by facilitating the hydrolysis of GTP to GDP, which in turns leads to the reassociation of the G-protein subunits and the termination of their activity. Multiple RGS isotypes have been described that interact selectively with different G-proteins[124–126]. RGS proteins also have been associated behaviorally with opioid tolerance[127].

Tolerance

Tolerance is a standard response to continued exposure to opioids, as discussed above. The mechanisms involved with tolerance are extensive, ranging from modifications of the receptor and/or its trafficking, to transduction systems, to general cellular effects and synaptic plasticity to diffuse changes in circuitry and interactions with other transmitters. Tolerance can be either homologous, in which the effects are limited only to opioid systems, or heterologous, in which similar actions are seen with other transmitters sharing the same effector systems. Desensitization of opioid receptor activity, which some consider a form of tolerance, can occur rapidly following opioid receptor occupation[118]. Slower processes, many of which require protein synthesis, include the up-regulation of adenylyl cyclase in response to chronic opioids[128–130].

It has been suggested that prolonged opioid receptor interactions reduce G-protein coupling[131]. Due to a combination of desensitization and changes in receptor levels resulting from endocytosis and trafficking, receptor desensitization occurs more rapidly than down-regulation, although they both are thought to require receptor phosphorylation[132]. Various kinases such as G-protein receptor kinases, protein kinase-A (PKA), protein kinase-C (PKC), calcium-calmodulin dependent protein kinase-II, tyrosine kinase can phosphorylate opioid receptors at the third intracellular loop and the C-terminal tail. which is thought to modulate the ability of the receptor to activate the G-proteins[133].

Modulation of receptor actions

Opioid function at the cellular level can be influenced by many factors. While all these actions have been clearly demonstrated experimentally, understanding and integrating them into a comprehensive understanding of behavior has not been easy. The major problem is one of relative importance and causality. These are the major questions to be addressed.

Opioid receptors are internalized after activation by an agonist. Removing the receptor from the surface sequesters it from further activation and may protect from additional enzymatic modifications. Internalization requires endocytosis and is dependent upon a variety of mechanisms, some of which involve β-arrestin, dynamin and G-protein receptor kinases[133–135]. Once internalized, the ligand can dissociate from the receptor, which can then be returned to the surface of the cell or the receptor can be degraded proteolytically. The significance of internalization on behavior has not been fully established. It is interesting that morphine does not induce internalization, which has suggested to some investigators a paradoxical relationship between internalization and tolerance in which failure to internalize leads to tolerance[136]. However, this concept remains quite controversial since a number of drugs that do internalize the receptor also produce tolerance.

A variety of kinases have been implicated in the neuroadaptive changes to opioid signal transduction following continued exposure to the drug[137]. When activated, kinases and phosphatases can have extensive effects on receptor function. Phosphorylation of opioid receptors has been associated with desensitization, while other receptors, such as the NMDA receptor which counter opioid responses, are activated[137].

Opioid/neurotransmitter interactions and tolerance

A number of transmitters and their receptors have been implicated in countering the actions of opioids, including glutamate and NMDA receptors, cholecystokinin (CCK), γ-aminobutyric acid (GABA), dopamine and nitric oxide[97,100,131,138]. Early studies suggested that CCK antagonists could block morphine tolerance, but subsequent studies suggested that this might simply reflect a potentiation of morphine responses in general without a direct effect on tolerance[139,140]. However, there does appear to be a direct involvement of NMDA receptors and nitric oxide systems in morphine tolerance, as noted earlier[96–99,101,141]. Blockade of NMDA receptors or nitric oxide synthase can prevent or reverse pre-established opioid tolerance.

Fully evaluating these systems is complex, since these systems can have opposing effects on opioid analgesia that depend upon the receptor location. For example, activation of NMDA systems within the rostral ventromedial medulla facilitate opioid analgesia by activating descending pain inhibitory tracts, which dampen dorsal horn neurotransmission. Conversely, NMDA receptors within the dorsal horn are considered to be pronociceptive[142,143]. GABA is antinociceptive within the dorsal horn, but within the periaqueductal gray, GABA counters analgesia by inhibiting 'off cells' , which are responsible for the descending inhibition of dorsal horn sensory processing. GABA-A receptor agonists, such as muscimol, produce hyperalgesia and hypersensitivity in the periaqueductal gray[144–147].

Opioid-induced hyperexcitability

Occasional patients receiving spinal opioids over a prolonged period of time develop hyperesthesia with high doses of morphine[148–150]. This paradoxical pain is associated with high doses of morphine[151]. These abnormal pain states initiated by opioids resemble neuropathic pain qualitatively and differ from the original pain for which the opioid was initiated. However, these pain states are not common and clinical importance remains a matter of debate. It has been suggested that opioid-induced pain, neuropathic pain and opioid analgesic tolerance share some of the same underlying neurophysiological mechanisms[148,150,152,153]. It is believed that this hyperalgesia may be related to the hyperexcitability seen in cells with low doses of morphine[119,120], but this is uncertain in view of the need for high spinal morphine doses, not low ones, to induce the syndrome.

Opioid dosing

The optimal dosing schedule for opioids is still unsettled. Many clinicians have long recommended 'around the clock' dosing, in which the opioids are given at fixed intervals without waiting for the pain to re-appear. This has many advantages, primarily in the fact that the patient does not need to suffer while waiting for their medication to act. Some investigators have suggested that intermittent opioids for chronic pain lead to 'mini-withdrawal' responses that interfere with opioid actions[154]. Persistent hyperalgesia also has been reported long after opioid withdrawal[155–157]. It has been suggested that both opioid withdrawal and naloxone increase spinal glutamate release and NMDA receptor activation, and may lead to more analgesic tolerance[158]. On the other hand, very low doses of naloxone sufficient to selectively block the excitatory effects of the drug are pro-analgesic. Thus, this remains a complex area of investigation with uncertain clinical implications. However, the advantages of maintaining the patient pain free along with the studies showing a decreased overall analgesic requirement with patient-controlled analgesia strongly support the concept of 'around the clock dosing'. Clinicians should be careful and be aware of the durations of the drugs they are using, particularly the long-lasting agents that may take several days to reach steady-state levels and yet not dose patients at intervals which allow a period of withdrawal.

Mu opioid receptor genetics

All three opioid receptor classes have been cloned and all are members of the G-protein coupled receptor family, with their traditional seven transmembrane domains[78,105,118,159,160]. The first coding exon of each encodes the N-terminus and the first transmembrane domain, while the second coding exon encodes the next three transmembrane domains and the third coding exon, the last three transmembrane domains and the C-terminus (Fig. 2.6). The only exception is MOR-1, which has an additional fourth coding exon at the 3'-end responsible for the last 12 amino acids in the intracellular C-terminus[118,161–164]. The three opioid receptors share 60% amino acid identity, predominantly in the transmembrane domains and receptor homology among species is very high, particularly the second, third and seventh transmembrane domains[165]. The second and third intracellular loops are also well conserved among

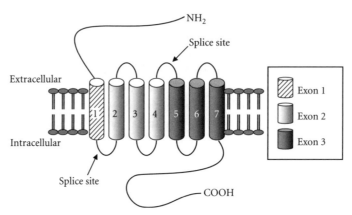

Fig. 2.6 Schematic structure of the DOR-1 and KOR-1 opioid receptors.

the three opioid receptors and are the principle sites for G-protein coupling[118]. The C-terminus tail is not well conserved among the major opioid receptors and has a number of putative phosphorylation sites.

Alternative splicing

Only one gene has been identified that encodes a mu receptor, leaving open the question of its relationship to the mu receptor subtypes implied from the pharmacological studies. Soon after the initial cloning, a splice variant was identified in a human cell line[52] and rat brain[57]. Subsequently, a host of splice variants were identified in mice (Fig. 2.7), with similar splicing patterns in rats and humans[53–56,166]. The most common pattern among the species involves splicing at the C-terminus (Fig. 2.8). This splicing is downstream from exon 3, which is interesting, since the kappa receptor KOR-1 and delta receptor DOR-1 both only have three coding exons. These C-terminus MOR-1 splice variants all contain identical transmembrane domains which are thought to comprise the binding pocket, but differ at the tip of their C-terminus (Fig. 2.8). Thus, it is not surprising that they all show similar affinities and selectivities for mu ligands (Table 2.4). Despite these similarities in binding affinities, the mu opioids can vary enormously in terms of their relative efficacies and potencies at these variants (Fig. 2.9), presumably due to the differences in the C-terminus. For example, the potency of fentanyl and DAMGO were quite similar for all the variants tested, while dynorphin A and β-endorphin varied markedly. The efficacy of the drugs also varied from variant to variant (Fig. 2.9B). Although methadone showed similar efficacies, as defined by the maximal stimulation of [^{35}S]GTPgS binding, β-endorphin showed a wide range. However, what makes these observations most interesting was the difference in rank order of the drugs from one variant to another. β-Endorphin was more efficacious than fentanyl in MOR-1E, but fentanyl was more efficacious in

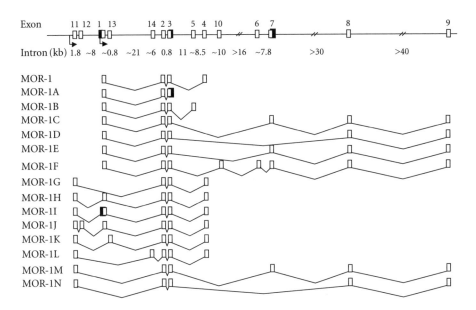

Fig. 2.7 Schematic of the alternative splicing in the mouse MOR-1 gene.

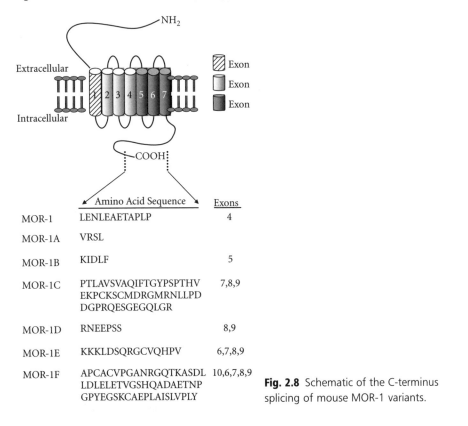

	Amino Acid Sequence	Exons
MOR-1	LENLEAETAPLP	4
MOR-1A	VRSL	
MOR-1B	KIDLF	5
MOR-1C	PTLAVSVAQIFTGYPSPTHV EKPCKSCMDRGMRNLLPD DGPRQESGEGQLGR	7,8,9
MOR-1D	RNEEPSS	8,9
MOR-1E	KKKLDSQRGCVQHPV	6,7,8,9
MOR-1F	APCACVPGANRGQTKASDL LDLELETVGSHQADAETNP GPYEGSKCAEPLAISLVPLY	10,6,7,8,9

Fig. 2.8 Schematic of the C-terminus splicing of mouse MOR-1 variants.

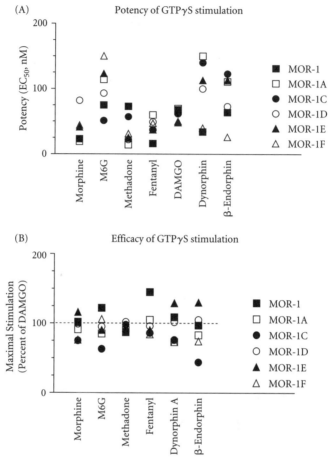

Fig. 2.9 Activation of the MOR-1 variants. The ability of the indicated drugs to active the receptors expressed in CHO cells was assessed by their ability to induce the binding of a stable GTP analog, [^{35}S]GTPgS. (A) The potency of the drugs was assessed by their ED$_{50}$ values. (B) Efficacy was determined by the maximal stimulation of the drug in each variant and expressed as a percentage of the maximal effect of DAMGO. From the literature[177].

MOR-1. Thus, the ability of the various mu opioids to activate these receptors varies markedly among the variants and among each other. These functional differences may help explain the variability among the drugs seen clinically.

Within the brain, the variants all have distinct regional distributions[167–170]. Even in areas that contain more than one variant, there is evidence indicating expression of each in distinct neurons. Thus, these variants display region- and cell-specific processing. At the ultrastructural level they also differ. For example, MOR-1 is localized both pre- and postsynaptically. In contrast, MOR-1C is almost exclusively localized presynaptically. Additional studies illustrate that the variants also are associated with different classes

Table 2.4 Affinity of opioids for MOR-1 variants

Ligand	K_i value (nM)					
	MOR-1	MOR-1A	MOR-1C	MOR-1D	MOR-1E	MOR-1F
Morphine	5.3 ± 2.5	3.1 ± 0.5	2.7 ± 0.8	1.6 ± 0.2	2.4 ± 0.6	3.0 ± 0.6
M6G	6.4 ± 2.4	5.0 ± 1.5	4.5 ± 1.8	4.8 ± 0.9	5.6 ± 0.9	9.6 ± 1.0
Methadone	1.4 ± 0.1	0.7 ± 0.1	0.5 ± 0.1	1.4 ± 0.1	0.7 ± 0.3	1.3 ± 0.2
Fentanyl	2.3 ± 1.0	1.5 ± 0.6	1.2 ± 0.4	3.3 ± 1.5	1.2 ± 0.5	1.7 ± 0.5
DAMGO	1.7 ± 0.4	1.0 ± 0.3	0.9 ± 0.2	0.8 ± 0.2	0.6 ± 0.2	1.1 ± 0.3
Dynorphin A	10.5 ± 0.7	8.2 ± 2.8	4.6 ± 1.1	2.7 ± 0.8	8.9 ± 1.1	12.1 ± 1.0
β-Endorphin	8.4 ± 4.9	4.3 ± 1.0	5.8 ± 0.5	1.7 ± 0.5	4.9 ± 1.2	6.0 ± 1.6
[Met]^{5}enkephalin-Arg^6-Phe^7	4.1 ± 1.0	3.5 ± 1.3	2.1 ± 0.7	3.7 ± 1.2	4.4 ± 0.9	3.9 ± 0.7
Endomorphin 1	2.1 ± 0.9	2.3 ± 0.3	1.1 ± 0.3	1.8 ± 0.3	2.3 ± 0.2	2.9 ± 1.1
Endomorphin 2	4.2 ± 2.3	3.9 ± 0.8	1.5 ± 0.2	2.0 ± 0.4	4.4 ± 1.0	4.1 ± 1.6
U50,488H	>500	>500	>500	>500	>500	>500
DPDPE	>500	>500	>500	>500	>500	>500

Receptor competition binding studies were performed on CHO cells stably transected with the indicated splice variant using the mu agonist ^{3}H-DAMGO. Results are from the literature[177].

of neurons. Whereas MOR-1C is associated with neurons containing CGRP at both the light and ultrastructural level, MOR-1 is not[170].

The mouse also has extensive splicing at the N-terminus. Exon 11 is located approximately 10 kb upstream from exon 1[53] and it has its own promoter independent from the promoter associated with exon 1[171]. While some of the variants generated by the exon 11 promoter encode truncated proteins of unknown significance, three of these exon 11 variants also encode the same protein as MOR-1 itself, leading to the question of why four different splice variants under the control of two different promoters generate the same identical protein.

Dimerization of opioid receptors

Receptor heterogeneity also can be achieved through receptor dimerization[118,172–174]. Both homo- and heterodimerization have been observed. Dimerization is common among G-protein receptors. It has been suggested that dimerization of opioid receptors requires interactions between transmembrane domain 5 in one receptor and transmembrane domain 6 in the other to form an interface between the two receptors within the lipid layer[175].

Opioid receptor dimerization can alter opioid receptor selectivity and trafficking[176]. Heterodimers may have different opioid binding profiles compared to monomers, as shown by the association of DOR-1 and KOR-1[176], to form a receptor consistent with the kappa$_2$ receptors first proposed from binding assays[58]. Perhaps the most prominent change in ligand selectivity within the opioid field is the dimerization of MOR-1 and the orphanin FQ receptor, ORL1 (KOR-3)[174]. The binding of orphanin FQ/nociceptin (OFQ/N) to its own receptor has very high affinity and insensitive to traditional opioids. Co-expression of the ORL1 (KOR-3) receptor with MOR-1changes this selectivity, with standard opioids competing OFQ/N binding quite potently.

Clinical relevance

The cardinal principle to pain management is the need to individualize therapy. Clinical observations have long documented a wide range of responses among individuals to different mu opioids, actions that can be recapitulated in animal models. Unfortunately, the choice of drug for an individual patient remains empiric. There is no way to anticipate which one will be optimal. Thus, the clinician is faced with the need to switch therapies until an effective one is found. Pure opioid agonists have no ceiling effect on pain control, so escalation of drug dose can enhance responses. However, dose escalation is often limited by side effects. With chronic dosing, all patients will become both tolerant and physically dependent. When the dose of the drug can no longer be increased, it is common to switch the patient to an alternative opioid, a concept termed 'opioid rotation'[103]. By changing the drug, it is often possible to restore analgesic effectiveness due to the presence of incomplete cross-tolerance. However, it is important to note that the relative potency of opioids changes in tolerant patients and the equivalent ratios commonly published for opioid naïve patients are not correct. Indeed, when switching drugs in a highly tolerant patient, it is common practice to reduce the anticipated dose of the second drug by 50% or even more to avoid overdosing the patient.

Despite the known benefits of opioids in controlling pain, opioids are rarely used alone in pain management. A wide range of adjuvant drugs are available and effective. These range from NSAIDS to antidepressants. NMDA antagonists also have the theoretical advantage of reducing tolerance, although this has not yet been demonstrated clinically. The wide range of responses among patients to adjuvant analgesics requires individualization of therapy.

Conclusions

Opioid pharmacodynamics are both unique and complex. Advances in molecular medicine have unraveled many of the mysteries behind the wide diversity of opioid responses between individuals, but many more remain. Our present understanding of opioid receptor genetics, and its molecular pharmacology opens new avenues in the design and development of new agents. Equally important, it provides a scientific foundation to support what clinicians have known for centuries. All patients and their pain are unique and so must be their treatments.

References

1 Beckett AH, Casy AF. Synthetic analgesics: stereochemical considerations. *J Pharm Pharmacol* 1954; **6**: 986–1001.

2 Portoghese PS, Mikhail AA, Kupferberg HJ. Stereochemical studies on medicinal agents. VI.[1] Bicyclic bases.[2] Synthesis and pharmacology of epimeric bridged analogs of meperidine, 2-methyl-5-carbethoxy-2-azabicyclo[2.2.1]heptane[3]. *J Med Chem* 1967; **11**: 219–25.

3 Martin WR. Opioid antagonists. *Pharmacol Rev* 1967; **19**: 463–521.

4 Pert CB, Snyder SH. Opiate receptor: demonstration in nervous tissue. *Science* 1973; **179**: 1011–14.

5 Terenius L. Stereospecific interaction between narcotic analgesics and a synaptic plasma membrane fraction of rat cerebral cortex. *Acta Pharmacol Toxicol* 1973; **32**: 317–20.

6 Simon EJ, Hiller JM, Edelman I. Stereospecific binding of the potent narcotic analgesic [^{3}H]etorphine to rat-brain homogenate. *Proc Natl Acad Sci USA* 1973; **70**: 1947–9.

7 Snyder SH, Pasternak GW. Historical review: opioid receptors. *Trends Pharmacol Sci* 2003; **24**: 198–205.

8 Martin WR, Eades CG, Thompson JA, *et al*. The effects of morphine and nalorphine-like drugs in the nondependent and morphine-dependent chronic spinal dog. *J Pharmacol Exp Ther* 1976; **197**: 517–32.

9 Chavkin C, Goldstein A. Specific receptor for the opioid peptide dynorphin: structure–activity relationships. *Proc Natl Acad Sci USA* 1981; **78**: 6543–7.

10 Goldstein A, Tachibana S, Lowney LI, *et al*. Dynorphin-(1–13), an extraordinarily potent opioid peptide. *Proc Natl Acad Sci USA* 1979; **76**: 6666–70.

11 Reisine T, Pasternak GW. Opioid analgesics and antagonists. In: Hardman JG, Limbird LE (Eds) *Goodman & Gilman's: the pharmacological basis of therapeutics*. Washington, DC: McGraw-Hill, 1996; pp. 521–56.

12 Akil H, Mayer DJ, Liebeskind JC. Antagonism of stimulation-produced analgesia by naloxone, a narcotic antagonist. *Science* 1976; **191**: 961–2.

13 Mayer DJ, Liebeskind JC. Pain reduction by focal electrical stimulation of the brain: an anatomical and behavioral analysis. *Brain Res* 1974; **68**: 73–93.

14 Snyder SH, Pert CB, Pasternak GW. The opiate receptor. *Ann Int Med* 1974; **81**: 534–40.

15 Hughes J. Isolation of an endogenous compound from the brain with pharmacological properties similar to morphine. *Brain Res* 1975; **88**: 295–308.

16 Pasternak GW, Goodman R, Snyder SH. An endogenous morphine like factor in mammalian brain. *Life Sci* 1975; **16**: 1765–9.

17 Terenius L. Wahlstrom A. Search for an endogenous ligand for the opiate receptor. *Acta Physiol Scand* 1975; **94**: 74–81.

18 Hughes J, Smith TW, Kosterlitz HW, *et al*. Identification of two related pentapeptides from the brain with potent opiate agonist activity. *Nature* 1975; **258**: 577–9.

19 Simantov R, Snyder SH. Isolation and structure identification of a morphine-like peptide 'enkephalin' in bovine brain. *Life Sci* 1976; **18**: 781–8.

20 Zadina JE, Hackler L, Ge LJ, *et al*. A potent and selective endogenous agonist for the μ-opiate receptor. *Nature* 1997; **386**: 499–502.

21 Evans CJ, Hammond DL, Frederickson RCA. The opioid peptides. In: Pasternak GW (Ed.) *The Opiate Receptors*. Clifton: Humana Press, 1988, pp. 23–74.

22 Li CH, Chung D, Doneen BA. Isolation, characterization and opiate activity of beta-endorphin from human pituitary glands. *Biochem Biophys Res Commun* 1976; **72**: 1542–7.

23 Li CH, Chung D. Primary structure of human β-lipotropin. *Nature* 1976; **260**: 622–4.

24 Pert CB, Pasternak GW, Snyder SH. Opiate agonists and antagonists discriminated by receptor binding in brain. *Science* 1973; **182:** 1359–61.

25 Pert CB, Pasternak GW, Snyder SH. Opiate agonists and antagonists discriminated by receptor binding in brain. *Proc Comm Drug Depend* 1974; 376–82.

26 Pasternak GW, Snowman AS, Snyder SH. Selective enhancement of [^{3}H]opiate agonist binding by divalent cations. *Mol Pharmacol* 1975; **11:** 478–84.

27 Pasternak GW, Snyder SH. Opiate receptor binding: enzymatic treatments and discrimination between agonists and antagonists. *Mol Pharmacol* 1975; **11:** 735–44.

28 Pasternak GW, Wilson HA, Snyder SH. Differential effects of protein-modifying reagents on receptor binding of opiate agonists and antagonists. *Mol Pharmacol* 1975; **11:** 340–51.

29 Wilson HA, Pasternak GW, Snyder SH. Differentiation of opiate agonist and antagonist receptor binding by protein-modifying reagents. *Nature* 1975; **256:** 448–50.

30 Childers SR, Snyder SH. Differential regulation by guanine nucleotides of opiate agonist and antagonist receptor interactions. *J Neurochem* 1980; **34:** 583–93.

31 Takemori AE, Larson DL, Portoghese PS. Irreversible narcotic antagonistic and reversible agonistic properties of the fumaramate methylester derivative of naltrexone. *Eur J Pharmacol* 1981; **70:** 445–51.

32 Ward SJ, Portoghese PS, Takemori AE. Use of the novel opiate, β-funaltrexamine (β-FNA) in the elucidation of receptor types involved in opiate-mediated respiratory depression, *Conference Proceeding*. Tokyo: Kodansha, Ltd, 1981; 229–32.

33 Pasternak GW, Childers SR, Snyder SH. Naloxazone, long-acting opiate antagonist: effects in intact animals and on opiate receptor binding *in vitro*. *J Pharmacol Exp Ther* 1980; **214:** 455–62.

34 Pasternak GW, Childers SR, Snyder SH. Opiate analgesia: evidence for mediation by a subpopulation of opiate receptors. *Science* 1980; **208:** 514–16.

35 Hahn EF, Pasternak GW. Naloxonazine, a potent, long-acting inhibitor of opiate binding sites. *Life Sci* 1982; **31:** 1385–8.

36 Pasternak GW. Insights into mu opioid pharmacology—the role of mu opioid receptor subtypes. *Life Sci* 2001; **68:** 2213–19.

37 Portoghese PS, Sultana M, Takemori AE. Naltrindole, a highly selective and potent non-peptide delta opioid receptor antagonist. *Eur J Pharmacol* 1988; **146:** 185–6.

38 Portoghese PS, Lipkowski AW, Takemori AE. Binaltorphimine and nor-binaltorphimine, potent and selective k-opioid receptor agonists. *Life Sci* 1987; **40:** 1287–92.

39 Martin WR. Opioid antagonists. *Pharmacol Rev* 1967; **19:** 463–521.

40 Lord JAH, Waterfield AA, Hughes J, *et al*. Multiple opiate receptors. In: International narcotic research club. **Opiates and endogenous peptides: proceedings of the International Narcotic Research Club meeting, Aberdeen, UK. 19–22 July 1976.** Amsterdam: North-Holland, 1976, pp. 275–80.

41 Lord JAH, Waterfield AA, Hughes J, *et al*. Endogenous opioid peptides: multiple agonists and receptors. *Nature* 1977; **267:** 495–9.

42 Chang K-J, Cooper BR, Hazum E, *et al*. Multiple opiate receptors: different regional distribution in the brain and differential binding of opiates and opioid peptides. *Mol Pharmacol* 1979; **16:** 91–104.

43 Wolozin BL, Pasternak GW. Classification of multiple morphine and enkephalin binding sites in the central nervous system. *Proc Natl Acad Sci USA* 1981; **78:** 6181–5.

44 Hahn EF, Carroll-Buatti M, Pasternak GW. Irreversible opiate agonists and antagonists: the 14-hydroxydihydromorphinone azines. *J Neurosci* 1982; **2:** 572–6.

45 Spiegel K, Kourides I, Pasternak GW. Prolactin and growth hormone release by morphine in the rat: different receptor mechanisms. *Science* 1982; **217:** 745–7.

46 Ling GSF, Pasternak GW. Spinal and supraspinal opioid analgesia in the mouse: the role of subpopulations of opioid binding sites. *Brain Res* 1983; **271:** 152–6.

47 Ling GSF, Spiegel K, Lockhart SH, *et al.* Separation of opioid analgesia from respiratory depression: evidence for different receptor mechanisms. *J Pharmacol Exp Ther* 1985; **232:** 149–55.

48 Ling GSF, Simantov R, Clark JA, *et al.* Naloxonazine actions *in vivo. Eur J Pharmacol* 1986; **129:** 33–8.

49 Paul D, Pasternak GW. Differential blockade by naloxonazine of two μ opiate actions: analgesia and inhibition of gastrointestinal transit. *Eur J Pharmacol* 1988; **149:** 403–4.

50 Pasternak GW, Bodnar RJ, Clark JA, *et al.* Morphine-6-glucuronide, a potent mu agonist. *Life Sci* 1987; **41:** 2845–9.

51 Paul D, Standifer KM, Inturrisi CE, *et al.* Pharmacological characterization of morphine-6β-glucuronide, a very potent morphine metabolite. *J Pharmacol Exp Ther* 1989; **251:** 477–83.

52 Bare LA, Mansson E, Yang D. Expression of two variants of the human μ opioid receptor mRNA in SK-N-SH cells and human brain. *FEBS Lett* 1994; **354:** 213–16.

53 Pan Y-X, Xu J, Mahurter L, *et al.* Generation of the mu opioid receptor (MOR-1) protein by three new splice variants of the Oprm gene. *Proc Natl Acad Sci USA* 2001; **98:** 14084–9.

54 Pan Y-X, Xu J, Mahurter L, *et al.* Identification and characterization of two new human mu opioid receptor splice variants, hMOR-1O and hMOR-1X. *Biochem Biophys Res Commun* 2003; **301:** 1057–61.

55 Pan YX, Xu J, Bolan EA, *et al.* Identification and characterization of three new alternatively spliced mu opioid receptor isoforms. *Mol Pharmacol* 1999; **56:** 396–403.

56 Pan YX, Xu J, Bolan EA, *et al.* Isolation and expression of a novel alternatively spliced mu opioid receptor isoform, MOR-1F. *FEBS Lett* 2000; **466:** 337–40.

57 Zimprich A, Simon T, Hollt V. Cloning and expression of an isoform of the rat μ opioid receptor (rMOR 1 B) which differs in agonist induced desensitization from rMOR1. *FEBS Lett* 1995; **359:** 142–6.

58 Zukin RS, Eghbali M, Olive D, *et al.* Characterization and visualization of rat and guinea pig brain kappa opioid receptors: evidence for kappa₁ and kappa₂ opioid receptors. *Proc Natl Acad Sci USA* 1988; **85:** 4061–5.

59 Gistrak MA, Paul D, Hahn EF, *et al.* Pharmacological actions of a novel mixed opiate agonist/antagonist, naloxone benzoylhydrazone. *J Pharmacol Exp Ther* 1990; **251:** 469–76.

60 Luke MC, Hahn EF, Price M, *et al.* Irreversible opiate agonists and antagonists: V. Hydrazone and acylhydrazone derivatives of naltrexone. *Life Sci* 1988; **43:** 1249–56.

61 Price M, Gistrak MA, Itzhak Y, *et al.* Receptor binding of ³H-naloxone benzoylhydrazone: a reversible kappa and slowly dissociable μ opiate. *Mol Pharmacol* 1989; **35:** 67–74.

62 Paul D, Levison JA, Howard DH, *et al.* Naloxone benzoylhydrazone (NalBzoH) analgesia. *J Pharmacol Exp Ther* 1990; **255:** 769–74.

63 Berzetei-Gurske IP, White A, Polgar W, *et al.* The *in vitro* pharmacological characterization of naloxone benzoylhydrazone. *Eur J Pharmacol* 1995; **277:** 257–63.

64 Clark JA, Liu L, Price M, *et al.* Kappa opiate receptor multiplicity: evidence for two U50,488-sensitive kappa₁ subtypes and a novel kappa₃ subtype. *J Pharmacol Exp Ther* 1989; **251:** 461–8.

65 Rothman RB, Bykov V, DeCosta BR, *et al.* Interaction of endogenous opioid peptides and other drugs with four kappa opioid binding sites in guinea pig brain. *Peptides* 1990; **11:** 311–17.

66 Jiang Q, Takemori AE, Sultana M, *et al.* Differential antagonism of opiate delta antinociception by [D-Ala², Cys⁶]enkaphalin and naltrindole-5'-isothiocyanate: evidence for subtypes. *J Pharmacol Exp Ther* 1991; **257:** 1069–75.

67 Mattia A, Vanderah T, Mosberg HI, *et al.* Lack of antinociceptive cross-tolerance between [D-Pen^2,D-Pen^5]enkephalin and [D-Ala^2]deltorphin II in mice: evidence for delta receptor subtypes. *J Pharmacol Exp Ther* 1991; **258**: 583–7.

68 Portoghese PS, Moe ST, Takemori AE. A selective δ_1 opioid receptor agonist derived from oxymorphone. Evidence for separate recognition sites for δ_1 opioid receptor agonists and antagonists. *J Med Chem* 1993; **36**: 2572–4.

69 Takemori AE, Portoghese PS. Enkephalin antinociception in mice is mediated by δ_1- and δ_2-opioid receptors in the brain and spinal cord, respectively. *Eur J Pharmacol* 1993; **242**: 145–50.

70 Janson W, Stein C. Peripheral opioid analgesia. *Curr Pharm Biotechnol* 2003; **4**: 270–4.

71 Schafer MK, Bette M, Romeo H, *et al.* Localization of kappa-opioid receptor mRNA in neuronal subpopulations of rat sensory ganglia and spinal cord. *Neurosci Lett* 1994; **167**: 137–40.

72 Stein C, Yassouridis A. Peripheral morphine analgesia. *Pain* 1997; **71**: 119–21.

73 Stein C. Mechanisms of disease: the control of pain in peripheral tissue by opioids. *N Engl J Med* 1995; **332**: 1685–90.

74 Stein C, Schäfer M, Hassan AHS. Peripheral opioid receptors. *Ann Med* 1995; **27**: 219–21.

75 Yaksh TL. Pharmacology and mechanisms of opioid analgesic activity. *Acta Anaesthesiol Scand* 1997; **41**: 94–111.

76 Dickenson AH. Spinal cord pharmacology of pain. *Br J Anaesth* 1995; **75**: 193–200.

77 Besse D, Lombard MC, Zajac JM, *et al.* Pre- and postsynaptic distribution of mu, delta and kappa opioid receptors in the superficial layers of the cervical dorsal horn of the rat spinal cord. *Brain Res* 1990; **521**: 15–22.

78 Uhl GR, Childers S, Pasternak GW. An opiate-receptor gene family reunion. *Trends Neurosci* 1994; **17**: 89–93.

79 Mansour A, Watson SJ, Akil H. Opioid receptors: past, present and future, *Trends Neurosci* 1995; **18**: 69–70.

80 Atweh SF, Kuhar MJ. Distribution and physiological significance of opioid receptors in the brain. *Br Med Bull* 1983; **39**: 47–52.

81 Rawlings W, Bynum TE, Pasternak GW. Pancreatic ascites: diagnosis of leakage site by endoscopic pancreatography. *Surgery* 1977; **81**: 363–5.

82 Mansour A, Fox CA, Akil H, *et al.* Opioid-receptor mRNA expression in the rat CNS: anatomical and functional implications. *Trends Neurosci* 1995; **18**: 22–9.

83 Mansour A, Fox CA, Burke S, *et al.* Mu, delta, and kappa opioid receptor mRNA expression in the rat CNS: an *in situ* hybridization study. *J Comp Neurol* 1994; **350**: 412–38.

84 Mansour A, Fox CA, Meng F, *et al.* Kappa 1 receptor mRNA distribution in the rat CNS: comparison to kappa receptor binding and prodynorphin mRNA. *Mol Cell Neurosci* 1994; **5**: 124–44.

85 Pert A, Yaksh TL. Sites of morphine induced analgesia in primate brain: relation to pain pathways. *Brain Res* 1974; **80**: 135–40.

86 Yeung JC, Rudy TA. Multiplicative interaction between narcotic agonisms expressed at spinal and supraspinal sites of antinociceptive action as revealed by concurrent intrathecal and intracerebroventricular injections of morphine. *J Pharmacol Exp Ther* 1980; **215**: 633–42.

87 Kolesnikov YA, Jain S, Wilson R, *et al.* Peripheral morphine analgesia: synergy with central sites and a target of morphine tolerance. *J Pharmacol Exp Ther* 1996; **279**: 502–6.

88 Kolesnikov Y, Pasternak GW. Topical opioids in mice: analgesia and reversal of tolerance by a topical N-methyl-D-aspartate antagonist. *J Pharmacol Exp Ther* 1999; **290**: 247–52.

89 Rossi GC, Pasternak GW, Bodnar RJ. Synergistic brainstem interactions for morphine analgesia. *Brain Res* 1993; **624**: 171–80.

90 Wilson SG, Smith SB, Chesler EJ, *et al*. The heritability of antinociception: common pharmacogenetic mediation of five neurochemically distinct analgesics. *J Pharmacol Exp Ther* 2003; **304:** 547–59.

91 Lariviere WR, Wilson SG, Laughlin TM, *et al*. Heritability of nociception. III. Genetic relationships among commonly used assays of nociception and hypersensitivity. *Pain* 2002; **97:** 75–86.

92 Flores CM, Mogil JS. The pharmacogenetics of analgesia: toward a genetically-based approach to pain management. *Pharmacogenomics* 2001; **2:** 177–94.

93 Pick CG, Cheng J, Paul D, *et al*. Genetic influences in opioid analgesic sensitivity in mice, *Brain Res* 1991; **556:** 295–8.

94 Chang A, Emmel DW, Rossi GC, *et al*. Methadone analgesia in morphine-insensitive CXBK mice. *Eur J Pharmacol* 1998; **351:** 189–91.

95 Rossi GC, Brown GP, Leventhal L, *et al*. Novel receptor mechanisms for heroin and morphine-6β -glucuronide analgesia. *Neurosci Lett* 1996; **216:** 1–4.

96 Elliott K, Minami N, Kolesnikov YA, *et al*. The NMDA receptor antagonists, LY274614 and MK-801, and the nitric oxide synthase inhibitor, NG-nitro-L-arginine, attenuate analgesic tolerance to the mu-opioid morphine but not to kappa opioids. *Pain* 1994; **56:** 69–75.

97 Pasternak GW, Kolesnikov YA, Babey AM. Perspectives on the N-methyl-D-aspartate nitric oxide cascade and opioid tolerance. *Neuropsychopharmacology* 1995; **13:** 309–13.

98 Trujillo KA, Akil H. Inhibition of morphine tolerance and dependence by the NMDA receptor anagonist MK-801. *Science* 1991; **251:** 85–7.

99 Ben-Eliyahu S, Marek P, Vaccarino AL, *et al*. The NMDA receptor antagonist MK-801 prevents long-lasting non-associative morphine tolerance in the rat. *Brain Res* 1992; **575:** 304–8.

100 Babey AM, Kolesnikov Y, Cheng J, *et al*. Nitric oxide and opioid tolerance. *Neuropharmacology* 1994; **33:** 1463–70.

101 Kolesnikov YA, Pick CG, Pasternak GW. N^G-nitro-L-arginine prevents morphine tolerance. *Eur J Pharmacol* 1992; **221:** 339–40.

102 Pasternak GW. Incomplete cross-tolerance and multiple mu opioid peptide receptors. *Trends Pharmacol Sci* 2001; **22:** 67–70.

103 Cherny N, Ripamonti C, Pereira J, *et al*. Strategies to manage the adverse effects of oral morphine: an evidence-based report. *J Clin Oncol* 2001; **19:** 2542–54.

104 Pasternak GW. The molecular biology of mu opioid analgesia. In: Devor M, Rowbotham MC, Wiesenfeld-Hallin Z (Eds) *Proceedings of the 9th World Congress on Pain*, IASP Press, Seattle, 2000, pp. 147–62.

105 Pasternak GW. The pharmacology of mu analgesics: from patients to genes. *Neuroscientist* 2001; **7:** 220–31.

106 Paton WDM. The action of morphine and related substances on contraction and on acetylcholine output of coaxially stimulated guinea-pig ileum. *Br J Pharmacol* 1957; **12:** 119–24.

107 Schaumann W. Inhibiton by morphine of the release of acetylcholine from the intestine of the guinea-pig. *Br J Pharmacol* 1957; **12:** 115–18.

108 Dickenson AH. Central acute pain mechanisms. *Ann Med* 1995; **27:** 223–7.

109 Coderre TJ, Fundytus ME, McKenna JE, *et al*. The formalin test: a validation of the weighted-scores method of behavioural pain rating. *Pain* 1993; **54:** 43–50.

110 Dray A, Urban L, Dickenson A. Pharmacology of chronic pain. *Trends Pharmacol Sci* 1994; **15:** 190–7.

111 Dubner R, Ruda MA. Activity-dependent neuronal plasticity following tissue injury and inflammation. *Trends Neurosci* 1992; **15:** 96–103.

112 McMahon AP. Cell signalling in induction and anterior-posterior patterning of the vertebrate central nervous system. *Curr Opin Neurobiol* 1993; **3**: 4–7.

113 Williams JT, Christie MJ, Manzoni O. Cellular and synaptic adaptations mediating opioid dependence. *Physiol Rev* 2001; **81**: 299–343.

114 Ingram SL, Williams JT. Opioid inhibition of Ih via adenylyl cyclase. *Neuron* 1994; **13**: 179–86.

115 Henry DJ, Grandy DK, Lester HA, *et al*. Kappa-opioid receptors couple to inwardly rectifying potassium channels when coexpressed by *Xenopus oocytes*. *Mol Pharmacol* 1995; **47**: 551–7.

116 Ikeda K, Kobayashi T, Ichikawa T, *et al*. The untranslated region of μ-opioid receptor mRNA contributes to reduced opioid sensitivity in CXBK mice. *J Neurosci* 2001; **21**: 1334–9.

117 Liu JG, Prather PL. Chronic exposure to μ-opioid agonists produces constitutive activation of μ-opioid receptors in direct proportion to the efficacy of the agonist used for pretreatment. *Mol Pharmacol* 2001; **60**: 53–62.

118 Law PY, Wong YH, Loh HH. Molecular mechanisms and regulation of opioid receptor signaling. *Ann Rev Pharmacol Toxicol* 2000; **40**: 389–430.

119 Crain SM, Shen K-F, Chalazonitis A. Opioids excite rather than inhibit sensory neurons after chronic opioid exposure of spinal cord-ganglion cultures. *Brain Res* 1988; **455**: 99–109.

120 Shen K-F, Crain SM. Dual opioid modulation of the action potential duration of mouse dorsal root ganglion neurons in culture. *Brain Res* 1989; **491**: 227–42.

121 Standifer KM, Pasternak GW. G proteins and opioid receptor-mediated signalling. *Cell Signal* 1997; **9**: 237–48.

122 Prather PL, Loh HH, Law PY. Interaction of δ-opioid receptors with multiple G proteins: a nonrelationship between agonist potency to inhibit adenylyl cyclase and to activate G proteins. *Mol Pharmacol* 1994; **45**: 997–1003.

123 Prather PL, McGinn TM, Erickson LJ, *et al*. Ability of δ-opioid receptors to interact with multiple G-proteins is independent of receptor density. *J Biol Chem* 1994; **269**: 21293–302.

124 Tso PH, Wong YH. Molecular basis of opioid dependence: role of signal regulation by G-proteins. *Clin Exp Pharmacol Physiol* 2003; **30**: 307–16.

125 De Vries L, Zheng B, Fischer T, *et al*. The regulator of G protein signaling family. *Ann Rev Pharmacol Toxicol* 2000; **40**: 235–71.

126 Hunt TW, Fields TA, Casey PJ, *et al*. RGS10 is a selective activator of Gα$_i$ GTPase activity. *Nature* 1996; **383**: 175–7.

127 Garzon J, Rodriguez-Diaz M, Lopez-Fando A, *et al*. RGS9 proteins facilitate acute tolerance to mu-opioid effects. *Eur J Neurosci* 2001; **13**: 801–11.

128 Nestler EJ. Molecular mechanisms of opiate and cocaine addiction. *Curr Opin Neurobiol* 1997; **7**: 713–19.

129 Nestler EJ. Historical review: molecular and cellular mechanisms of opiate and cocaine addiction. *Trends Pharmacol Sci* 2004; **25**: 210–18.

130 Koob GF, Nestler EJ. The neurobiology of drug addiction. *J Neuropsychiat Clin Neurosci* 1997; **9**: 482–97.

131 Ueda H, Inoue M, Mizuno K. New approaches to study the development of morphine tolerance and dependence. *Life Sci* 2003; **74**: 313–20.

132 Harrison LM, Kastin AJ, Zadina JE. Opiate tolerance and dependence: receptors, G-proteins, and antiopiates. *Peptides* 1998; **19**: 1603–30.

133 Borgland SL. Acute opioid receptor desensitization and tolerance: is there a link? *Clin Exp Pharmacol Physiol* 2001; **28**: 147–54.

134 Finn AK, Whistler JL. Endocytosis of the mu opioid receptor reduces tolerance and a cellular hallmark of opiate withdrawal. *Neuron* 2001; **32:** 829–39.

135 Keith DE, Anton B, Murray SR, *et al*. μ-opioid receptor internalization: opiate drugs have differential effects on a conserved endocytic mechanism *in vitro* and in the mammalian brain. *Mol Pharmacol* 1998; **53:** 377–84.

136 Whistler JL, Chuang HH, Chu P, *et al*. Functional dissociation of μ opioid receptor signaling and endocytosis: implications for the biology of opiate tolerance and addiction. *Neuron* 1999; **23:** 737–46.

137 Liu JG, Anand KJ. Protein kinases modulate the cellular adaptations associated with opioid tolerance and dependence. *Brain Res Rev* 2001; **38:** 1–19.

138 Kolesnikov YA, Pan YX, Babey AM, *et al*. Functionally differentiating two neuronal nitric oxide synthase isoforms through antisense mapping: evidence for opposing NO actions on morphine analgesia and tolerance. *Proc Natl Acad Sci USA* 1997; **94:** 8220–5.

139 Watkins LR, Kinscheck IB, Mayer DJ. Potentiation of opiate analgesia and apparent reversal of morphine tolerance by proglumide. *Science* 1984; **224:** 395–6.

140 Bodnar RJ, Paul D, Pasternak GW. Proglumide selectively potentiates supraspinal μ₁ analgesia in mice. *Neuropharmacology* 1990; **29:** 507–10.

141 Kolesnikov YA, Pick CG, Ciszewska G, *et al*. Blockade of tolerance to morphine but not to kappa opioids by a nitric oxide synthase inhibitor. *Proc Natl Acad Sci USA* 1993; **90:** 5162–6.

142 Heinricher MM, Schouten JC, Jobst EE. Activation of brainstem N-methyl-D-aspartate receptors is required for the analgesic actions of morphine given systemically. *Pain* 2001; **92:** 129–38.

143 Ren K, Dubner R. Descending modulation in persistent pain: an update. *Pain* 2002; **100:** 1–6.

144 Stamford JA. Descending control of pain. *Br J Anaesth* 1995; **75:** 217–27.

145 Ingram SL, Vaughan CW, Bagley EE, *et al*. Enhanced opioid efficacy in opioid dependence is caused by an altered signal transduction pathway. *J Neurosci* 1998; **18:** 10269–76.

146 Baba H, Ji RR, Kohno T, *et al*. Removal of GABAergic inhibition facilitates polysynaptic A fiber-mediated excitatory transmission to the superficial spinal dorsal horn. *Mol Cell Neurosci* 2003; **24:** 818–30.

147 Guan Y, Terayama R, Dubner R, *et al*. Plasticity in excitatory amino acid receptor-mediated descending pain modulation after inflammation. *J Pharmacol Exp Ther* 2002; **300:** 513–20.

148 Wegert S, Ossipov MH, Nichols ML, *et al*. Differential activities of intrathecal MK-801 or morphine to alter responses to thermal and mechanical stimuli in normal or nerve-injured rats. *Pain* 1997; **71:** 57–64.

149 Arner S, Rawal N, Gustafsson LL. Clinical experience of long-term treatment with epidural and intrathecal opioids—a nationwide survey. *Acta Anaesthesiol Scand* 1988; **32:** 253–9.

150 Ossipov MH, Lai J, Vanderah TW, *et al*. Induction of pain facilitation by sustained opioid exposure: relationship to opioid antinociceptive tolerance. *Life Sci* 2003; **73:** 783–800.

151 Stillman MJ, Moulin DE, Foley KM. Paradoxical pain following high dose spinal morphine. *Pain* 2004; **30:** 4.

152 Vanderah TW, Suenaga NM, Ossipov MH, *et al*. Tonic descending facilitation from the rostral ventromedial medulla mediates opioid-induced abnormal pain and antinociceptive tolerance. *J Neurosci* 2001; **21:** 279–86.

153 McNally GP. Pain facilitatory circuits in the mammalian central nervous system: their behavioral significance and role in morphine analgesic tolerance. *Neurosci Biobehav Rev* 1999; **23:** 1059–78.

154 Laulin JP, Celerier E, Larcher A, *et al*. Opiate tolerance to daily heroin administration: An apparent phenomenon associated with enhanced pain sensitivity. *Neuroscience* 1999; **89:** 631–6.

155 **Crain SM, Shen KF.** Ultra-low concentrations of naloxone selectively antagonize excitatory effects of morphine on sensory neurons, thereby increasing its antinociceptive potency and attenuating tolerance dependence during chronic cotreatment. *Proc Natl Acad Sci USA* 1995; **92:** 10540–4.

156 **Crain SM, Shen K-F.** Chronic morphine-treated sensory ganglion neurons remain supersensitive to the excitatory effects of naloxone for months after return to normal culture medium: an *in vitro* model of 'protracted opioid dependence'. *Brain Res* 1995 Oct 2; **694**(1–2): 103–10.

157 **Doverty M.,** White JM, Somogyi AA, *et al*. Hyperalgesic responses in methadone maintenance patients. *Pain* 2001; **90:** 91–6.

158 **Dunbar SA, Karamian IG.** Periodic abstinence enhances nociception without significantly altering the antinociceptive efficacy of spinal morphine in the rat. *Neurosci Lett* 2003; **344:** 145–8.

159 **Kieffer BL.** Opioids: first lessons from knockout mice. *Trends Pharmacol Sci* 1999; **20:** 19–26.

160 **Zaki PA, Bilsky EJ, Vanderah TW, *et al*.** Opioid receptor types and subtypes: the δ receptor as a model. *Ann Rev Pharmacol Toxicol* 1996; **36:** 379–401.

161 **Chen Y, Mestek A, Liu J, *et al*.** Molecular cloning and functional expression of a μ-opioid receptor from rat brain. *Mol Pharmacol* 1993; **44:** 8–12.

162 **Eppler CM, Hulmes JD, Wang J-B, *et al*.** Purification and partial amino acid sequence of a μ opioid receptor from rat brain. *J Biol Chem* 1993; **268:** 26447–51.

163 **Thompson RC, Mansour A, Akil H, *et al*.** Cloning and pharmacological characterization of a rat μ opioid receptor. *Neuron* 1993; **11:** 903–13.

164 **Wang JB, Imai Y, Eppler CM, *et al*.** μ opiate receptor: cDNA cloning and expression. *Proc Natl Acad Sci USA* 1993; **90:** 10230–4.

165 **Reisine T, Bell GI.** Molecular biology of opioid receptors. *Trends Neurosci* 1993; **16:** 506–10.

166 **Pasternak DA, Pan L, Xu J, *et al*.** Identification of three new alternatively spliced variants of the rat mu opioid receptor gene: dissociation of affinity and efficacy. *J Neurochem* 2004; in press.

167 **Abbadie C, Pan Y-X, Pasternak GW.** Differential distribution in rat brain of mu opioid receptor carboxy terminal splice variants MOR-1C and MOR-1-like immunoreactivity: evidence for region-specific processing. *J Comp Neurol* 2000; **419:** 244–56.

168 **Abbadie C, Pan Y-X, Drake CT, *et al*.** Comparative immunhistochemical distributions of carboxy terminus epitopes from the mu opioid receptor splice variants MOR-1D, MOR-1 and MOR-1C in the mouse and rat central nervous systems. *Neurosci* 2000; **100:** 141–53.

169 **Abbadie C, Gultekin SH, Pasternak GW.** Immunohistochemical localization of the carboxy terminus of the novel mu opioid receptor splice variant MOR-1C within the human spinal cord, *Neuroreport* 2000; **11:** 1953–7.

170 **Abbadie C, Pasternak GW, Aicher SA.** Presynaptic localization of the carboxy-terminus epitopes of the mu opioid receptor splice variants MOR-1C and MOR-1D in the superficial laminae of the rat spinal cord. *Neuroscience* 2001; **106:** 833–42.

171 **Pan YX.** Identification and characterization of a novel promoter of the mouse mu opioid receptor gene (Oprm) that generates eight splice variants. *Gene* 2002; **295:** 97–108.

172 **Cvejic S, Devi LA.** Dimerization of the delta opioid receptor: implication for a role in receptor internalization. *J Biol Chem* 1997; **272:** 26959–64.

173 **George SR, Fan T, Xie Z, *et al*.** Oligomerization of mu- and delta-opioid receptors. Generation of novel functional properties. *J Biol Chem* 2000; **275:** 26128–35.

174 **Pan Y-X, Bolan EA, Pasternak GW.** Dimerization of morphine and orphanin FQ/nociceptin receptors: generation of a novel opioid receptor subtype. *Biochem Biophys Res Commun* 2002; **297**(3): 659–63.

175 **Portoghese PS.** From models to molecules: opioid receptor dimers, bivalent ligands, and selective opioid receptor probes. *J Med Chem* 2001; **44:** 2259–69.

176 **Jordan BA, Devi LA.** G-protein-coupled receptor heterodimerization modulates receptor function. *Nature* 1999; **399:** 697–700.

177 **Bolan EA, Pasternak GW.** Functional analysis of MOR-1 splice variants of the mu opioid receptor gene, Oprm. *Synapse* 2004; **51:** 11–18.

Chapter 3

Opioid pharmacokinetics

Kenneth C. Jackson II

The appropriate use of opioid analgesics requires clinicians to have knowledge of both the pharmacodynamic and pharmacokinetic properties of this class of medication. In simple terms, this means that clinicians must understand how these agents produce their pharmacological effects, i.e. pharmacodynamic activity, as well as understand what happens to the drug within the body from the time of administration to the point in time where the drug no longer resides in the body, i.e. pharmacokinetic activity. A basic understanding of the pharmacodynamics of opioid analgesics reveals three distinct classes of analgesics that maintain diversity in their pharmacological actions; full agonists, partial agonists and mixed agonist-antagonists[1]. While these three classes of opioids are commonly considered useful across a variety of clinical practice settings, in the context of cancer pain only the full opioid agonists (e.g. morphine) maintain an ability to provide analgesia over the full spectrum of cancer pain presentations[2]. Within the scope of this chapter, basic concepts and principles related to full opioid agonist pharmacokinetics will be presented and explored. Specific pharmacokinetic information and parameters will be further defined and delineated in chapters dedicated to specific opioid analgesics.

The exact interplay between pharmacodynamic and pharmacokinetic parameters remains difficult in the context of opioid-based analgesia[3]. While pharmacokinetic monitoring has become a mainstay in a variety of other medical endeavors, e.g. aminoglycoside dosing and anticonvulsant monitoring, the correlation between serum drug levels and analgesia remains difficult to ascertain. Instead, clinicians must focus their efforts on monitoring analgesic response via patient report and physical assessment. This is not to say that an understanding of pharmacokinetic parameters is unnecessary. Quite the contrary is true, it is vital that clinicians be vigilant, possibly more so, of these very properties because of this situation.

In the most basic of terms, opioid pharmacokinetics can be viewed as the disposition of an individual opioid from the point of initial administration to a patient. Four distinct phases are considered within the scope of pharmacokinetics: absorption, distribution, metabolism and elimination. Of note, these parameters impact the effectiveness of opioids and other analgesics when administered via any route currently used to provide analgesia. While not unique to opioids, the availability of a variety of elegantly formulated controlled release dosage preparations adds an additional dimension for consideration (Table 3.1).

Table 3.1 Long-acting opioids

Pharmaceutically long-acting opioids	Inherently (pharmacologically) long-acting opioids
Fentanyl transdermal delivery system (Duragesic)	Levorphanol
Hydromorphone controlled-release (Dilaudid-CR, Palladone) (*pending FDA approval)	Methadone
Morphine sustained-release or controlled release (Avinza, Kadian, MS Contin, Oramorph SR, Roxanol SR and others)	
Oxycontin controlled-release (Oxycontin)	

Absorption

Most opioids can be administered orally and absorbed from the gastrointestinal tract. Oral administration is convenient, simple, inexpensive and preferred whenever possible. Oral administration requires that an agent be absorbed across the gastrointestinal lining into the vasculature. In the case of opioids, this is a passive system and does not require an active transport mechanism. Once administered via the oral or other enteral route, opioids remain subject to substantial first pass hepatic metabolism. This explains the larger doses required of orally administered opioids when compared with the parenteral route. Most immediate-release oral opioid preparations have an onset of analgesic activity between 20 and 40 min, with a peak analgesic effect normally 30–60 min following oral administration. Some newer formulations have a quicker onset of duration and accordingly a shorter peak effect. Alternatively, initial effect and peak effects can be delayed in certain patients or with certain medication formulations[4]. It is interesting to note that oral formulations are often effective in managing breakthrough pain, despite the delays in peak serum concentrations following oral administration[4].

Most orally available opioids can be administered rectally when the oral route is no longer viable. Rectal administration avoids the hepatic first pass effect if the dosage form is administered correctly. Three sets of veins are responsible for rectal blood return: the superior, middle and inferior rectal veins. The superior vein is responsible for the upper portion of the rectum (approximately 15–20 cm high) and returns blood to the portal vein that leads to immediate hepatic metabolism. The middle and inferior rectal veins return blood to the inferior vena cava. Drug administration into the lower rectal vault allows for larger amounts of the parent drug to reach the systemic circulation without being effected by the first pass effect[5,6]. Hydromorphone, morphine and oxymorphone are commercially available as rectal suppositories. Controlled release morphine tablets have been used rectally with good results at essentially the same doses as are used orally[7].

Lipophilicity favors absorption across biological surfaces including the skin and oral mucosa. In terms of assessing lipophilicity, a partition coefficient of octanol to water can be used to gauge relative affinity[8] (Table 3.2). Lipophilic opioids such as fentanyl

Table 3.2 Pharmacokinetic and physicochemical variables for opioid analgesics

Drug	Vc (L/kg)	Vd (L/kg)	Cl (mL/min/kg)	T1/2β (min)	Partition coefficient (octanol/water)
Morphine	0.23	2.8	15.5	134	1
Hydromorphone	0.34	4.1	22.7	15	1
Meperidine	0.6	2.6	12	180	21
Methadone	0.15	3.4	1.6	23hr	115
Levorphanol		10	10.5	11hr	
Alfentanil	0.12	0.9	7.6	94	130
Fentanyl	0.85	4.6	21	186	820
Sufentanil	0.1	2.5	11.3	149	1750
Buprenorphine	0.2	2.8	17.2	184	10,000
Nalbuphine	0.45	4.8	23.1	222	
Butorphanol		5	38.6	159	
Dezocine		12	52	156	

Vc, central volume of distribution; Vd, volume of distribution; Cl, clearance; T1/2β, elimination half-life.
From Katz (1996)[8].

maintain a higher partition coefficient, and are known to more easily and quickly pass across cellular surfaces. The partition coefficient for fentanyl is 820, compared with 1 for morphine[8]. Lipophilic agents can also facilitate transdermal delivery, and thereby permit simple and convenient administration of drug to patients unable to take opioids orally or rectally. The transdermal delivery of an opioid occurs via release of the lipophilic opioid from a gel matrix, located in a topical patch, into subcutaneous fat tissue. The patient's adipose tissue serves as an *in vivo* drug reservoir from which the lipophilic opioid can be released into the vascular compartment. Following patch removal, the opioid continues to move into the vascular compartment serum from the subcutaneous fat depot. Currently, fentanyl is the only FDA approved transdermal opioid delivery system. After application, transdermal fentanyl takes an average of 15–20 h to reach steady state serum levels[9]. Following the removal of a transdermal fentanyl patch, effects may continue for 12–24 h. These factors can make transdermal fentanyl a poor option for patients with rapidly changing opioid requirements or patients who have poor adipose tissue stores.

The parenteral route of administration provides a useful alternative for patients where enteral or transdermal administration of an opioid is not possible or desirable. Intravenous (i.v.) administration of opioids does not require an absorptive process and by definition is considered to maintain 100% bioavailability. Intramuscular (i.m.) and subcutaneous (s.c.) opioid administration provide similar bioavailability to i.v. administration[10]. However, the time to peak effect for both i.m. and s.c. administration is delayed since both administration routes require absorption across physiological surfaces to gain entry into the vascular compartment. Absorption of opioids from the i.m. or s.c. route is a rate-limiting step, for which lipophilicity is a major factor. As with transdermal delivery, the more lipophilic opioid compounds provide their pharmacodynamic effect more rapidly following parenteral administration. Intramuscular injections are generally not recommended due to the pain and possible tissue damage they can inflict[11]. Absorption from i.m. and s.c. injections can be erratic, and is generally considered to be less effective than oral, rectal and i.v. administration.

Neuraxial opioid administration provides for drug application to tissues within the central nervous system. Since the bulk of opioid activity occurs within the central nervous system (CNS), neuraxial transmission bypasses the absorption processes required by other routes of administration. Enteral and parenteral administration require transport into the CNS, across the blood–brain barrier. Principally, there are two modes of neuraxial administration, via the epidural or intrathecal route. In the case of epidural administration, opioids must still be absorbed across a biological surface, i.e. the dura matter, into the subarachnoid space. Lipophilic compounds cross this surface readily and are available for use by spinal opioid receptors faster than more hydrophilic compounds. Epidural administration also supplies the drug to the epidural plexus for systemic redistribution. The drug taken up by the epidural plexus can drain into the inferior vena cava, via the azygos vein, or can be transferred directly to the cerebral venous system. The drug flow to the cerebral venous system may account for both analgesic and adverse effects by providing drug directly to supraspinal centers[12,13]. In contrast, intrathecal administration bypasses this absorption phase by placing opioids directly into the subarachnoid space. Once in the intrathecal space, opioids can be available to interact with opioid receptors.

Distribution

Opioid distribution within the vascular compartment following absorption is a function of plasma protein binding and drug lipophilicity. Morphine, a hydrophilic opioid, is moderately protein bound. Plasma protein binding associated with morphine generally ranges from 30 to 35% and does not appear to be influenced greatly by displacement. In addition, morphine does not remain redistributed within extravascular tissues for an extended period of time. In contrast, fentanyl is both highly protein bound (80–85%) and lipophilic. The free fraction of fentanyl increases in cases of acidosis. Fentanyl readily distributes to adipose tissue throughout the body, from where it redistributes very slowly into the systemic circulation.

Lipophilicity affects both epidural and IT administration. Once the drug gains access to the subarachnoid space, lipophilicity determines both onset of analgesia and duration of action. Lipophilic substances tend to act quickly, but do not provide prolonged levels of analgesia. Additionally, highly lipophilic compounds may be more beneficial in cases where segmental analgesia is required. Hydrophilic medications such as morphine provide a slower onset, but consequently also provide longer duration of analgesic effect[14]. Morphine can provide analgesia up to 24 h after spinal administration[15]. Drug distribution within the subarachnoid area is governed by cerebrospinal fluid (CSF) flow, as well as lipophilicity. Once an opioid diffuses into the CSF, the drug is distributed in two directions. CSF, and consequently medication, move primarily in a rostral fashion, i.e. to the brain. CSF can also move passively toward the base of the spine, i.e. caudal movement. Minimal amounts of spinal medications follow this caudal movement.

Hydrophilic compounds are prone to rostral or cephalad spread, and tend to remain within the CSF for long periods of time as a result of their slow clearance from the subarachnoid space. Clearance involves uptake into the dorsal horn, as well as some slow vascular absorption. Rostral spread often accounts for the late onset of CNS-related adverse effects, such as respiratory depression and somnolence. Lipophilic opioids appear not to be effected by rostral spread to the same degree as hydrophilic agents.

The volume of medication administered appears to influence the distribution of opioids within the subarachnoid space[13,16]. Moulin and Coyle assert that the larger the volume of an intrathecal injection, the higher the incidence of central side effects[13]. This is more problematic for hydrophilic compounds, such as morphine. Lipophilic compounds delivered in larger volumes may actually produce an increased dermatomal spread with a result of enhanced analgesia[17,18]. However, dermatomal spread may not be affected by volumes of up to 2.5 ml[18]. Because of the small volume of CSF found in the spine, administration of large medication volumes may disrupt both the volume of distribution and CSF flow rates.

Metabolism (biotransformation) and elimination (excretion)

Opioids are generally not readily eliminated by the kidneys in the parent form and require metabolism to more water-soluble metabolites. The liver is the principle organ associated with opioid metabolism. Hepatic biotransformation allows for modification of the parent opioid analgesic compounds via numerous processes that facilitate elimination. These processes include dealkylation, glucoronidation, hydrolysis and oxidation. Once metabolized, renal elimination accounts for approximately 90% of the excretion of an opioid (parent drug and metabolites) via urine. Fecal elimination is a minor pathway and accounts for less than 10% of total opioid excretion. Clinically, it is necessary to understand the metabolic fate of opioid analgesics for proper selection of a therapeutic regimen (Table 3.3)[19].

Certain opioid metabolites are associated with neurotoxicity and may displace more active opioid compounds from the opioid receptors[20]. Patients with impaired renal function, or those receiving high dose or long-term opioid therapy should be monitored carefully when these opioids are used. This is especially germane in older patient populations.

Morphine-3-glucuronide (M3G) and morphine-6-glucuronide (M6G) are the two major morphine metabolites[21]. As much as 50% of the parent morphine drug may be eliminated in the form of M3G, while M6G accounts for approximately an additional 5%[22]. Both glucuronide metabolites depend on renal elimination for clearance. The M3G metabolite appears to have antinociceptive properties, and has been associated with hyperalgesia and neurotoxicities, including myoclonus[20,23]. Interestingly,

Table 3.3 Opioid metabolites

Parent drug (% excreted unchanged)	Analgesic duration (h)	Metabolites (% if known)	Metabolite half-lives (h)	Metabolite elimination route	Comments
Morphine (~7.2%—iv) (~3.7%—po)	4–6				Elimination of morphine is not affected by renal failure; however, Vd may be smaller, resulting in increased plasma concentrations; enterohepatic circulation of morphine and glucuronides occur
		Morphine-3-glucuronide (57–74)	2.8–4	Renal	Half life is 41–141 h in renal failure; 5–20 time more potent than morphine in causing hyperalgesia, EEG spiking, agitation, seizures in a nim animals; possibly by a non-opioid receptor mechanism
		Morphine-6-glucuronide (4.7–1.2)	Duration of action 2 times longer than parent drug	Renal	Half life is 89–136 h in renal failure; may be responsible for narcosis in patients with renal failure; by IT administration is 100 times more potent than morphine; accumulates with chronic dosing
		Morphine-3-ethereal sulfate (5–10)			
		Normorphine (3.5)			May have toxic effects (myoclonus, allodynia)
		Morphine-N-oxide			
Codeine 11.1%[5]	4–6	Codeine-6-glucuronide			Primary elimination pathway; profound narcosis has occurred in chronic renal failure
		Norcodeine		Renal	Equipotent to codeine in analgesic activity
		Morphine (10)			May account for analgesic activity of codeine
Fentanyl (<10%)	1–2				May be extensively liver metabolized
		Norfentanyl		Renal, hepatic	Metabolized to despropionyl fentanyl, may cause neurotoxic side effects, structurally similar to normeperidine
		4-N-anilinopiperidine			

Drug	Half-life (h)	Metabolite	Clearance route	Clearance dependent on hepatic blood flow
Hydromorphone (5.6%)		Hydromorphonw-3-glucuronide		Shown to accumulate in renal failure in one patient
		Hydromorphonw-6-glucuronide	Renal	Formed from intermediate metabolites, dihydroisomorphine and dihydromorphine
		Nor-metabolites		Significance not known
Levorphanol	6–8	Levorphanol glucuronide	Renal	Liver metabolized by glucuronide conjugation
Methadone 21% (acidic urine increases the fraction of elimination[f_e])	4–6 initially; 6–12 after steady state (1–2 days)			In one anephric patient, 98% of methadone was found in feces as metabolite, suggesting a shift in metabolism from renal to fecal urinary excretion of methadone and metabolites is dose dependent and is the major route of elimination in doses >55 mg/day; 10–45% of methadone is eliminated in feces as metabolites
		1,5-demethyl-2-ethyl-3,3-iphenyl-1-pyrroline	Renal, biliary	Unpredictable half-life with chronic dosing long-term analgesia is 10 times that of morphine; major metabolite f_e =0.30
		2-ethyl-5-methyl-3,3-diphenyl-1-pyrroline	Renal, biliary	Minor metabolite
		Methadone-N-oxide		Minor metabolite
Oxycodone	3–6	Noroxymorphone		Renally excreted, primarily as metabolites
		Oxymorphone	Hepatic, renal	Active metabolite; renally excreted as oxymorphone-glucuronide
		Noroxycodone		

the M6G metabolite possesses analgesic properties and appears to be significantly more potent than morphine on an mg-to-mg basis. Accumulation of both glucuronide metabolites, as a function of poor renal status or dehydration, predisposes patients to toxicity, as well poor pain control.

Normorphine, a desmethyl metabolite of morphine, may also contribute to the toxic effects seen with high dose or long-term morphine use. However, reports of normorphine accumulation have been associated with elevated M3G and M6G levels[24]. Whether normorphine accumulation independently contributes to the toxicity profile remains unclear.

It remains unclear what role other opioid metabolites play in the management of opioid based analgesia, especially for patients with impaired renal elimination. It has been suggested that hydromorphone may have a similar metabolic pathway to morphine, yielding 3 and 6 glucuronide metabolites with a profile similar to their morphine counterparts[25,26]. Fentanyl has a desmethyl metabolite, which may prove problematic in some patients[21,27]. Oxycodone has only an active analgesic metabolite oxymorphone, which may make oxycodone safer for some elderly and renally impaired patients[28–30].

Conclusion

Appropriate utilization of opioid analgesics requires a thorough understanding of pharmacodynamic activity and pharmacokinetic parameters. Most opioid analgesics maintain short half-lifes that necessitate frequent dosing to provide adequate analgesia. Modern developments in pharmaceutical manufacturing have provided dosage formulations that allow these short-acting compounds to be used in a manner that promotes better analgesia and patient compliance. Inherently long-acting opioids, such as levorphanol and methadone, also play a role in the management of cancer pain, but use is often complicated by the unpredictable nature of these agents' half-lifes. This is especially true for patients with poor renal elimination or who have an unstable pain process.

References

1 Hare B. The opioid analgesics: rational selection of agents for acute and chronic pain. *Hosp Formul* 1987; **22:** 64–86.

2 **American Pain Society.** *Principles of Analgesic Use in the Treatment of Acute Pain and Cancer Pain,* 5th edn. Glenview: American Pain Society, 2003.

3 Suri A, Estes KS, Geisslinger G, *et al.* Pharmacokinetic-pharmacodynamic relationships for analgesics. *Int J Clin Pharmacol Ther* 1997; **35(8):** 307–23.

4 Cleary J. Pharmacokinetic and pharmacodynamic issues in the treatment of breakthrough pain. *Semin Oncol* 1997; **24:** 13–19.

5 Rusho W. Clinical issues and concerns in the use of extemporaneously compounded medications. *J Pharm Care Pain Sympt Contr* 1996; **4:** 5–20.

6 Warren D. Practical use of rectal medications in palliative care. *J Pain Sympt Manag* 1996; **11:** 378–87.

7 Kaiko R, Fitzmartin R, Thomas G, *et al.* The bioavailability of morphine in controlled-release 30-mg tablets per rectum compared with immediate-release 30-mg rectal suppositories and controlled-release 30-mg oral tablets. *Pharmacotherapy* 1992; **12:** 107–13.

8 Katz J. Opioids and nonsteroidal anti-inflammatory analgesics. In: Raj P (Ed.) *Pain Medicine.* St Louis: Mosby, 1996, pp. 126–140.

9 Korte W, Stoutz N, Morant R. Day-to-day titration to initiate transdermal fentanyl in cancer patients: short and long term experience in a prospective study of 39 patients. *J Pain Sympt Manag* 1996; **11:** 139–46.

10 Moulin D, Kreeft J, Murray-Parsons N, *et al.* Comparison of continuous subcutaneous and intravenous hydromorphone infusion for management of cancer pain. *Lancet* 1991; **337:** 465–8.

11 Jacox A, Carr DB, Payne R, *et al. Management of Cancer Pain,* Clinical Practice Guideline No. 9, AHCPR Publication No. 94–0592. Rockville: Agency for Health Care Policy and Research, US Department of Health and Human Services, Public Health Service, 1994.

12 Cousins M, Mather L. Intrathecal and epidural administration of opioids. *Anesthesiology* 1984; **61:** 276–310.

13 Moulin D, Coyle N. Spinal opioid analgesics and local anesthetics in the management of chronic cancer pain. *J Pain Sympt Manag* 1986; **1:** 79–86.

14 de Leon-Casasola O, Lema M. Postoperative epidural opioid analgesia: what are the choices? *Anesth Analg* 1996; **83:** 867–75.

15 Krames E. Intrathecal infusion therapies for intractable pain: patient management guidelines. *J Pain Sympt Manag* 1993; **8:** 36–46.

16 Finley R. Pain management with spinally administered opioids. *Am J Hosp Pharm* 1990; **47:** S14–17.

17 Birnbach D, Johnson M, Arcario T, *et al.* Effect of diluent volume on analgesia produced by epidural fentanyl. *Anesth Analg* 1989; **68:** 808–10.

18 Gwirtz K. Single-dose intrathecal opioids in the management of acute postoperative pain. In: Sinatra R, Hord A, Ginsberg B, *et al.* (Eds) *Acute Pain Mechanisms and Management.* St Louis: Mosby-Yearbook, 1992; 253–68.

19 Lipman AG, Jackson KC. Opioids. In: Warfield C, Bajwa Z (Eds) *Principles and Practice of Pain Management,* 2nd edn. New York: McGraw-Hill, 2004.

20 Pereira J, Bruera E. Emerging neuropsychiatric toxicities of opioids. *J Pharm Care Pain Sympt Contr* 1997; **5:** 3–29.

21 Christrup L. Morphine metabolites. *Acta Anaesthesiol Scand* 1997; **41:** 116–22.

22 Forman W. Opioid analgesic drugs in the elderly. *Clin Geriat Med* 1996; **12:** 489–500.

23 Sjogren P, Jensen N, Jensen T. Disappearance of morphine-induced hyperalgesia after discontinuing or substituting other opioid agonists. *Pain* 1994; **59:** 313–16.

24 Glare P, Walsh T, Pippenger C. Normorphine, a neurotoxic metabolite? *Lancet* 1990; **335:** 725–6.

25 Smith MT. Neuroexcitatory effects of morphine and hydromorphone: evidence implicating the 3-glucuronide metabolites. *Clin Exp Pharmacol Physiol* 2000; **27(7):** 524–8.

26 Wright AW, Mather LE, Smith MT. Hydromorphone-3-glucuronide: a more potent neuro-excitant than its structural analogue, morphine-3-glucuronide. *Life Sci* 2001; **69(4):** 409–20.

27 Steinberg R, Gilman D, Johnson F. Acute toxic delirium in a patient using transdermal fentanyl. *Anesth Analg* 1992; **75:** 1014–16.

28 **Heiskanen T, Olkkola KT, Kalso E.** Effects of blocking CYP2D6 on the pharmacokinetics and pharmacodynamics of oxycodone. *Clin Pharmacol Ther* 1998; **64(6):** 603–11.

29 **Heiskanen T, Olkkola KT, Kalso E.** Effects of blocking CYP2D6 on the pharmacokinetics and pharmacodynamics of oxycodone. *Clin Pharmacol Ther* 1998; **64(6):** 603–11.

30 **Heiskanen TE, Ruismaki PM, Seppala TA,** *et al.* Morphine or oxycodone in cancer pain? *Acta Oncol* 2000; **39(8):** 941–7.

Chapter 4

Codeine

Janet R. Hardy

Codeine (methylmorphine) is a naturally occurring derivative of an opium alkaloid. Along with morphine and thebaine, it is a true 'opiate', i.e. a natural product and not a synthetic derivative of opium as are many of the 'opioids' used in every-day practice. It is a relatively weak analgesic, used most commonly in mild to moderate pain, either alone or in combination with non-opioids, such as aspirin, paracetamol or non-steroidal anti-inflammatory drugs (NSAIDs). There has been considerable debate about the relative contribution of the parent compound and its metabolites to both the beneficial effects, i.e. pain relief, and the undesirable effects, such as constipation and nausea, but its major analgesic effect is thought to result from its partial biotransformation to morphine. Codeine also has an important role as an antitussive and antidiarrheal.

Pharmacokinetics and pharmacodynamics

Codeine is well absorbed after administration by mouth. It is usually given orally and has a bioavailability similar to that of oral morphine, ranging from 12 to 84% (mean 40%). The plasma half-life of codeine has been documented from 1.8 to 4.5 h (median about 2.5 h) and a similar figure has been demonstrated for its major metabolite codeine-6-glucuronide (C6G)[1]. Parent drug and metabolites are relatively highly protein bound—54, 32 and 46%, respectively, for codeine, C6G and morphine. The maximum plasma concentration is higher after multiple doses than a single dose[2]. Renal clearance for codeine and C6G is similar, at around 1 ml/min/kg[3]. Codeine is excreted via a tubular cation mechanism and C6G via glomerular filtration, and possibly a tubular anion mechanism[3]. Renal impairment leads to increased half lives of both codeine and C6G[4], but as the renal clearance of codeine contributes to only a small degree of overall clearance (approximately 4%), this is of little clinical consequence[3]. The area under the curve (AUC) of C6G is about 10 times higher than that of codeine and it unclear whether this is an important factor in efficacy. The AUC of morphine is only about 3% that of codeine and is now thought to be largely responsible for the drug's analgesic activity.

Metabolism

Glucuronidation to C6G is the primary route of metabolism of codeine. Minor metabolic pathways are O-demethylation to morphine and N-demethylation to norcodeine. Thus, codeine has six major metabolites: C6G (81%), norcodeine (2%), morphine (0.6%), M3G (2%), M6G (0.8%) and normorphine (2.4%)[3]. Of more importance than renal function on the pharmacological effectiveness of codeine is its metabolism. This provides a classic example of the application of pharmacogenomic principles to drug use[5]. Metabolism to morphine is dependent on O-demethylation that is subject to individual and ethnic variation as a result of polymorphisms in the cytochrome P450 enzyme system. CYP2D6 is responsible for the conversion of codeine to morphine. Genetic variation leads to a group of 'poor metabolizers' (PM) in whom demethylation occurs only to a limited extent and 'extensive metabolizers' (EM) in whom morphine is easily detected following administration. Approximately 7–10% of Caucasians are poor metabolizers due to homozygosity for non-functional CYP2D6 mutant alleles[6,7]. This accounts for the wide variation in adequacy of pain relief seen when a standard dose of codeine is delivered. Pretreatment with quinidine (a potent inhibitor of CYP2D6) also markedly impairs the analgesic effect of codeine[8]. This variation in codeine metabolism occurs not only between individuals, but also between different racial groups[9,10]. CYP2D6 polymorphism also affects the metabolism of other drugs often used in combination with analgesics such as phenothiazines, mexiletine, paroxetine and propranalol[5].

Clinical use

Codeine is a relatively weak analgesic. Although codeine and its primary metabolite C6G have been shown to bind to the mu receptor, their affinity for the receptor is much less than that of morphine[2]. It is likely that the analgesic effect is mediated via morphine and its active metabolites following O-demethylation of codeine. Codeine can therefore be seen as a pro-drug. The NNT (number of patients who need to receive drug at least once to achieve at least 50% pain relief) of 60 mg codeine is 16.7[11]. This compares with an NNT of 5.6 for paracetamol 500 mg and 2.3 for diclofenac 50 mg in single dose placebo-controlled studies.

In single dose studies, codeine is approximately one-tenth to one-twelfth as potent as morphine when given parenterally, and one-third to one-quarter as potent as morphine when given by mouth[2]. However, potency ratios change with repeated dosing. Codeine is generally given orally in doses of 30–60 mg, 4–6-hourly. There is a linear dose–response curve in doses up to 360 mg i.m., but higher doses have not been tested[2]. The oral to parenteral potency is around 2.3, i.e. about double that of morphine. Its onset of analgesic action is 30–60 min and the duration of effect similar to that of morphine, about 4–6 h. It is commonly given as a compound preparation in combination with paracetamol (see below).

Codeine is frequently recommended as an antitussive. Several studies have found codeine (10–120 mg/day) to be effective in relieving the frequency and intensity of cough, and to be superior to a placebo[12]. There is little evidence in favor of using codeine in preference to any other opioid however, all having a similar side effect profile at effective antitussive doses[13]. Being a weak analgesic, codeine is a logical choice, unless a stronger opioid, such as morphine, is required for the co-treatment of pain or dyspnoea. The most likely mode of action is central, via direct action on the cough center in the medulla or via brain stem respiratory centers. Mu receptor stimulation may reduce mucous production or increase mucociliary clearance, and hence the need to cough[13]. There have been reports of opioid binding sites in both human and rat pulmonary tissue, but the characteristics of these receptors are not typical of mu opioid receptors[14].

Another common use is as an antidiarrheal agent. In animal studies, the relative specificities for antidiarrheal as opposed to analgesic effects for codeine, morphine, diphenoxylate and loperamide were 5.24, 6.45, 23.7 and 552, respectively[15]. Loperamide given orally does not cross the blood–brain barrier significantly and thus has very few adverse effects. Codeine is more likely to cause side effects, but is cheap. Some have suggested that the individual response to opioids for diarrhea can be as idiosynchratic as that for pain and that, in some patients, codeine has superior antidiarrheal properties to other opioids without causing excess nausea or drowsiness[16]. However, there is no evidence to support this premise. Codeine's usefulness as a treatment for diarrhea might explain why it is considered by many to be more constipating than other opioids, but animal studies suggest that it is no more constipating than morphine[15]. Both drugs reduce gut motility via the activation of mu receptors, both centrally and peripherally in the gastrointestinal tract.

Codeine can be supplied as tablets (15, 30 and 60 mg), an oral syrup (25 mg/5 ml) and as a linctus (15 mg/5 ml). A parenteral preparation has been produced, but is not recommended. There are many combination preparations available, combining codeine at low (8 mg) or higher doses (30 mg) with paracetamol or aspirin.

Evidence

A number of studies have assessed the analgesic potential of single dose codeine. In acute postoperative pain, a single dose of 60 mg is superior to placebo, and 120 mg is superior to either 60 mg or 650 of aspirin[17]. In chronic cancer pain the effectiveness of 60 mg has been demonstrated[18] and 120 mg appeared to be superior to 60 mg [19]. In a non-randomized study of 944 patients with chronic cancer pain resistant to non-opioids, 107 were changed to dextroproxyphene, 321 to oxycodone, 234 to buprenorphine, 139 to pentazocine and 132 to codeine (60 mg). Of the latter group, 24% remained on this drug beyond 4 weeks at a median dose of 206 mg/day, 28% changed to oral morphine and 27% to parenteral analgesia[20]. Similar results, including side effect profile, was seen for each of the drugs, thus validating (according to the authors) the use of these drugs at step 2 of the analgesic ladder.

Effectiveness of combination treatment

In a study by Houde and colleagues in patients with cancer pain, it was not possible to distinguish between 32 mg codeine and 650 mg aspirin, although both were better than placebo[21]. Taken together, an additive effect was seen supporting the practice of combining codeine with aspirin, paracetamol and, more recently, NSAIDs. Many combination preparations have since been developed. In 1996, the Dutch Cochrane Centre performed a systematic review of studies evaluating codeine/paracetamol combinations[22]. Twenty-four trials of acute non-cancer pain were included: 21 postsurgery, one postpartum, one in osteoarthritis and one in induced pain scenarios. Doses ranged from 400 to 1000 mg paracetamol and 10–60 mg codeine. Both efficacy and toxicity were evaluated. It was concluded that the benefit over codeine alone was modest, i.e. a 5% increase in efficacy (95% CI 4.9–6.2). Only three studies involved multidosing and a clear increase in toxicity was noted with the combination preparations compared with paracetamol alone, namely dizziness, drowsiness, nausea, vomiting and constipation. Late efficacy data were not available for the multidose studies, except in one in pain associated with osteoarthritis that suggested the early benefit of the combination was lost with time. No dose relationship was found when comparing 1000/60 versus 600/60 versus variable/30 paracetamol/codeine combinations. No controlled trial of 8 mg codeine added to paracetamol has been reported[22], but it would seem unlikely to have any benefit over paracetamol alone. No pharmacokinetic interactions have been reported between codeine and paracetamol[23,24].

In a cross-over study in patients with degenerative joint disease, codeine 20 mg plus ibuprofen 400 mg and paracetamol 500 mg was better than ibuprofen alone[25].

A comparison of diclofenac (50 mg) combined with placebo, codeine (40 mg) or imipramine in cancer pain of longer than 10 days duration failed to show any difference between the arms with regard to failure rate or observer assessment of pain[26].

There is concern that many combination preparations only add potential toxicity with little increased benefit over the use of the individual agents given alone.

Role of slow release preparations

Single and multidose studies of controlled release codeine preparations have shown equivalent bioavailability to intermediate dose preparations and a pharmacokinetic profile indicating that 12-hourly administration would be appropriate[17]. A randomized study has assessed the dose effect of controlled release codeine at 100, 200 and 300 mg given 12-hourly compared with paracetamol/codeine (600/60 mg) given 6-hourly[17]. Analgesic efficacy was assessed at days 1 and 4. The maximum effect was seen with 300 mg codeine, but this dose also produced the most side effects. Regression analysis of total pain relief with dose showed that 150 mg of controlled release codeine was equivalent to 600/60 paracetamol/codeine.

Two studies have evaluated slow release (SR) codeine with placebo in chronic cancer and non-cancer pain. The first was in patients with a range of musculoskeletal disorders. The dose of codeine was based on the consumption of paracetamol/codeine in the previous 7 days. Patients were randomized to placebo or SR codeine. The primary end points of the study were pain intensity and the need for break through pain analgesia. There were significantly lower pain scores and need for breakthrough analgesia in the SR codeine arm. Although constipation, somnolence, nausea/vomiting and pruritis scores were higher on SR codeine, this was only significant for nausea[27].

A randomized double blind study against placebo in cancer patients used similar endpoints, but included a cross-over after 7 days[28]. Again, there was a significantly lower Pain Intensity and Pain Disability index for SR codeine compared with placebo. The daily requirement for breakthrough analgesia (paracetamol/codeine) was significantly lower for SR codeine, whereas nausea and somnolence were significantly more common. Eighty per cent of patients and 73% of investigators preferred SR codeine to placebo.

Toxicity

The side effects of codeine are similar to those of other opioids: constipation, sedation, dizziness, nausea, miosis, dry mouth and pruritis. There is no evidence that codeine is more constipating than any other opioid. Side effects occur in both extensive and poor metabolizers of the drug. Thus, up to 10% of patients given codeine will develop side effects without any beneficial analgesic effects[7]. The adverse effects seem dose related i.e. increase with increasing dose[17].

Conclusion

Codeine is a relatively weak opioid. It is given most commonly in combination with a non-opioid, such as paracetamol. Its well established role as an antitussive and antidiarrheal agent will probably ensure its continued use.

References

1 Persson K, Hammarlund-Udenaes M, Mortimer O, *et al.* The post-operative pharmacokinetics of codeine. *Eur J Clin Pharm* 1992; **42:** 63–6.

2 Twycross R. Weak opioids. In: Twycross R (Ed.) *Pain Relief in Advanced Cancer.* Edinburgh: Churchill Livingston, 1994 pp. 233–54.

3 Vree T, Versey-Van Wissen C. Pharmacokinetics and metabolism of codeine in humans. *Biopharm Drug Disposit* 1992; **13:** 445–60.

4 Guay D, Awni W, Findlay J, *et al.* Pharmacokinetics and pharmacodynamics of codeine in end-stage renal disease. *Clin Pharmacol Ther* 1988; **43:** 63–71.

5 Fagerlund T, Braaten O. No pain relief from codeine . . . ? An introduction to pharmacogenomics. *Acta Anaesth Scand* 2001; **45:** 140–9.

6 Yue Q, Hasselstrom J, Svensson J, *et al.* Pharmacokinetics of codeine and its metabolites in Caucasian healthy volunteers: comparison between extensive and poor hydroxylators of debrisoquine. *Br J Pharmacol* 1991; **31:** 635–42.

7 Eckhardt K, Li S, Ammon S, *et al.* Same incidence of adverse events after codeine administration irrespective of the genetically determined differences in morphine formation. *Pain* 1998; **76:** 27–33.

8 Sindrup S, Arendt-Nielsen L, Brosen K, *et al.* The effect of quinidine on the analgesic effect of codeine. *Eur J Clin Pharm* 1992; **42:** 587–92.

9 Caraco Y, Sheller J, Wood A. Impact of ethnic origin and quinidine coadministration on codeine's disposition and pharmacodynamic effects. *J Pharmacol Exp Therapeut* 1999; **290:** 413–22.

10 Yue Q, Svensson J, Alm C, *et al.* Interindividual and interethnic differences in the demethylation and glucuronidation of codeine. *Br J Clin Pharmacol* 1989; **28:** 629–37.

11 McQuay H, Moore R. *An Evidence-based Resource for Pain Relief.* Oxford: Oxford University Press, 1998.

12 Homsi J, Walsh D, Nelson K. Important drugs for cough in advanced cancer. *Support Care Cancer* 2001; **9:** 565–74.

13 Fuller R, Jackson D. Physiology and treatment of cough. *Thorax* 1990; **45:** 425–30.

14 Cabot P, Dodd P, Cramond T, *et al.* Characterisation of non-conventional opioid binding sites in rat and human lung. *Eur J Pharmacol* 1994; **268:** 247–55.

15 Awouters F, Niemeegers C, Janssen P. Pharmacology of antidiarrheal drugs. *Ann Rev Toxicol Pharm* 1983; **23:** 279–301.

16 Sykes N. Constipation and diarrhea. In: Doyle D, Hanks G, MacDonald N (Eds) *Oxford Textbook of Palliative Medicine*, 2nd edn. Oxford: Oxford University Press, 1998, pp. 513–26.

17 Chary S, Goughnour B, Moulin D, *et al.* The dose–response relationship of controlled-release codeine (codeine contin) in chronic cancer pain. *J Pain Sympt Manag* 1994; **9:** 363–71.

18 Stambaugh J, McAdams J. Comparison of the analgesic efficacy and safety of oral ciramadol, codeine and placebo in patients with chronic cancer pain. *J Clin Pharmacol* 1987; **27:** 162–6.

19 Jochimsen P, Noyes R. Appraisal of codeine as an analgesic in older patients. *J Am Geriatric Soc* 1978; **11:** 521–3.

20 De Conno F, Ripamonti C, Sbanotto A, *et al.* A clinical study on the use of codeine, oxycodone, dextropropoxyphene, buprenorphine and pentazocine in cancer pain. *J Pain Sympt Manag* 1991; **6:** 423–7.

21 Houde R, Wallenstein S, Beaver W. Evaluation of analgesics in patients with cancer pain. In: Lasagna L (Ed.) *Clinical Pharmacology. International Encyclopaedia of Pharmacology and Therapeutics.* Oxford: Pergamon Press, 1966.

22 De Craen A, Giulio G, Lampe-Schoenmaeckers A, *et al.* Analgesic efficacy and safety of paracetamol-codeine combinations versus paracetamol alone: a systemic review. *Br Med J* 1996; **313:** 321–5.

23 Sonne J, Enghusen Poulsen H, Loft S, *et al.* Therapeutic doses of codeine have no effect on acetaminophen clearance or metabolism. *Eur J Clin Pharmacol* 1988; **35:** 109–11.

24 Somogyi A, Bochner F, Chen Z. Lack of effect of paracetamol on the pharmacokinetics and metabolism of codeine in man. *Eur J Clin Pharmacol* 1991; **41:** 379–82.

25 Vlok G, Van Vuren J. Comparison of a standard ibuprofen treatment with a new ibuprofen/paracetamol/codeine combination in chronic osteo-arthritis. *S Afr Med J* 1987; Suppl: 1–6.

26 Minotti V, de Angelis V, Righetti E, *et al.* Double-blind evaluation of short-term analgesic efficacy of orally administered diclofenac, diclofenac plus codeine and diclofenac plus imiprmine in chronic cancer pain. *Pain* 1998; **74:** 133–7.

27 Arkinstall W, Sandler A, Goughnour B, *et al.* Efficacy of controlled-release codein in chronic non-malignant pain: a randomised, placebo-controlled clinical trial. *Pain* 1995; **62:** 169–78.

28 Dhaliwal H, Sloan P, Arkinstall W. Randomised evaluation of controlled-release codeine and placebo in chronic cancer pain. *J Pain Sympt Manag* 1995; **10:** 612–23.

Chapter 5

Hydrocodone

Mellar P. Davis

Introduction

Hydrocodone (dihydrocodeinone) is a semi-synthetic congener of codeine, which is highly selective for mu opioid receptor (MOR). Hydrocodone has not been directly compared with morphine in humans and its comparison with other opioids is clouded by the non-steroidal anti-inflammatory drug (NSAID) and acetaminophen combination product. Hydrocodone titration is also limited by availability in only the combination products. Hydrocodone and oxycodone possess almost identical potencies and very similar pharmacokinetics. Oxycodone studies have been published in cancer pain, but hydrocodone, have not. Hydrocodone has been used for, dental, postoperative and acute musculoskeletal pain.

Pharmacodynamics

Hydrocodone is more potent than codeine, but reported to be less potent than morphine by receptor affinity and competitive binding assays with 3H-DAMGO. Binding affinity for the MOR is 10 times greater for morphine (K_i 1.2 nM) compared with hydrocodone (K_i 19.9 nM)[1]. The relative analgesic potency of hydrocodone as compared with morphine has been reported to be 0.59[2]. The difference between hydrocodone's binding affinity and analgesic potency is either due to an active hydrocodone metabolites or to the intrinsic efficacy receptor activation, which is more efficient than morphine. Hydrocodone does have active metabolites, which include hydromorphone, 6-beta hydromorphol and 6-alpha hydromorphol[2]. As a general rule, metabolic conversion of most codeine congeners leads to the formation of metabolites, which will have a greater affinity for opioid receptors than the parent drug. On the other hand, O-demethylation of hydrocodone to its major metabolite, hydromorphone, is not necessary for analgesia in experimental animals nor does it appear to be necessary in humans[3–5]. In rhesus monkeys the analgesic potency of hydrocodone is 3.3 times that of morphine as measured in the tail withdrawal latency test (ED_{50} 1.09 + 0.23 mg/kg versus 3.61 + 0.52 mg/kg) and is not blocked by quinidine, which would inhibit hydrocodone conversion to hydromorphone[5].

Both MOR and delta opioid receptor (DOR) activate G proteins of the Gi/o subclass for agonist efficacy. This process requires guanine triphosphate (GTP) binding. GTP binding can be measured by radio-labeled (^{35}S) GTP-gamma-S[6–8]. Maximum stimulation of (^{35}S) GTP-gamma-S binding by an agonist correlates with an intrinsic efficacy and receptor activation, but does not necessarily correlate with opioid receptor affinity[6]. Hydrocodone has a greater efficacy for G-protein activation as measured by (^{35}S) GTP gamma-S than codeine and closely matches the efficacy of oxycodone[9]. Intrinsic efficacy explains in part the potency differences between codeine (which requires conversion to morphine to activate MOR) and oxycodone and hydrocodone[9]. This also explains the high clinical analgesic potency despite the relative weak MOR receptor binding of hydrocodone[1]. O-demethylated metabolites of hydrocodone have an increased binding affinity to DOR, but do not play a major role in hydrocodone induced analgesia[9]. Analgesic synergy occurs between hydrocodone and ibuprofen (as measured in the inflammatory rodent heat tail flick assay). Ibuprofen in general is ineffective in this animal model, but at low doses and with a fixed ratio of hydrocodone increases the pain relief 4-fold as compared with hydrocodone alone[10]. This is not due to ibuprofen induced interference with hydrocodone metabolism or excretion. Ibuprofen is metabolized through CYP2C9 (90%) and does not compete for hydrocodone clearance[11].

Drugs that enhance γ-aminobutyric acid (GABA) activity also enhance hydrocodone analgesia in animal models[12].

Hydrocodone is only weakly porphyrinogenic unlike tramadol and fentanyl. Hydrocodone can therefore be used in patients with genetic porphyrin metabolism defects. It is particularly useful in patients with acute porphyrias[13].

Pharmacokinetics

Hydrocodone is said to be well absorbed. However, one source quotes an oral bioavailability of only 25%. Hydrocodone undergoes O-demethylation by CPY2D6 to hydromorphone. Demethylation of norhydrocodone presumably occurs through CYP2D6 and also via 6-keto reduction to 6-alpha and 6-beta hydroxy metabolites[2]. Even though hydrocodone does not undergo glucuronidation, the active metabolite, hydromorphone, and the glucuronidated metabolite, 6-hydroxymorphanol, can be conjugated[2]. Approximately 50% of the total dose is recovered in the urine and urinary hydrocodone accounts for 11% of the total administered dose[2]. There are wide individual differences in the recovery of hydrocodone metabolites in the urine. The excretion of hydrocodone in the urine per dose can range from 6 to 20% of the total dose and norhydrocodone can range from 2 to 14% of the total dose[2]. Reduced hydrocodone (hydrocodol) excretion is fairly consistent and accounts for only 1–3% of the total dose[2]. In humans, the metabolite ratio of hydrocodone to hydromorphone highly correlates with the O-demethylation ratios for dextromethorphan, a marker of CYP2D6 activity[4]. The median values for partial metabolic clearance by O-demethylation in single dose studies are 28.1 + 10.3 ml/h/kg for extensive metabolizers,

3.4 + 2.4 ml/h/kg for poor metabolizers (persons containing two defective CYP2D6 genes) and 5.0 + 3.6 ml/h/kg for extensive metabolizers on quinidine, a CYP2D6 blocker[4]. Extensive metabolizers given CYP2D6 blockers will have mild increases in hydrocodone serum levels[5].

Differences in CYP23D6 genetics have limited influences on hydrocodone pain responses, indicating that conversion to hydromorphone is not critical for analgesia[4,5,14]. Paroxetine and fluoxetine reduce hydrocodone conversion to hydromorphone, but do not influence analgesia. Extensive metabolizers are reported to have a more rapid onset to pain relief compared with slow metabolizers, but not a greater duration or extent of relief[4]. Ultra-rapid metabolizers (those with more than two active CYP2D6 genes) have been reported to have more CNS side effects with hydrocodone[15]. This may be related to the accumulation of an O-demethylated metabolite.

Norhydrocodone is derived from CYP3A4 metabolism and may have some analgesic properties[2,15].

Hydrocodone's half-life is 3.8 h, although analgesic responses can be longer in duration than the parent drug half-life[16]. Hydrocodone's metabolism closely matches that of oxycodone. Both are active analgesics, both are metabolized through CYP2D6 and have potent active metabolites (hydromorphone and oxymorphone). As previously mentioned, both activate the MOR with the same degree of efficacy.

Routes of administration

Hydrocodone is available only for oral administration. There are no parenteral preparations. Its absorption per rectum is unknown, although there is no reason to believe that it is less well absorbed than other opioids.

Drug interactions and toxicity

There are very few reports of drug interactions with hydrocodone. Drug interactions are less than those associated with codeine and tramadol, since both of the latter two drugs require conversion to an active metabolite before pain relief can occur. Opioids may potentiate acetaminophen toxicity by delaying gastric emptying and prolonging absorption, and hydrocodone is no exception. Delayed gastric emptying has been associated with persistent elevated acetaminophen serum levels[17]. Hydrocodone will cause the usual opioid side effects. In addition, hydrocodone combinations have been associated with recurrent panic attacks in predisposed individuals[18]. By case report hydrocodone can cause recurrent hiccups[19].

Patients dying from hydrocodone cough preparations have been found to have high concentrations of hydromorphone in their bile[20]. Deaths have also occurred in the pediatric population when hydrocodone cough preparations were used to suppress cough due to viral respiratory illnesses[21].

Hydrocodone is a commonly abused opioid in the United States. The 'at risk' population appears to be middle class females[22]. Hydrocodone can be prescribed by telephone and is easily obtained through some insurance plans[22]. Hydrocodone is considered a 'weak' opioid by many, and does not carry the addiction stigmata of oxycodone, morphine or methadone[22]. Unlike codeine, blocking the conversion of hydrocodone to hydromorphone does reduce its abuse liability[15]. Hydrocodone is a minor metabolite of codeine and can be detected along with codeine in the urine of patients receiving codeine alone. As a result physicians may be led into believing that patients are using or abusing multiple opioids[23]. Hydrocodone serum levels seen with fatal overdoses are 0.4 mg/l (range 0.12–1.6 mg/l), which is quite similar to fatal oxycodone levels, 0.43 mg/l (range 0.12–8.0 mg/l)[24]. Hydrocodone is associated with polysubstance abuse[25]. Overuse or abuse of hydrocodone can be associated with rapidly progressive sensory neural hearing loss[26,27].

Dosing and special populations

There is very little published on hydrocodone in hepatic and renal failure. Since oxycodone and hydrocodone are metabolized and excreted in a very similar fashion, it can be anticipated that hydrocodone metabolism with heptic failure and elimination in renal failure will be reduced[28,29]. There are no studies regarding hydrocodone use in the elderly population. Like oxycodone, it is probable that age will not be a major factor in hydrocodone metabolism and elimination[30]. Gender has been reported to play a role in the clearance of oxycodone (and perhaps hydrocodone), since CYP2D6 levels were originally thought to be reduced in women[31,32]. Other reports have shown that the median dextromethorphan to dextrophan ratios are actually lower in females indicating greater CYP2D6 activity compared with men[33,34]. Overall gender differences in CYP2D6 (and CYP3A4) will not significantly influence drug metabolism or response[35].

Evidence-based use of hydrocodone in cancer pain

Hydrocodone combination analgesics have been reported for dental, postoperative, orthopedic and acute musculoskeletal pain, but not cancer pain (Table 5.1). Most if not all patients treated with hydrocodone, have had acute inflammatory pain. The results of these studies are influenced (and biased) by the NSAID or acetaminophen in the combination. These studies demonstrated that potent NSAIDs (ketorolac) and selective Cox2 inhibitors are as effective, if not more so, than hydrocodone plus acetaminophen for acute inflammatory pain. Hydrocodone appears to be more potent than codeine and tramadol and slightly less potent than oxycodone (Tables 5.1 and 5.2).

Although there are no reports of hydrocodone combination analgesics for cancer pain, there is no reason to believe that hydrocodone will be less effective than other opioids and, despite the lack of published clinical experience with hydrocodone with cancer pain, it is being used regularly in practice. There are certain advantages to

Table 5.1 Summary of hydrocodone equivalents

Type of pain	Analgesic response
Dental	
Ziccardi[41]	Hydrocodone 15 mg/ibuprofen 400 mg > codeine 60 mg/acetaminophen 600 mg
Tucker[42]	Etodolac 300 mg = hydrocodone/acetaminophen
Reed[43]	Ketoprofen 50 mg = hydrocodone 10 mg/acetaminophen 1000 mg
Fricke[44]	Tramadol 75 mg/acetaminophen 650 mg = hydrocodone 7.5 mg/acetaminophen 650 mg
Fricke[45]	Ketorolac 10 mg > hydrocodone 10 mg acetaminophen 1000 mg
Forbes[46]	Hydrocodone 7.5 mg/acetaminophen 500 mg > codeine 30 mg/acetaminophen 300 mgß
Orthopedic	
Barber[47]	Ketorolac 10 mg > hydrocodone 10 mg/acetaminophen 1000 mg
Gimbel[48]	Celecoxib 200 mg > hydrocodone 10 mg/acetaminophen 1000 mg
White[49]	Ketorolac 10 mg = hydrocodone 7.5 mg/acetaminophen 750 mg
Postoperative	
Wideman[50]	Hydrocodone 15 mg/ibuprofen 400 mg > hydrocodone 15 mg = ibuprofen 400 mg
Sunshine[51]	Hydrocodone 15 mg/ibuprofen 400 mg > hydrocodone 7.5 mg/ibuprofen 200 mg
Palangio[52]	Hydrocodone 15 mg/ibuprofen 400 mg > hydrocodone 7.5 mg/ibuprofen 200 mg
Palangio[53]	Hydrocodone 15 mg/ibuprofen 400 mg = oxycodone 10 mg/acetaminophen 650 mg
Beaver[54]	Hydrocodone 10 mg/acetaminophen 1000 mg > codeine 60 mg
	Hydrocodone 10 mg > codeine 60 mg
	Acetaminophen 1000 mg > codeine 60 mg
Acute musculoskeletal pain	
Marshall[55]	Hydrocodone 5 mg/acetaminophen 500 mg > tramadol 100 mg
Palangio[56]	Hydrocodone 7.5 mg/ibuprofen 2000 mg = oxycodone 5 mg/acetaminophen 325 mg
Turturro[57]	Hydrocodone 5 mg/acetaminophen 500 mg = codeine 30 mg/acetaminophen 500 mg

Table 5.2 Hydrocodone equivalents

Opioid	Dose equivalent (mg)
Hydrocodone	10 mg
Codeine	60–100 mg
Tramadol	75–100 mg
Oxycodone	6 mg

hydrocodone. Individuals on medications that block CYP2D6 activity will not respond to codeine and tramadol. In addition, tramadol when combined with selective serotonin reuptake inhibitors (SSRI) will precipitate a serotonin syndrome. Hydrocodone analgesia is not subject to CYP2D6 activity or reported to interact with

Table 5.3 Hydrocodone combinations hydrocodone/
acetaminophen combinations

Hydrocodone	Acetaminophen
2.5 mg	500 mg
5 mg	400, 500 mg
7.5 mg	400, 500, 650, 740 mg
10 mg	325, 400, 650, 660 mg
Hydrocodone	Ibuprofen
7.5 mg	200 mg
Hydrocodone	Homatropine
5 mg	1.5 mg

SSRIs. On the other hand, there are probably no particular advantages of hydrocodone over oxycodone combinations in this setting unless non-cross tolerance or better tolerance (fewer side effects) can be demonstrated.

Combination products improve convenience but limit hydrocodone dose titration due either to the ceiling dose of ibuprofen and acetaminophen. Hydrocodone's dosing is limited to oral, although patient compliance may improve with fewer number of tablets taken daily due to the combination[36–38]. A risk for prescribing the combination is prolonged acetaminophen clearance due to delayed gastric emptying. However, this is not particular to hydrocodone. Patients may inadvertently take additional acetaminophen or ibuprofen, while on hydrocodone combined analgesics resulting in NSAID toxicity, while not being aware that the combination product contains a NSAID.

Dose and route

Safe acetaminophen doses are 4 g daily and should not exceed 6 g. Ibuprofen has a ceiling dose of 2.4 g/day. There is an extensive range of hydrocodone-acetaminophen combinations, which are commercially available (Table 5.3). Hydrocodone doses are possible up to 120 mg/day with an acetaminophen combination and 90 mg/day with the ibuprofen combination. Hydrocodone is available as a combination with homatropine for cough and is limited to 15 mg of hydrocodone every 4 h as a single dose due to homatropine[39,40].

References

1 Chen ZR, Irvine RJ, Somogyi AA, *et al.* Mu receptor binding of some commonly used opioids and their metabolites. *Life Sci* 1991; **44(22):** 2165–71.

2 Cone EJ, Darwin WD, Gorodetzky CW, *et al.* Comparative metabolism of hydrocodone in man, rat, guinea pig, rabbit, and dog. *Drug Metab Disposit* 1978; **6(4):** 488–93.

3 Tomkins DM, Otton SV, Joharchi N, *et al.* Effect of cytochrome P450 2D1 inhibition on hydrocodone metabolism and its behavioral consequences in rats. *J Pharmacol Exp Ther* 1997; **280(3):** 1374–82.

4 Otton SV, Schadel M, Cheung SW, *et al.* CYP2D6 phenotype determines the metabolic conversion of hydrocodone to hydromorphone. *Clin Pharmacol Ther* 1993; **54(5)**: 463–72.

5 Lelas S, Wegert S, Otton SV, *et al.* Inhibitors of cytochrome P450 differentially modify discriminative-stimulus and antinociceptive effects of hydrocodone and hydromorphone in rhesus monkeys. Drug Alc Depend 1999; **54**: 239–49.

6 Selley DE, Liu Q, Childers SR. Signal transduction correlates of mu opioid agonist intrinsic efficacy: receptor-stimulated [35S]GTPgS binding in mMOR-CHO cells and rat thalamus. *J Pharmacol Exp Ther* 1998; **285**: 496–505.

7 Remmers AE, Clark MJ, Alt A, *et al.* Activation of G protein by opioid receptors: role of receptor number and G-protein concentration. *Eur J Pharmacol* 2000; **396(2–3)**: 67–75.

8 Harrison C, Traynor JR. The [^{35}S]GTPgS binding assay: approaches and applications in pharmacology. *Life Sci* 2003; **74**: 489–508.

9 Thompson C, Wojno H, Greiner E, *et al.* Activation of G-proteins by morphine and 3-methooxymorphine congeners: insights to the relevance of O- and N-demethylated metabolites at {micro} and {delta} opioid receptors. *J Pharmacol Exp Ther* 2004; **308(2)**: 547–54.

10 Kolesnikov YA, Wilson RS, Pasternak GW. The synergistic analgesic interactions between hydrocodone and ibuprofen. *Anesth Analg* 2003; **97(6)**: 1721–3.

11 McGinnity DF, Parker AJ, Soars M, *et al.* Automated definition of the enzymology of drug oxidation by the major human drug metabolizing cytochrome P450s. *Drug Metab Dispos* 2000; **28(11)**: 1327–34.

12 Zakusov VV, Ostrovskaya RU, Bulayev VM. GABA-opiates interactions in the activity of analgesics. *Arch Int Pharmacodyn Ther* 1983; **265(1)**: 651–75.

13 Lambrecht RW, Gildemeister OS, Williams A, *et al.* Effects of selected antihypertensives and analgesics on hepatic porphyrin accumulation: implications for clinical porphyria. *Biochem Pharmacol* 1999; **58(5)**: 887–96.

14 Kaplan HL, Busto UE, Baylon GJ. Inhibition of cytochrome P450 2D6 metabolism of hydrocodone to hydromorphone does not importantly affect abuse liability. *J Pharmacol Exp Ther* 1997; **281(1)**: 103–8.

15 De Leon J, Dinsmore L, Wedlund P. Adverse drug reactions to oxycodone and hydrocodone in CYP2D6 ultrarapid metabolizers. *J Clin Psychopharmacol* 2003; **23(4)**: 420–1.

16 McEvoy GK, Miller JL, Snow EK, *et al.* (Eds). *AHFS Drug Information*. 2002.

17 Spiller HA. Persistently elevated acetaminophen concentrations for two days after an initial four-hour non-toxic concentration. *Vet Hum Toxicol* 2001; **43(4)**: 218–19.

18 Sansone RA, Sansone LA. Exacerbation of panic disorder symptoms following vicodin exposure. *Gen Hosp Psychiat* 2002; **24**: 448–54.

19 Lauterbach EC. Hiccup and apparent myoclonus after hydrocodone: review of the opiate-related hiccup and myoclonus literature. *Clin Neuropharmacol* 1999; **22(2)**: 87–92.

20 Park JI, Nakamura GR, Greisemer EC, *et al.* Hydromorphone detected in bile following hydrocodone ingestion. *J. Forensic Sci.* 1982; **27(1)**: 223–4.

21 Morrow PL, Faris EC. Death associated with inadvertent hydrocodone overdose in a child with a respiratory tract infection. *Am J Forens Med Pathol* 1987; **8(1)**: 60–3.

22 Mitka M. Abuse of prescription drugs: is a patient ailing or addicted? *J Am Med Ass* 2000; **283(9)**: 1126–9.

23 Oyler JM, Cone EJ, Joseph RE Jr, *et al.* Identification of hydrocodone in human urine following controlled codeine administration. *J Anal Toxicol* 2000; **24(7)**: 530–5.

24 Spiller HA. Postmortem oxycodone and hydrocodone blood concentrations. *J Forens Sci* 2003; **48(2)**: 429–31.

25 Meeker JE, Som CW, Macapagal EC, *et al.* Zolpidem tissue concentrations in a multiple drug related death involving ambien. *J Anal Toxicol* 1995; **19(6):** 531–4.

26 Freidman RA, House JW, Luxford WM, *et al.* Profound hearing loss associated with hydrocodone/acetaminophen abuse. *Am J Otol* 2000; **21(2):** 188–91.

27 Oh AK, Ishiyama A, Baloh RW. Deafness associated with abuse of hydrocodone/acetaminophen. *Neurology* 2000; **54(12):** 2345.

28 Kirvela M, Lindgren L, Seppala T, *et al.* The pharmacokinetics of oxycodone in uremic patients undergoing renal transplantation. *J Clin Anesth* 1996; **8:** 13–18.

29 Tallgren M, Olkkola KT, Seppala T, *et al.* Pharmacokinetics and ventilatory effects of oxycodone before and after liver transplantation. *Clin Pharmacol Ther* 1997; **61(6):** 655–61.

30 Davis MP, Varga J, Dickerson D, *et al.* Normal-release and controlled-release oxycodone: pharmacokinetics, pharmacodynamics, and controversy. *Support Care Cancer* 2003; **11(2):** 84–92.

31 Kaiko RF, Benziger DP, Fitzmartin RD, *et al.* Pharmacokinetic-pharmacodynamic relationships of controlled release oxycodone. *Clin Pharmacol Ther* 1996; **59(1):** 52–61.

32 Rademaker M. Do women have more adverse drug reactions? *Am J Dermatol* 2001; **2(6):** 349–51.

33 Hagg S, Spigset O, Dahlqvist R. Influence of gender and oral contraceptives on CYP2D6 and CYP2C19 activity in healthy volunteers. *Br J Clin Pharmacol* 2001; **51(2):** 169–73.

34 Meibohm B, Beirele I, Derendorf H. How important are gender differences in pharmacokinetics? *Clin Pharmacokinet* 2002; **41(5):** 329–42.

35 McCune JS, Lindley LC, Decker JL, *et al.* Lack of gender differences and large intrasubject variability in cytochrome P450 activity measured by phenotyping with dextromethorphan. *J Clin Pharmacol* 2001; **41(7):** 723–31.

36 Armstrong SC, Cozza KL. Pharmacokinetic drug interactions of morphine, codeine, and their derivatives: theory and clinical reality, part I. *Psychosomatics* 2003; **44:** 167–71.

37 Armstrong SC, Cozza KL. Pharmacokinetic drug interactions of morphine, codeine, and their derivatives: theory and clinical reality, part II. *Psychosomatics* 2003; **44:** 515–20.

38 Armstrong TA, Rohal GM. Potential danger from too much acetaminophen in opiate agonist combination products. *Am J Hlth Syst P* 1999; **56(17):** 1774–5.

39 Homsi J, Walsh D, Nelson KA. Important drugs for cough in advanced cancer. *Support Care Cancer* 2001; **9(8):** 565–74.

40 Homsi J, Walsh D, Nelson KA, *et al.* Hydrocodone for cough in advanced cancer. *Am J Hospice Palliat Care* 2000; **17(5):** 342–6.

41 Ziccardi VB, Desjardins PJ, Daly-DeJoy E, *et al.* Single-dose vicoprofen compared with acetaminophen with codeine and placebo in patients with acute postoperative pain after third molar extractions. *J Oral Maxillofac Surg* 2000; **58(6):** 622–8.

42 Tucker PW, Smith JR, Adams DF. A comparison of 2 analgesic regimens for the control of postoperative peridontal discomfort. *J Periodont* 1996; **67(2):** 125–9.

43 Reed KL, Smith JR, Lie T, *et al.* A pilot study comparing ketoprohen and acetaminophen with hydrocodone for the relief of postoperative periodontal discomfort. *Anesth Prog* 1997; **44(2):** 49–54.

44 Fricke JR Jr, Karim R, Jordan D, *et al.* A double-blind, single-dose comparison of the analgesic efficacy of tramadol/acetaminophen combination tablets, hydrocodone/acetaminophen combination tablets, and placebo after oral surgery. *Clin Therapeut* 2002; **24(6):** 953–68.

45 Fricke J, Halladay SC, Bynum L, *et al.* Pain relief after dental impaction surgery using ketorolac, hydrocodone plus acetaminophen, or placebo. *Clin Therapeut* 1993; **15(3):** 500–9.

46 Forbes JA, Bowser MW, Calderazzo JP, *et al.* An evaluation of the analgesic efficacy of three opioid-analgesic combinations in postoperative oral surgery pain. *J Oral Surg* 1981; **39(2):** 108–12.

47 Barber FA, Gladu DE. Comparison of oral ketorolac and hydrocodone for pain relief after anterior cruciate ligament reconstruction. *Arthroscopy* 1998; **14(6):** 605–12.

48 Gimbel JS, Brugger A, Zhao W, *et al.* Efficacy and tolerability of celecoxib versus hydrocodone/acetaminophen in the treatment of pain after ambulatory orthopedic surgery in adults. *Clin Therapeut* 2001; **23(2):** 228–41.

49 White P, Joshi GP, Carpenter RL, *et al.* A comparison of oral ketorolac and hydrocodone for analgesia after ambulatory surgery: arthroscopy versus laparoscopic tubal ligation. *Anesth Analg* 1997; **85(1):** 37–43.

50 Wideman GL, Keffer M, Morris E, *et al.* Analgesic efficacy of a combination of hydrocodone with ibuprofen in postoperative pain. *Clin Pharmacol Ther* 1999; **65(1):** 66–76.

51 Sunshine A, Olson NZ, O'Niell E, *et al.* Analgesic efficacy of a hydromorphone with ibuprofen combination compared with ibuprofen alone for the treatment of acute postoperative pain. *J Clin Oncol* 1997; **37(10):** 908–15.

52 Palagino M, Wideman GL, Keffer M, *et al.* Dose response effect of combination hydrocodone with ibuprofen in patients with moderate to severe postoperative pain. *Clin Ther* 2000; **22(8):** 990–1002.

53 Palagino M, Wideman GL, Keffer M, *et al.* Combination hydrocodone and ibuprofen versus combination oxycodone and acetaminophen in the treatment of postoperative obstetric or gynecologic pain. *Clin Ther* 2000; **22(5):** 600–12.

54 Beaver WT, McMillan D. Methodological considerations in the evaluation of analgesic combinations: acetaminophen (paracetamol) and hydrocodone in postpartum pain. *Br J Clin Pharmacol* 1980; **10(Suppl 2):** 215S–23S.

55 Marshall RC. Tramadol or hydrocodone-acetaminophen for acute musculoskeletal pain? *J Family Pract* 1998; **47(5):** 330–1.

56 Palagino M, Morris E, Doyle RT, *et al.* Combination hydrocodone and ibuprofen versus combination oxycodone and acetaminophen in the treatment of moderate or severe acute low back pain. *Clin Therapeut* 2002; **24(1):** 87–99.

57 Turturro MA, Paris PM, Yealy DM, *et al.* Hydrocodone versus codeine in acute musculoskeletal pain. *Annl Emerg Med* 1991; **20(10):** 1100–3.

Chapter 6

Tramadol

Mellar P. Davis

Introduction

Tramadol is a synthetic 4-phyenyl-piperdine analogue of codeine. It has been available in Germany since 1977 and in the United States since 1995[1]. Tramadol is the most frequently used step II opioid worldwide and is marketed in over 100 countries. Over 50 million people have received tramadol[2]. Tramadol has a unique multiple receptor agonist profile, which differs from other 'step II' opioids.[3]

Pharmacology

Pharmacodynamics

Tramadol's affinity for the mu opioid receptor (MOR) is 10-fold less than codeine, 100-fold less than dextropropoxyphene and 6,000-fold less than morphine[2,4,5]. However, affinity for the MOR does not account for its relative analgesic potency, which is much greater[6]. Tramadol blocks monoamine re-uptake at the same concentrations that MOR binding occurs[6,7]. It does not bind to alpha adrenoreceptors, 5HT2 receptors, NMDA, benzodiazepine receptors, nor is it a Cox inhibtor[4,7,8]. Tramadol also has a local anesthetic activity, which is weaker than lidocaine[9]. Because of its influence on monoamines analgesic properties, tramadol is only partially blocked by naloxone[2,6,10–12]. Unlike morphine the adrenoreceptor antagonist, yohimbine and serotonin receptor antagonist, ulancerin, blocks tramadol's pain relief[4,13]. It's binding affinity for re-uptake sites is two orders of magnitude less than that of imipramine[6]. Tramadol competes with desipramine and norephinephrine re-uptake binding sites. Tramadol enhances serotonin and norephinephrine production[2,6,14–18].

Tramadol consists of two enantiomers. The positive enantiomer of tramadol binds MOR and, to a lesser extent, delta opioid receptor (DOR) and kappa opioid receptor (KOR). Its negative enantiomer has a 10-fold less binding affinity for MOR, but a greater affinity for KOR and DOR compared with the positive enantiomer[6,19]. The negative enantiomer stimulates release of norepinephrine, the positive enantiomer increases serotonin efflux[4,20]. Overall, the positive enantiomer of tramadol is a more potent analgesic than the negative enantiomer, but the combination is even a more potent analgesic[4,21].

Tramadol is metabolized into two active metabolites. The first metabolite is O-desmethyl tramadol (M1) and is formed as a result of demethylation by the cytochrome CYP2D6[19,22]. Compared with the parent drug, M1 has a 700-fold greater affinity for MOR. The second metabolite, di N, O-desmethyl tramadol (M5), has a 24-fold greater affinity for MOR than the parent opioid[23]. Although the parent opioid binds to MOR, it does not activate the receptor site unlike the metabolites, M1 and M5. The intrinsic efficacy of M1 is between that of morphine and fentanyl[23]. The M5 metabolite has a much lower intrinsic efficacy than M1. CYP2D6 activity, by forming M1 and M5, influences analgesia by some studies, but not by other studies[6,14,23–25]. M1 has a reduced monoamine re-uptake inhibition compared with that of tramadol[6]. The M1 metabolite to a lesser degree binds weakly to KOR and to DOR[19].

Pharmacokinetics

Absorption

Single dose studies of tramadol demonstrate its oral bioavailability at 70%. Thirty per cent is cleared by first pass through the liver. Absorption is therefore nearly 100% from the small bowel[2,6]. Oral absorption is not influenced by food[14,26]. Tramadol's metabolism is saturable and has increased bioavailability with multiple dosing. Oral bioavailability is increased with age, and with impaired hepatic and renal function. Rectal tramadol has a bioavailability of 78%[14]. The delayed onset of tramadol's monoamine re-uptake inhibition with saturable metabolism account for increased analgesia, with chronic dosing compared with single dose studies[27]. Young and healthy patients will have detectable plasma levels within 15–45 min of oral dosing[14]. Tramadol has similar oral and parenteral pharmacokinetics, including drug half-life. The half-life is 5–7 h and time to peak plasma is 3.1 h[28]. Tramadol is 20% protein bound. The half-life of M1 is slightly longer than the parent drug. M1 concentrations are 12.6% of tramadol with peak concentrations occurring 3 h after oral administration[2,6]. Tramadol's large volume of distribution (ranging between 306 and 203 l) is due to extensive tissue binding[14]. Steady state levels are obtained with 2 days of 4 h dosing.

Ten per cent of tramadol is eliminated in the bile. Ninety per cent is excreted in the urine, either as the parent drug or a metabolite. Fifteen to 30% of tramadol is excreted unchanged in the urine and 60% as metabolites[10,14,29,30]. Therefore, enterohepatic circulation is unlikely to be important as a factor in tramadol kinetics. Two major urinary metabolites, O-desmethyl tramadol (M1) and N-demethylation (M2), are by products of CYP2D6 and CYP3A4 metabolism. Both are conjugated, accounting for four of the known major metabolites[8,9]. There is a stereoselective cytochrome metabolism of tramadol and metabolites with uncertain clinical significance[2,31,32]. Neither tramadol nor its metabolites preferentially accumulate in kidney or liver tissues[33]. There are ethnic differences to the metabolism of tramadol as demonstrated in a study of the Nigerian population. Ninety-six per cent of tramadol is excreted unchanged in the urine in this population compared with 30% in the Caucasian population[34]. The prevalence of CYP2D6 #17 in African populations, and the CYP2D6 #10 gene in Oriental populations may alter tramadol metabolism and, thus, its ability to act as an analgesic[35,36]. Tramadol conversion to O-desmethyl tramadol requires CYP2D6 activity. The tramadol to O-desmethyl tramadol urine ratios in poor metabolizers results in diminished analgesia[31,37,38].

Routes of administration

Oral tramadol is available in most countries. Sustained release tramadol can be formed by combining tramadol in a glyceryl behenate matrix with lactose as an enhancer[7,39,40]. Bioavailability of sustained release tramadol is similar to normal release[2,41]. Tramadol is also available in some countries in parenteral form. In fact, the original formulation developed in Germany was parenteral. Adult and pediatric suppositories are available in a number of countries and well absorbed[2]. Tramadol can be given epidurally, but there appears to be little advantage to this route of administration[2].

Equianalgesia

In the largest retrospective studies of tramadol involving cancer patients, the morphine to tramadol equivalent ratios was 1 : 10[42–44]. A second smaller study found a ratio of 1 : 4. This study, although prospective in design, involved only 20 patients[45]. Such differences are perhaps related to the CYP2D6 genotype of the study populations[46]. Three-hundred milligrams of tramadol per day is equivalent to 0.6 mg of buprenophine/day[28]. Two postoperative studies using parenteral tramadol and morphine found that 50 mg of tramadol were equivalent to 5 mg morphine. In a second, larger study, 100 mg of parenteral tramadol was found to be equivalent to 5 mg of parenteral morphine[47]. Epidural tramadol is said to be one-thirtieth as potent as epidural morphine[48,49].

Oral tramadol's potency is equivalent to oral meperidine and pentazocine[47,50,51]. Most studies have found that 100 mg of oral tramadol were equal to 50 mg of parenteral meperidine[52–54].

Tramadol is more potent than dextropropoxyphene per milligram in chronic arthritis patients and more potent than codeine per milligrams for chronic non-malignant pain[55–57]. Geriatric patients with multiple pain syndromes found that 200–250 mg of tramadol produced the same degree of pain relief as 140 mg of codeine plus 1400 mg of acetaminophen. Combinations of tramadol plus acetaminophen produced the equivalent pain relief as codeine plus acetaminophen per milligram. One-hundred-and-fifty milligrams of tramadol is better than destroproxyphene 100 mg plus acetaminophen 650 mg for postoperative pain[57]. The combination of tramadol plus acetaminophen is better than tramadol alone[58,59,60]. Tramadol 75 mg plus acetaminophen 650 mg is equivalent to hydrocodone 10 mg plus equivalent acetaminophen[6,61]. Dihydrocodeine 120 mg is equivalent to tramadol 200 mg[62].

Tramadol is half as potent as diclofenac in milligrams[63]. Other studies have shown that tramadol and diclofenac are equally potent for chronic non-malignant pain[64]. Parenteral tramadol 100 mg produces relief of pain equivalent to ketorolac 30 mg for patients undergoing maxillary surgery[65]. Four-hundred milligrams of ibuprofen is equivalent to tramadol 75 mg plus acetaminophen 650 mg for postoperative pain[60]. Finally, parenteral dipyrone 2.5 mg is superior to 100 mg of tramadol for renal colic[66–68].

Drug interactions

Tramadol analgesia is reduced by ondansetron due to competitive inhibition through CYP2D6[69]. Ondansetron also blocks tramadol's enhanced serotonin activity by blocking serotonin receptors. Ondansetron does not decrease the nausea or vomiting associated with tramadol unlike morphine[25,69]. Both selective serotonin re-uptake inhibitors (SSRIs) and tramadol increase serotonin within synapses, and leads to a significant risk for the serotonin syndrome[70–77]. Olanzapine and resperidone both selectively block 5HT2 receptors, and facilitate serotonin neurotransmission through 5HT1A. These drugs, with tramadol, may also cause the serotonin syndrome[78]. In the same light, monoamine oxidase inhibitors or the antidepressants, venlafaxine and buspirone may do the same[79,80]. Carbamazepine stimulates tramadol clearance through CYP3A4 N-demethylation and to it's inactive metabolite. The dose of tramadol may need to be doubled if patients are on 800 mg or more of carbamazepine[3,14,26]. Cimetidine increases tramadol and M1 half-life, respectively, by 19 and 25%, but does not significantly alter drug kinetics nor are dose adjustments necessary[4]. There are favorable analgesic responses with magnesium or ketamine and tramadol in patients experiencing postoperative pain[81]. Combinations of the antidepressant mianserin plus tramadol improves psychological dysfunction and reduces pain at lower doses than achieved by tramadol alone. Mianserin like mirtazapine is not a serotonin re-uptake inhibitor and does not block CYP2D6[36,82].

Toxicity

The side effects associated with tramadol are usually mild, but can vary widely in frequency from study to study. Side effects of tramadol are dose-dependent[55]. Overall, approximately 15% of patients will have side effects[83,84]. A post-marketing survey involving over 1300 patients recorded nausea in 5%, dizziness in 5%, vomiting in 1%, sedation in 2% and dry mouth in 3%. The prevalence of urinary difficulties is similar to other opioids[85]. The adverse effects of sustained release tramadol are equivalent to normal release tramadol[2]. The side effect profile with tramadol is due to opioid-related adverse side effects (dyspepsia, nausea, vomiting, tiredness, drowsiness) and monominergic effects (headache, dizziness, sweating)[2,5]. Tramadol is associated with less respiratory depression than other opioids[2]. Tolerance to side effects occurs, which can be further minimized by starting with low doses. Nausea and vomiting respond to phenothiazines, dexamethasone and metoclopramide[2,4,5,85]. Tramadol-induced nausea appears to be associated with peak plasma concentrations[4]. Unlike other opioids, tramadol has very little influence on gastric emptying, oral-cecal transit time and sphincter of oddi function[2,14,86]. Constipation occurs in 22–35% with tramadol alone compared with 58% with codeine plus acetaminophen, 49% with codeine plus aspirin, and 41% with oxycodone and acetaminophen[2,49,87,88]. Hepatic toxicity has not been reported with tramadol[10].

Tramadol induced seizures occur in three different at risk populations:[89]

- those who are on high doses of tramadol;
- those who are predisposed to seizures;
- those who are on medications that reduce seizure thresholds[2].

Otherwise, the incidence of seizures is low (1 in 7000). Idiopathic seizures in non-predisposed individuals on standard doses are unusual[90].

Tramadol does not induce a withdrawal reaction when given to patients receiving morphine or methadone; nor does it prevent withdrawal when substituted for potent opioids[2]. Unlike other opioids, tapering doses of tramadol are not necessary to avoid withdrawal[90].

Tramadol does not influence the thermoregulatory thresholds for sweating. It does not produce fever and, in fact, has been effective in relieving postoperative shivers[4,91–96].

Tramadol does not reduce renal blood flow. Insignificant changes in blood pressures occur after parenteral tramadol of 100 mg or with a dose of 1.5 mg/kg, despite increasing norephinephrine serum levels[14]. Despite increased norephinephrine, patients with coronary artery disease may safely receive tramadol, since there is no influence on heart rate, aortic pressure or peripheral arterial resistance. Tramadol has a mild negative inotropic effect, which may be problematic for patients with heart failure[4,57,95]. Other studies have demonstrated dose-dependent increases in systolic and diastolic pressures, increased heart rate and a 25% increases in peripheral resistance[14]. Tramadol does decrease pulmonary artery resistance.

Respiratory depression will occur in normal volunteers without pain at doses of 1–1.5 mg tramadol/kg weight[96]. Postoperative and chronic pain patients do not have significant changes in arterial O_2 saturations, respiratory function, minute ventilation or increase arterial CO_2 with tramadol as they do with equianalgesic doses of morphine, pentazocine and meperidine[4,14,51]. Tramadol can culminate in renal failure and cause respiratory depression with standard doses[97].

Tramadol does not impair hand-eye coordination. Tramadol reduces experimentally-induced cough. Unlike morphine, tramadol does not cause histamine release and has a reduced risk for pruritus[14].

Tramadol overdoses produce central nervous system depression, respiratory depression, muscle spasm and opisthotonos. Overdoses are rarely associated with fatality and, if fatality does occur, it is usually due to comedications, such as sedatives[98]. Respiratory depression is only partially reversed by naloxone and seizures are not responsive to opioid antagonists. Fatality is reported with doses of 300–350 mg/kg[2].

Abuse

The incidence of tramadol abuse is less than with other opioids. It is still recommended that tramadol be prescribed with caution to individuals with a history of substance abuse[5,99]. The overall incidence for psychological dependence is 1–6.9/1000 persons treated/year[100]. A German survey demonstrated abuse in 0.323/million single dose units compared with 0.38/million for dextropropoxyphene, 7.9/million for codeine and 10/million for dihydrocodeine. In the United States, abuse, dependency, withdrawal or overdose have been reported in 115 out of 5 million patients treated[26]. Most of these patients had a history of substance abuse and the occurrence was within isolated pockets around the country[14]. Most tramadol abuse is associated with polysubstance use and only 4.3% of the abuse is due to tramadol as a single agent[4]. Parenteral tramadol cannot be recognized as a opioid by individuals with a history of drug dependency[4,101,102].

Dose modification

Renal failure

Renal insufficiency with a creatinine clearance range of 5–80 ml/min increases tramadol half-life by a factor of 1.5–2. Only 7% of this drug is removed in a standard 4 h hemodialysis session[5]. It is recommended that if the creatinine clearance is less than 30 ml/min, dose intervals should be extended to 12 h and patients should receive a maximum dose of 200 mg/day[2,5,14].

Liver failure

Hepatic impairment or cirrhosis increases tramadol half-life by 2–3 times. Patients with significant liver disease or cirrhosis should receive no more than 50 mg every 12 h[2,5,14].

Elderly

Tramadol half-life and oral bioavailability increase with age. Maximum doses in patients 75 years or older with good renal and hepatic function are 300 mg/day[3,5].

Evidence-based use of tramadol for cancer pain

Retrospective, prospective and open-labeled studies, as well as randomized prospective trials, have been performed in cancer patients with pain.

A non-blinded, non-randomized study of high dose tramadol (300 mg or greater) in 810 patients was compared with low-dose morphine (less than 60 mg/day) in 848 cancer patients. The mean daily tramadol dose was 428 + 101 mg and morphine does was 42 + 13 mg. High dose tramadol produced equivalent analgesia to low dose morphine. Constipation, neuropsychiatric symptoms and pruritus were more frequent with morphine. Tramadol discontinuation was usually related to uncontrolled severe pain requiring greater than the maximum doses allowable within the study[42].

An observational trial involving 51 patients used either oral or intramuscular tramadol. Patients received a mean daily dose of 300 mg for between 2 weeks and 14 months duration. Neither pain scale nor assessment frequency were standardized. Tramadol relieved 83% of bone pain, 61% of visceral pain and 33% of neuropathic pain[103].

A 290-patient cohort was treated with a mean tramadol dose of up 394 + 139 mg to a maximum of 600 mg daily pre-study non-opioid adjuvants were continued on study. Seventy-eight per cent had mild to no pain while on tramadol and 15% were able to continue tramadol throughout the course of their disease[4]. Adverse effects requiring discontinuation occurred in 4%.

In a small open-labeled trial, 86% of patients had good to excellent pair response with 200 mg of oral tramadol daily[104].

Sustained release tramadol was initiated in 146 cancer patients and 90 completed a 6-week trial. Naproxen 1000 mg per day was continued while patients were started on tramadol. Average and maximum daily pain were progressively reduced through the first 4 days of the trial. Good to complete pain relief was achieved in 43% the first week and in 71% at week six. The maximum daily tramadol dose was 650 mg. Seventy per cent of patients required less than 400 mg a day during the 6 weeks of the study. Adverse effects occurred in one out of four patients. Fatigue, dizziness, and constipation decreased in frequency over the 6 weeks of the trial. The incidence of nausea, vomiting and sweating did not change with time. Sixty-two per cent of the patients were deemed responders. No cardiovascular side effects nor analgesic tolerance were noted. The mean daily dose throughout the trail was 374 + 139 mg[88].

A post-marketing phase IV study of tramadol involved 154 patients with cancer pain. The mean daily dose on the trial was 160 mg with a maximum daily dose of 400 mg and an average 2-week duration on study. Eighty-eight per cent of patients responded with satisfactory pain relief[105].

Prospective trials

A prospective randomized comparison between tramadol and morphine included 119 patients. The mean tramadol dose was 368 mg and daily morphine doses ranged between 69 and 96 mg per day. Tramadol had less adverse effects in the first 3 months, but morphine produced better analgesia, particularly for severe pain. Both sleep patterns and activities improved with tramadol[106]. Overall improvement was reported in 73% of the patients.

A prospective cross-over trial with a two by two design compared morphine and tramadol. Three-hundred-and-seventy-five milligrams of oral tramadol was equivalent to 101 mg of oral morphine. Tramadol had less nausea and constipation[45].

In a multicenter prospective trial, 100 mg of sustained released tramadol every 8–12 h had better analgesia than doses of sublingual buprenorphine 0.2 mg every 6–8 h[28].

A prospective 7-day cross-over trial involving 60 patients compared buprenorphine 0.6 mg with 300 mg tramadol per day. Analgesia was equivalent, but tramadol had greater patient acceptance. One patient discontinued tramadol for side effects, whereas 18 patients discontinued buprenorphine because of side effects[107].

A prospective double-blind cross-over randomized trial compared tramadol and morphine. The mean daily morphine doses by day 4 was 101 + 58 mg and for tramadol was 375 + 135 mg. Tramadol pain scores were inferior on days 1 and 2, but equivalent by day 4. Side effects were lower for tramadol. More patients dropped out for reasons of side effects with morphine and for lack of pain relief with tramadol. Patient's preferences were 40% for morphine and 15% for tramadol[108].

A prospective double-blind randomized trial compared 100 mg of flupirtine with 50 mg of tramadol at a fixed dose schedule. Verbal rating scales were performed weekly. Flupirtine reduced pain in 63% and tramadol in 46% by week 4. More rescue analgesia was needed with tramadol. Nineteen per cent of tramadol-treated patients and 6% of flupirtine-treated patients had adverse drug reactions[109].

A prospective multicenter trial compared parenteral tramadol with an experimental agent AP.237 (a non-opioid). Eighty-two per cent of patients responded to tramadol and 62% to AP.237. Side effects with tramadol were experienced by 21% of the patients[110,111].

The evidence for the use of tramadol in cancer pain is relatively strong. Large open-labeled non-randomized trials, prospective randomized trials and cross-over trials demonstrate tramadol analgesia in advanced cancer pain. Uncontrolled variables include placebo effects in open label trials and the variable intensity of pain in patients with previous opioid exposure, differences in dosing strategy and total allowable daily dose. The individual differences of predicted equianalgesia between morphine and tramadol is quite significant. In most reported experiences, tramadol is better used for moderate than for severe pain.

Dose and routes

Oral normal release tramadol is available in the United States in 50 and 100 mg tablets, and usual dosing is every 4–6 h with a maximum recommended dose of 400 mg/day. Greater than 400 mg/day doses have been used without toxicity and have produced greater analgesia than lower doses. [Oral drops (20 drops equal to 50 mg), ampules of 100 mg preservative free, dispersible 50-mg preparations and sustained release (100, 150 and 200 mg) are available in some countries.] Also rectal suppositories are available for adults (100 mg) and children (15, 30 and 50 mg) in some countries.

Initial oral doses of tramadol are 50 mg every 4–6 h titrated to pain relief or side effects. Sustained release tramadol every 12 h may improve compliance. Parenteral dosing is equivalent to oral dosing. Continuous tramadol infusions are started at

37.5 mg/h. For severe pain, a loading dose of 150–250 mg to a maximum of 600 mg over 24 h is initiated. Patient controlled analgesia starts with a 40-mg loading dose and 20 mg as needed per hour[50,51]. Pediatric single doses are usually 1–2 mg/kg for ages greater than 12 months and 1 mg/kg for age less than 12 months. Alternatively, tramadol drops at a dose of 1.5 mg/kg may be used[2]. Parenteral tramadol is compatible with midazolam, haloperidol, hyoscine butylbromide and metoclopramide for those who need a broaden range of symptoms treated[112].

Summary

Tramadol is an effective step II opioid with reduced side effects as compared with morphine and buprenorphine. Dose ratios range between 1 : 10 and 1 : 4 (morphine to tramadol). Tramadol has a unique receptor profile and greater potency than predicted, based upon the MOR binding affinity. Tramadol is avoided with serotonin re-uptake inhibitors, tricyclic antidepressants and perhaps atypical antipsychotics. Dose will need to be adjusted for age, renal and hepatic function. The abuse potential for tramadol is low. Tramadol is an important opioid in countries where there is limited access to potent opioids.

References

1 Rose JB, Finkel JC, Arquedas-Mohs A, *et al.* Oral tramadol for the treatment of pain of 7–30 days' duration in children. *Anesth Analg* 2003; **96**(1): 78–81.

2 Shipton EA. Tramadol—present and future. *Anaesth Intens Care* 2000; **28**: 363–74.

3 Gibson TP. Pharmacokinetics, efficacy, and safety of analgesia with a focus on tramadol HCl. *Am J Med* 1996; **101**(Suppl 1A): 47S–53S.

4 Radbruch L, Grond S, Lehmann KA. A risk-benefit assessment of tramadol in the management of pain. *Drug Safety* 1996; **15**(1): 8–29.

5 Lewis KS, Han N. Tramadol: a new centrally acting analgesic. *Am J Hlth Pharm* 1997; **54**(6):643–52.

6 Raffa RB. A novel approach to the pharmacology of analgesics. *Am J Med* 1996; **101**(1A): 40S–46S.

7 Raffa RB, Haslego ML, Maryanoff CA, *et al.* Unexpected antinociceptive effect on the N-oxide (RWJ 38705) of tramadol hydrochloride. *J Pharmacol Exp Ther* 1996; **278**(3): 1098–104.

8 Lai J, Ma SW, Porreca F, *et al.* Tramadol, M1 metabolite and enantiomer affinities for cloned human opioid receptors expressed in transfected HN9.10 neuroblastoma cells. *Eur J Pharmacol* 1996; **316**(2–3): 369–72.

9 Mert T, Gunes Y, Guven M, *et al.* Comparison of nerve conduction blocks by an opioid and a local anesthetic. *Eur J Pharmacol* 2002; **439**: 77–81.

10 Dayer P, Collart L, Desmeules J. The pharmacology of tramadol. *Drugs* 1994; **47**(Suppl 1): 3–7.

11 Raffa RB, Friderichs E, Reimann W, *et al.* Opioid and nonopioid components independently contribute to the mechanism of action of tramadol, an 'atypical' opioid analgesic. *J Pharmacol Exp Ther* 1992; **260**(1): 275–85.

12 Raffa RB, Friderichs E, Reimann W, *et al.* Complementary and synergistic antinociceptive interaction between the enantiomers of tramadol. *J Pharmacol Exp Ther* 1993; **267**(1): 331–40.

13 **Desmeules JA, Piguet V, Collart L,** *et al.* Contribution of nonaminergic modulation to the analgesic effect of tramadol. *Br J Clin Pharmacol* 1996; **41(1):** 7–12.

14 **Lee CR, McTavish D, Sorkin EM.** Tramadol: A preliminary review of it pharmacodynamic and pharmacokinetic properties, and therapeutic potential in acute and chronic pain states. *Drugs* 1993; **46(2):** 313–40.

15 **Sagata K, Minami K, Yanagihara N,** *et al.* Tramadol inhibits norepinephrine transporter function at desipramine-binding sites in cultured bovine adrenal medullary cells. *Anesth Analg* 2002; **94(4):** 901–6.

16 **Hopwood SE, Owesson CA, Callado LF,** *et al.* Effects of chronic tramadol on pre- and post-synaptic measures of monoamine function. *J Psychophamacol* 2001; **15(3):** 147–53.

17 **Bamigbade TA, Davidson C, Langford RM,** *et al.* Actions of tramadol, its enantiomers and principal metabolite, O-desmethyltramadol, on serotonin (5-HT) efflux and uptake in the rat dorsal raphe nucleus. *Br J Anaesth* 1997; **79(3):** 352–6.

18 **Reimann W, Schneider F.** Induction of 5-hydroxytryptamine release by tramadol, fenfluramine and reserpine. *Eur J Pharmacol* 1998; **349:** 199–203.

19 **Lai J, Shou-wu M, Porreca F,** *et al.* Tramadol, M1 metabolite and enantiomer affinities for cloned human opioid receptors expressed in transfected HN9.10 neuroblastoma cells. *Eur J Pharmacol* 1996; **316:** 369–72.

20 **Halfpenny DM, Callado LF, Hopwood SE,** *et al.* Effects of tramadol stereoisomers on norephinephrine efflux and uptake in the rat locus coeruleus measured by real time voltammetry. *Br J Anaesth* 1999; **83(6):** 909–15.

21 **Grond S, Meuser T, Uragg H,** *et al.* Serum concentrations of tramadol enantiomers during patient-controlled analgesia. *Br J Clin Pharmacol* 1999; **48(2):** 254–7.

22 **Subrahmanyam V, Renwick AB, Walters DG,** *et al.* Identification of cytochrome P-450 isoforms responsible for cis-tramadol metabolism in human liver microsomes. *Drug Metabol Disp* 2001; **29(8):** 1146–55.

23 **Gillen C, Haurand M, Kobelt DJ,** *et al.* Affinity, potency and efficacy of tramadol and its metabolites at the cloned human m-opioid receptor. *Naunyn-Schmied Arch Pharmacol* 2000; **362:** 116–21.

24 **Poulsen L, Aredlnt-Nielsen L, Brosen K,** *et al.* The hypoalgesic effect of tramadol in relation to CYP2D6. *Clin Pharmacol Therapeut* 1996; **60(6):** 636–44.

25 **Arcioni R, della Rocca M, Romano S,** *et al.* Ondansetron inhibits the analgesic effects of tramadol: a possible 5-HT3 spinal receptor involvement in acute pain in humans. *Anesth Analg* 2002; **94(6):** 1553–7.

26 **Williams HJ.** Tramadol hydrochloride: something new in oral analgesic therapy. *Curr Therapeut Res* 1997; **58(4):** 215.

27 **Wilder-Smith CH, Hill L, Osler W,** *et al.* Effect of tramadol and morphine on pain and gastrointestinal motor function in patients with chronic pancreatitis. *Digest Dis Sci* 1999; **44(6):** 1107–16.

28 **Bono AV, Cuffari S.** Effectiveness and tolerance of tramadol in cancer pain. A comparative study with respect to buprenorphine. *Drugs* 1997; **53(Suppl 2):** 40–9.

29 **Collart L, Luthy C, Favario-Constantin C,** *et al.* Duality of the analgesic effect of tramadol in humans. *Schweiz Med Wochenschr* 1993; **123(47):** 2241–3.

30 **Tao Q, Stone DJ, Borenstein MR,** *et al.* Differential tramadol and O-desmethyl metabolite levels in brain vs plasma of mice and rats administered tramadol hydrochloride orally. *J Clin Pharmacol Therapeut* 2002; **27(2):** 99–106.

31 **Paar WD, Frankus P, Dengler HJ.** High-performance liquid chromatographic assay for the simultaneous determination of tramadol and its metabolites in microsomal fractions of human liver. *J Chromatogr* 1996; **686:** 221–7.

32 Soetebeer UB, Schierenberg MO, Schulz H, *et al.* Direct chiral assay of tramadol and detection of the phase II metabolite O-demethyl tramadol glucuronide in human urine using capillary electrophoresis with laser-induced native fluorescence detection. *J Chromatogr* 2001; **765**(1): 3–13.

33 Levine B, Ramcharitar V, Smialek JE. Tramadol distribution in four postmortem cases. *Forens Sci Int* 1997; **86**: 43–8.

34 Ogunleye DS. Investigation of racial variations in the metabolism of tramadol. *Eur J Drug Metab Pharmacokinet* 2001; **26**(1–2): 95–8.

35 Gan SH, Ismail R, Wan Adnan WA, *et al.* Correlation of tramadol pharmacokinetics and CYP2D6*10 genotype in Malaysian subjects. *J Pharmaceut Biomed Anal* 2002; **30**: 189–95.

36 Davis MP, Homsi J. The importance of cytochrome P450 monooxygenase CYP2D6 in palliative medicine. *Support Care Cancer* 2001; **9**(6): 442–51.

37 Abdel-Rahman SM, Leeder JS, Wilson JT, *et al.* Concordance between tramadol and dextromethorphan parent/metabolite ratios: the influence of CYP2D6 and non-CYP2D6 pathways on biotransformation. *J Clin Pharmacol* 2002; **42**(1): 24–9.

38 Paar WD, Poche S, Gerloff J, *et al.* Polymorphic CYP2D6 mediates O-demethylation of the opioid analgesic tramadol. *Eur J Clin Pharmacol* 1997; **53**: 235–9.

39 Obaidat AA, Obaidat RM. Controlled release of tramadol hydrochloride from matrices prepared using glyceryl behenate. *Eur J Pharmaceut Biopharmaceut* 2001; **52**(2): 231–5.

40 Raffa RB. Pharmacology of oral combination analgesics: rational therapy for pain. *J Clin Pharm Therapeut* 2001; **26**(4): 257–64.

41 Raber M, Hofmann S, Junge K, *et al.* Analgesic efficacy and tolerability of tramadol 100 mg sustained-release capsules in patients with moderate to severe chronic low back pain. *Clin Drug Invest* 1999; **17**(6): 415–23.

42 Grond S, Radbruch L, Meuser T, *et al.* High-dose tramadol in comparison to low-dose morphine for cancer pain relief. *J Pain Sympt Manag* 1999; **18**(3): 174–9.

43 Vergion M, Degesves S, Garcet L, *et al.* Tramadol, an alternative to morphine for treating posttraumatic pain in the prehospital situation. *Anesth Analg* 2001; **92**(6): 1543–6.

44 Wilder-Smith CH, Hill L, Wilkins J, *et al.* Effects of morphine and tramadol on somatic and visceral sensory function and gastrointestinal motility after abdominal surgery. *Anesthesiology* 1999; **91**(3): 639.

45 Brema F, Pastorino G, Martini MC, *et al.* Oral tramadol and buprenorphine in tumour pain. An Italian multicentre trial. *Int J Clin Pharmacol Res* 1996; **16**(4–5): 109–16.

46 Stamer UM, Lehnen K, Hothker F, *et al.* Impact of CYP2D6 genotype on postoperative tramadol analgesia. *Pain* 2003; **105**(1–2): 231–8.

47 Vickers MD, Paravicini D. Comparison of tramadol with morphine for post-operative pain following abdominal surgery. *Eur J Anaesthesiol* 1995; **13**(4): 416–18.

48 Chrubasik S, Chrubasik J. Treatment of postoperative pain with peridural administration of opioids. *Anaesthesiol Reanim* 1995; **29**(1): 16–25.

49 Bloch MB, Dyer R, Heijke SA, *et al.* Tramadol infusion for postthoracotomy pain relief: a placebo controlled comparison with epidural morphine. *Anesth Analg* 2002; **94**(3): 523–8.

50 Lehmann KA. Tramadol for the management of acute pain. *Drugs* 1994; **47**(Suppl 1): 19–32.

51 Vickers MD, O'Flaherty D, Szekely SM, *et al.* Tramadol: pain relief by an opioid without depression of respiration. *Anaesthesia* 1992; **47**(4): 291–6.

52 Kainz C, Joura E, Obwegeser R, *et al.* Effectiveness and tolerance of tramadol with or without an antiemetic and pethidine in obstetric analgesia. *Z Geburtshilfe Perinatol* 1992; **196**(2): 78–82.

53 Van den Berg AA, Halliday E, Lule EK, *et al.* The effects of tramadol on postoperative nausea, vomiting and headache after ENT surgery. A placebo-controlled comparison with equipotent doses of nalbuphine and pethidine. *Acta Anesthesiol Scand* 1999; **43(1)**: 28–33.

54 Eray O, Cete Y, Oktay C, *et al.* Intravenous single-dose tramadol versus meperidine for pain relief in renal colic. *Eur J Anaesthesiol* 2002; **19(5)**: 368–7.

55 Moore RA, McQuay HJ. Single-patient data meta-analysis of 3453 postoperative patients: oral tramadol versus placebo, codeine and combination analgesics. *Pain* 1997; **69**: 287–94.

56 McQuay HJ, Moore RA. *Oral Tramadol Versus Placebo, Codeine, and Combination Analgesics in an Evidence-based Resource for Pain Relief.* New York: Oxford University Press, 1998, pp. 138–46.

57 Sunshine A. New clinical experience with tramadol. *Drugs* 1994; **47(Suppl 1)**: 8–18.

58 Mullican WS, Lacy JR. Tramadol/acetaminophen combination tablets and codeine/acetaminophen combination capsules for the management of chronic pain: a comparative trial. *Clin Therapeut* 2001; **23(9)**: 1429.

59 Sunshine A, Olson NZ, Zighelboim I, *et al.* Analgesic oral efficacy of tramadol hydrochloride in postoperative pain. *Clin Pharmacol Ther* 1992; **51(6)**: 740–6.

60 Edwards JE, McQuay HJ, Moore RA. Combination analgesic efficacy: individual patient data meta-analysis of single dose oral tramadol plus acetaminophen in acute postoperative pain. *J Pain Sympt Manag* 2002; **23(2)**: 121–30.

61 Fricke JR, Karim R, Jordan D, *et al.* A double-blind, single-dose comparison of the analgesic efficacy of tramadol/acetaminophen combination tablets, hydrocodone/acetaminophen combination tablets and placebo after oral surgery. *Clin Therapeut* 2002; **24(6)**: 953.

62 Wilder-Smith CH, Hill L, Spargo K, *et al.* Treatment of severe pain from osteoarthritis with slow-release tramadol or dihydrocodeine in combination with NSAIDs: a randomised study of comparing analgesia, antinociception and gastrointestinal effects. *Pain* 2001; **91**: 23–31.

63 Pavelka K, Peliskova Z, Stehlikova H, *et al.* Intraindividual differences in pain relief and functional improvement in osteoarthritis with diclofenac or tramadol. *Clin Drug Invest* 1998; **16(6)**: 421–9.

64 Pagliara L, Tornago S, Metastasio J, *et al.* Tramadol compared with diclofenac in traumatic musculoskeletal pain. *Curr Therapeut Res* 1997; **58(8)**: 473.

65 Zackova M, Taddei S, Calo P, *et al.* Ketorolac vs tramadol in the treatment of postoperative pain during maxillofacial surgery. *Minerva Anesthesiol* 2001; **67(9)**: 641–6.

66 Stanov G, Schmieder G, Zerle G, *et al.* Double-blind study with dipyrone versus tramadol and butylscopolamine in acute renal colic pain. *World J Urol* 1994; **12(3)**: 155–61.

67 Lehmann KA, Kratzenberg U, Schroeder-Bark B, *et al.* Postoperative patient-controlled analgesia with tramadol: analgesic efficacy and minimum effective concentrations. *Clin J Pain* 1990; **6(3)**: 212–20.

68 Gibson TP. Pharmacokinetics, efficacy, and safety of analgesia with a focus on tramadol HCI. *Am J Med* 1996; **101(1A)**: 47S–53S.

69 De Witt JL, Schoenmaekers B, Sessler DI, *et al.* The analgesic efficacy of tramadol is impaired by concurrent administration of ondansetron. *Anesth Analg* 2001; **95(5)**: 1319–21.

70 Gaudino W, Weiss L. Serotonin syndrome in a patient taking tramadol and nefazodone concomitantly: a case report. *Arch Phys Med Rehabil* 2003; **84(9)**: E23.

71 Sauget D, Franco PS, Amaniou M, *et al.* Possible serotonergic syndrome caused by combination of tramadol and sertraline in an elderly woman. *Ther* 2002; **57(3)**: 309–10.

72 Lange-Asschenfeldt C, Weigmann H, Hiemke C, *et al.* Serotonin syndrome as a result of fluoxetine in a patient with tramadol abuse: plasma level correlated symptomatology. *J Clin Psychopharmacol* 2002; **22(4)**: 440–1.

73 Gonzalez-Pinto A, Imaz H, De Heredia J, *et al.* Mania and tramadol-fluoxetine combination. *Am J Psychiat* 2001; **158(6):** 964–5.

74 Kesavan S, Sobala GM. Serotonin syndrome with fluoxetine plus tramadol. *J Roy Soc Med* 1999; **92(9):** 474–5.

75 Lantz MS, Buchalter EN, Giambanco V. Serotonin syndrome following the administration of tramadol with paroxetine. *Int J Geriat Psychiat* 1998; **13(5):** 343–5.

76 Egberts AC, tér Borgh J, Brodie-Meijer CC. Serotonin syndrome attributed to tramadol addition to paroxetine therapy. *Int Clin Psychopharmacol* 1997; **12(3):** 181–2.

77 Mason BJ, Blackburn KH. Possible serotonin syndrome associated with tramadol and sertraline coadministration. *Annl Pharmacother* 1997; **31(2):** 175–7.

78 Duggal HS, Fetchko J. Serotonin syndrome and atypical antipsychotics. *Am J Psychiat* 2002; **159(4):** 672–3.

79 Sagata K, Minami K, Tanagihara N, *et al.* Tramadol inhibits norephinephrine transporter function at desipramine-binding sites in cultured bovine adrenal medullary cells. *Anesth Analg* 2002; **94(4):** 901–6.

80 Devulder J, De Laat M, Dumoulin K, *et al.* Nightmares and hallucinations after long-term intake of tramadol combined with antidepressants. *Acta Clin Belg* 1996; **51(3):** 184–6.

81 Unlugenc H, Gunduz M, Ozalevli M, *et al.* A comparative study on the analgesic effect of tramadol, tramadol plus magnesium, and tramadol plus ketamine for postoperative pain management after major abdominal surgery. *Acta Anesth Scand* 2002; **46(8):** 1025–30.

82 Davis MP, Khawam E, Pozuelo L, *et al.* Management of symptoms associated with advanced cancer: olanzapine and mirtazapine. A World Health Organization Project. *Expert Rev Anticancer Ther* 2002; **2(4):** 365–76.

83 Houmes RJ, Voets MA, Verkaaik A, *et al.* Efficacy and safety of tramadol versus morphine for moderate and severe postoperative pain with special regard to respiratory depression. *Anesth Analg* 1992; **74(4):** 510–4.

84 Tuncer S, Bariskaner H, Yosunkaya A, *et al.* Influence of dexamethasone on nausea and vomiting during patient-controlled analgesia with tramadol. *Clin Drug Invest* 2002; **22(8):** 547–52.

85 Anon. Urinary disorders on tramadol. *Prescrire Int* 2001; **10(55):** 152.

86 Crighton IM, Martin P, Hobbs GJ, *et al.* A comparison of the effects of intravenous tramadol, codeine, and morphine on gastric emptying in human volunteers. *Anesth Analg* 1998; **87(2):** 445–9.

87 Budd K. Chronic pain—challenge and response. *Drugs* 1994; **47(Suppl 1):** 33–8.

88 Petzke F, Radbruch L, Sabatowski R, *et al.* Slow-release tramadol for treatment of chronic malignant pain–an open label multicenter trial. *Support Care Cancer* 2000; **9:** 48–54.

89 Murphy K, Delanty N. Drug-induced seizures: general principles in assessment, management and prevention. *CNS Drugs* 2000; **14(2):** 135–46.

90 Belgrade MJ. How to taper tramadol dose. *Postgrad Med* 2002; **111(2):** 111.

91 Alfonsi P. Postanaesthetic shivering: epidemiology, pathophysiology, and approaches to prevention and management. *Drugs* 2001; **61(15):** 2193–205.

92 Bilotta F, Pietropaoli P, Sanita R, *et al.* Nefopam and tramadol for the prevention of shivering during neuraxial anesthesia. *Reg Anesth Pain Med* 2002; **27(4):** 380–4.

93 Tsai Y, Chu K. A comparison of tramadol, amitriptyline, and merperidine for postepidural anesthetic shivering in parurients. *Anesth Analg* 2001; **93(5):** 1288–92.

94 Mathews S, Al Mulla A, Varghese PK, *et al.* Postanesthetic shivering—a new look at tramadol. *Anaesthesia* 2002; **57:** 387–403.

95 Mildh LH, Leino KA, Kirvela OA. Effects of tramadol and meperidine on respiration, plasma catecholamine concentrations, and hemodynamics. *J Clin Anesth* 1999; **11:** 310–16.

96 Nieuwenhuijs D, Bruce J, Drummond GB, *et al.* Influence of oral tramadol on the dynamic ventilatory response to carbon dioxide in healthy volunteers. *Br J Anaesth* 2001; **87(6):** 860–5.

97 Barnung SK, Treschow M, Borgbjerg FM. Respiratory depression following oral tramadol in a patient with impaired renal function. *Pain* 1997; **71:** 111–12.

98 Reeves RR, Liberto V. Abuse of combinations of carisoprodol and tramadol. *Sth Med J* 2001; **94(5):** 512–14.

99 Brinker A, Bonnell R, Beitz J. Abuse, dependence or withdrawal associated with tramadol. *Am J Psychiat* 2002; **159(5):** 881.

100 Knisley JS, Campbell ED, Dawson KS, *et al.* Tramadol post-marketing surveillance in health care professionals. *Drug Alc Depend* 2002; **68:** 15–22.

101 Cicero TJ, Adams EH, Geller A, *et al.* A postmarketing surveillance program to monitor Ultram® (tramadol hydrochloride) abuse in the United States. *Drug Alc Depend* 1999; **57:** 7–22.

102 Aronson MD. Nonsteroidal anti-inflammatory drugs, traditional opioids, and tramadol: contrasting therapies for the treatment of chronic pain. *Clin Therapeut* 1997; **19(3):** 420.

103 Rodrigues N, Rodrigues Pereira E. Tramadol in cancer pain. *Curr Therapeut Res* 1989; **46:** 1142–8.

104 Lenzhofer R, Moser K. Analgesic effect of tramadol in patients with malignant diseases. *Wien Med Wochenschr* 1984; **134(8):** 199–202.

105 Crossman M, Wilsmann KM. Effect and side-effects of tramadol. An open phase IV study with 7198 patients. *Therapiewoche* 1987; **37:** 3475–85.

106 Osipova NA, Novikov GA, Beresnev VA, *et al.* Analgesic effect of tramadol in cancer patients with chronic pain: a comparison with prolonged-action morphine sulfate. *Curr Therapeut Res* 1991; **50:** 812–21.

107 Wilder-Smith CH, Schimke J, Osterwalder B, *et al.* Oral tramadol, a m-opioid agonist and monoamine re-uptake-blocker, and morphine for strong cancer-related pain. *Annl Oncol* 1994; **5:** 141–6.

108 Tawfik MO, Elborolossy K, Nasr F. Tramadol hydrochloride in the relief of cancer pain: a double-blind comparison against sustained release morphine. *Pain* 1990; **Suppl 5:** S377.

109 Luben V, Muller H, Lobisch M, *et al.* Treatment of tumor pain with fluirtine. Results of a double-blind study versus-tramadol. *Fortschr Med* 1994; **112(19):** 282–6.

110 Wu GQ. Effects of tramadol hydrochloride injection in relief of cancer pain. *Zhonghua Zhong Liu Za Zhi* 1993; **15(4):** 303–6.

111 Wu GQ. Pain-relief effect of tramadol HCL capsule for moderate and severe cancer pain. *Zhonghua Zhong Liu Za Zhi* 1992; **14(3):** 219–21.

112 Negro S, Azuara M, Sanchez Y, *et al.* Physical compatibility and *in vivo* evaluation of drug mixtures for subcutaneous infusion to cancer patients in palliative care. *Support Care Cancer* 2002; **10:** 65–70.

Chapter 7

Dextropropoxyphene

Paul Glare

Pharmacology

Dextropropoxyphene (DPP), known as propoxyphene in the USA, is a synthetic opioid analgesic of the diphenylpropylamine class and derived from the synthetic strong opioid methadone. DPP is a base, with a pKa of 6.3.

As an analgesic, DPP is controversial. It is a widely used and popular painkiller that was taken by the Apollo XI astronauts to the moon[1]. Recently, it has earned a poor reputation in some quarters as an over-prescribed, minimally effective and potentially dangerous analgesic[2–4] and much has been made of its abuse in suicides[5]. Despite this, DPP still has its advocates who hold that it is effective, well-tolerated and liked by patients[6]. They argue that it belongs on the second rung of the analgesic ladder. In Britain, it has been the weak analgesic of choice in most hospices because it is believed to be less constipating than codeine[7]. It is widely used for cancer pain management in Italy[8].

DPP is generally prescribed in combination with aspirin (Doloxene) or paracetamol (Distalgesic in Britain; Digesic in Australia). In the USA, it is used both alone (Darvon) and in combination (Darvocet, Wigesic). Its analgesic properties reside in the d-isomer. Its l-isomer, levoPP, is not analgesic and is marketed in the USA as a cough suppressant under the trade name Novrad.

Pharmacodynamics

DPP is a weak mu agonist with low receptor affinity similar to that of codeine. Weight-for-weight, it is said to be equal to codeine in analgesic effect with repeated administration. As with the other weak opioid, it is said that DPP shows a 'ceiling effect' in relation to analgesia. This is an over-simplification: unlike agonist-antagonist drugs such as pentazocine, which have a true ceiling effect, the maximum effective dose of DPP is arbitrary. At higher doses, there are progressively more side effects, which outweigh the small gains in analgesia. The formulation of tablets or capsules also limits how much of the drug can be given. Onset of action is 20–30 min. Peak effect is achieved by 1.5–2 h and the duration of action is somewhere been 3 and 6 h.

Generally speaking, DPP is well tolerated, with the same side effects as morphine. In a few patients it causes unacceptable central nervous system (CNS) side effects (muzziness, lightheadedness, dysphoria and confusion). Acute CNS effects that have been reported include seizures and ataxia. In usual therapeutic doses, DPP may cause more cognitive impairment than oral morphine may, but neither opioid has substantial effects on cognition and psychomotor function when compared with lorazepam[9]. There is no way of predicting such patients. As with other opioids, constipation is a common side effect, although usually not as troublesome as with codeine/dihydrocodeine. Occasionally patients experience nausea and vomiting.

In addition to its opioid side effects, DPP may occasionally induce hepatotoxicity[10]. Early studies in animals demonstrated that acute cardiovascular effects of norpropoxyphene included decreased heart rate, contractility and mean blood pressure in addition to electrocardiogram abnormalities (increased PR interval, prolonged QRS duration). It appears that the cardiotoxicity of DPP is a non-opioid effect, as it is not reversed by naloxone[11]. Consequently, DPP has received much adverse publicity about its lethal potential, especially when it is in such widespread use in countries such as the UK and Scandinavia. Recently, there has been concern about its use for committing suicide in the general population, being the second most common prescribed drug that people use to commit suicide in England and Wales, and the sole method in 18% of all drug-related suicides and 5% of all total suicides[5]. In the opioid-naïve population, death can result from an overdose with relatively few tablets, especially when alcohol is also taken. However, it is generally believed that there is little evidence that is inherently less safe (or more effective) than other weak opioids. DPP is also a weak N-methyl-D-aspartate receptor antagonist, but this property is not thought to be clinically relevant[12].

The older cancer pain literature states that repeated administration of low dose DPP (65 mg every 4 h) does not produce serious adverse effects or physical dependence, but that, at high doses (>600 mg/day), produces CNS side effects such as hallucinations, confusion and a mild degree of physical dependence[13].

Kinetics[14]

Absorption

DPP is readily absorbed from the gastrointestinal tract over a 2–3-h period. Its oral bioavailability is 40%, with onset of action in 20–30 min.

Elimination

DPP is 78% protein bound. Its volume of distribution is 189 l. Clearance occurs at 66 l/h. It is excreted as norpropoxyphene (NPP) in the urine, with very little unchanged drug being excreted. Breast milk concentrations of up to 50% of the corresponding plasma level may be attained; theoretically, a dose of 1 mg/day might be ingested by the nursing infant[15]. However, insignificant amounts of DPP are normally found in the breast milk following normal doses and no harmful effects have been reported[16].

Nevertheless, it may be prudent to instruct the nursing mother to wait 4–6 h after taking DPP or other opioid analgesic before breast feeding[15].

Half-life

DPP has two half lives of 2.7 and 12 h. The half-life may be markedly prolonged in the elderly.

Metabolism

DPP undergoes extensive first pass metabolism. An unusual property of DPP is that its first pass metabolism is dose-dependent, so that its systemic availability increases with increasing doses[17]. There are three metabolic pathways: N-demethylation (major), aromatic hydroxylation (minor) and ester hydrolysis (minor). N-desmethylpropoxyphene, the major metabolite, is also known as NPP. *n*-demethylation of DPP to NPP occurs in the liver. NPP is pharmacologically active as an analgesic. As it crosses the blood–brain barrier to a lesser extent than DPP, NPP has a substantially less analgesic or central depressant effect. NPP has longer half-life than DPP (24–36 h). Thus, with regular administration of escalating doses there is enhanced bioavailability and some accumulation[18]. With multi-dosing, DPP reaches steady state plasm concentrations 5–7 times greater than those achieved with a single dose. This accumulation is not usually clinically significant at the standard doses used. It may explain the CNS syndrome (including tremulousness and seizures) seen in some patients.

Routes of administration

DPP is only available in oral formulations, either alone or in combination with acetaminophen/paracetamol or aspirin. Injections are painful, and have a destructive effect on soft tissues and veins.

Drug interactions and toxicity

DPP can inhibit the CYP2D6 enzyme of the CYP450 system. It can therefore interfere with the metabolism of many drugs used in the management of patients with advanced cancer, which are substrates for this enzyme. These include other analgesics (codeine, oxycodone), haloperidol, tricyclic antidepressants, domperidone and phenothoazines[19]. Perhaps the best known interaction clinically is between DPP and carbamazepine. DPP is thought to inhibit the oxidation of carbamazepine to CBZ-epoxide, resulting in increased carbamazepine levels, resulting in headache, dizziness, ataxia, nausea and tiredness[20]. This is particularly the case in the elderly[21]. DPP may also interfere with warfarin, causing elevated warfarin levels.

DPP is classified as Category C for teratogenicity by the US Food and Drug Administration and Category D if used for prolonged periods[22]. Possible congenital malformations with DPP have been reported[23,24]. Newborn infants can experience withdrawal symptoms if their mothers take DPP during pregnancy.

Dosing in special populations

Liver failure

The oxidation of DPP to NPP is reduced in patients with hepatic cirrhosis, resulting in both decreased drug clearance and increased oral bioavailability caused by a reduced first-pass metabolism. The consequence of reduced drug metabolism is the risk of accumulation in the body, especially with repeated administration[25]. Lower doses or longer administration intervals should be used to remedy this risk. DPP concentrations were appreciably higher and NPP concentrations were much lower in cirrhosis patients than in the normal subjects[26]. Most of the patients, unlike the normal subjects, experienced considerable sedation after propoxyphene. These results are probably due to increase systemic availability of orally administered propoxyphene in patients with hepatic cirrhosis and possibly to increased receptor response to the drug by these patients. It is concluded that propoxyphene should be administered cautiously and in reduced doses to patients with hepatic dysfunction. Special risks are known for dextropropoxyphene, for which several cases of hepatotoxicity have been reported.

Renal failure

DPP is not recommended for use in patients with renal failure as both it and its active metabolite NPP accumulate in renal failure. After a single dose of 130 mg of propoxyphene, the area under the curve for propoxyphene was an average of 76% greater in the anephric patients[27]. The corresponding maximal serum concentration was increased by 88%. The exact doses that produce toxicity in a hemodialysis patient, however, remain unclear.

Neither DPP nor NPP is adequately removed by conventional dialysis and the accumulation of NPP can occur[28]. The effects of high-flux dialysis on NPP removal are less clear. In dialysis patients, NPP accumulation has been implicated in producing CNS alterations, respiratory depression and cardiotoxicity. In addition to the potential toxicity from accumulation of NPP, there is evidence that propoxyphene clearance is reduced in dialysis patients. An early study compared the pharmacokinetics of propoxyphene in anephric patients with normal controls.

Elderly

DPP is considered by many authorities to be an inappropriate drug to use in the elderly. It was the consensus of 13 nationally recognized experts that all use of propoxyphene should be avoided in the elderly, since other analgesics are safer and more effective[29]. The drug is not mentioned in the recently published American Geriatric Society guideline for the management of pain in the elderly[30]. The plasma half-life increases from 6–12 h to >50 h in the elderly[31].

Evidence-based use for cancer pain

There have been few studies of DPP in the cancer pain population[8,32], even though it is widely used in this group[6].

In the acute and chronic pain literature, there has been controversy about the efficacy of the DPP component of DPP-containing compound analgesics. This resulted from a single dose study in the early 1970s that showed that DPP- aspirin compounds were less potent than codeine and no more effective than aspirin alone[33]. This has led some authorities to classify DPP on Step 1 of the analgesic ladder, limiting its role to mild pain, even though it is an opioid [34].

Despite these data, there is extensive clinical experience to the contradictory that DPP is effective for moderate pain and belongs on Step 2 of the analgesic ladder. This contradictory finding has been explained by the pharmacokinetics of DPP, and the differences obtained between single doses and repeated administration, analogous to the controversy about the oral: parenteral potency of morphine.

The controversy has been rekindled recently with a systematic review finding that in both head to head and indirect comparisons of paracetamol and the popular combination of paracetamol (650 mg) with DPP hydrochloride (32.5 mg), the combination was no better than paracetamol on its own. The total number of patients in the few published head-to-head comparisons was modest and the authors concluded that small differences in effect cannot be excluded, but these are unlikely to be of clinical importance[35]. Again, the review only included single dose studies. DPP in doses of 65 mg and higher has been shown to have a definite analgesic effect in several RCT trials[36] and a dose–response curve has been established[18]. The more recent Cochrane review of DPP in surgical pain found that single dose DPP 65 mg has a number-needed-to-treat (NNT) for at least 50% pain relief of 7.7 (95% CI 4.6–22) when compared with placebo over 4–6 h[37]. For the equivalent dose of DPP combined with paracetamol 650 mg the NNT was 4.4 (3.5–5.6) when compared with placebo. There was an increased incidence of CNS adverse effects for DPP plus paracetamol compared with placebo. The combination of DPP 65 mg with paracetamol 650 mg showed similar efficacy to tramadol 100 mg for single dose studies in postoperative pain, but with a lower incidence of adverse effects. The same dose of paracetamol combined with 60 mg codeine appears more effective, but with the slight overlap in the 95% confidence intervals, this conclusion is not robust. Adverse effects of both combinations were similar. Ibuprofen 400 mg has a lower (better) NNT than both DPP 65 mg plus paracetamol 650 mg and tramadol 100 mg.

A large Italian survey of various weak opioids in cancer pain management evaluated the use of a DPP 90 mg-paracetamol 325 mg combination over a 4-week period[8]. The survey showed that approximately one-third of patients treated in this way achieved pain relief with 2 or 3 doses of the compound per day. By 4 weeks, approximately 75% of patients' pain was no longer controlled with DPP. Dry mouth, drowsiness and constipation were the commonest reported side effects of the compound in that study (all >20%). It is noteworthy that the incidence of constipation was almost identical for DPP and codeine.

A recent small randomized controlled trial in patients with terminal cancer (median survival approximately 10 weeks) and a moderate degree of pain compared DPP 120–240 mg/day with low dose MS Contin (20 mg b.d.) for 10 days[32]. Similar levels of analgesia were achieved with relatively lower doses of DPP (using a standard opioid equipotency table) and less side effects. Most patients in the study treated with DPP eventually required strong opioid as pain escalated prior to death.

Doses and routes

Marketed as either the hydrochloride salt or napsylate. DPP napsylate 100 mg being equivalent to DPP hydrochloride 65 mg, the difference relating to the molecular weight of the two salts.

References

1 Dahl J. Darvon, A drug with dubious distinction. *Focus Pain* 1998; **Summer:** 3. Available at: www.wisc.edu/wcpi/ (accessed 26 January 2004).

2 Owen M, Hills LJ. How safe is dextropropoxyphene. *Med J Am* 1980; **1:** 617–18.

3 Haigh S. 12 years on: coproxamol revisited. *Lancet* 1996; **347:** 1840–41.

4 Perin ML, Pasero C. Problems with propoxyphene. *Am J Nurs* 2000; **100(6):** 22.

5 Hawton K, Simkin S, Deeks J. Co-proxamol and suicide: a study of national mortality statistics and local non-fatal self poisonings. *Br Med J* 2003; **326:** 1006–8.

6 Sykes JV, Hanks GW, Forbes K. Coproxamol revisited. *Br Med J* 1996; **348:** 408.

7 Twycross RG, Lack SA. *Therapeutics in Terminal Cancer*. Edinburgh: Churchill Livingstone, 1990.

8 de Conno F, Ripamonti C, Sbanotto A, *et al*. A clinical study of the use of codeine, oxycodone, dextropropoxyphene, buprenorphine and pentazocine in cancer pain. *J Pain Sympt Manag* 1991; **6:** 423–7.

9 O'Neill WM, Hanks GW, Simpson P, *et al*. The cognitive and psychomotor effects of morphine in healthy subjects: a randomized controlled trial of repeated (four) oral doses of dextropropoxyphene, morphine, lorazepam and placebo. *Pain* 2000; **85(1–2):** 209–215.

10 Rosenberg WMC, Ryley NG, Trowell JM, *et al*. DPP induced hepatotoxicity: a report of 9 cases. J Hepatol 1993; **19:** 470–4.

11 Hantson P, Evenepoel M, Ziade D, *et al*. Adverse cardiac manifestations following DPP OD: can naloxone be helpful? J Ann Emerg Med 1995; **25:** 263–6.

12 Ebert B, Anderson S, Hjeds H, *et al*. Dextropropoxyphene acts as a noncompetitive N-methyl D-aspartate antagonist. *J Pain Sympt Manag* 1998; **15:** 269–274.

13 Bonica JJ. Cancer pain. In: Bonica JJ (Ed.) *The Management of Pain*, 2nd edn. Philadelphia: Lea & Febiger, 1990, p. 425.

14 Inturrisi CE, Colburn WA, Vereby K, *et al*. PP and NPP kinetics after single and repeated doses of propoxyphene. *Clinical Pharmacol Ther* 1982; **31:** 157–672.

15 Anderson PO. Drugs and breast feeding—a review. *Drug Intell Clin Pharm* 1977; **11:** 208.

16 Kunka RL, Venkataramanan R, Stern RM *et al*. Excretion of propoxyphene and norpropoxyphene in breast milk. *Clin Pharmacol Ther* 1984; **35**: 675–80.

17 Perrier D, Gibaldi M. Influence of the first-pass effect on the systemic availability of propoxyphene. *J Clin Pharmacol* 1972; **12**: 449–52.

18 Beaver WT. Analgesic efficacy of DPP and DPP containing compounds: a review. *Hum Toxicol* 1984; **3**: 191s–220s.

19 Bernard SA, Bruera E. Drug interactions in palliative care. *J Clin Oncol* 2000; **18**: 1780–99.

20 Dam M, Christiansen J. Interaction of propoxyphene with carbamazepine. *Lancet* 1977; **II**: 509.

21 Bergendal L, Friberg A, Schaffrath AM, *et al*. The clinical relevance of the interaction between carbamazepine and dextropropoxyphene in elderly patients in Gothenburg, Sweden. *Eur J Clin Pharmacol* 1997; **53(3–4)**: 203–6.

22 Briggs GG, Freeman RK, Yaffe SJ. *Drugs in Pregnancy and Lactation*, 2nd edn. Baltimore: Williams & Wilkins, 1994.

23 Barrow MV, Souder DE. Propoxyphene and congenital malformations. *J Am Med Ass* 1971; **217**: 1551.

24 Schardein JL. *Drugs as Teratogens*. Cleveland: CRC Press, Inc, 1976.

25 Tegeder I, Lotsch J, Geisslinger G. Pharmacokinetics of opioids in liver disease. *Clin Pharmacokinet* 1999; **37(1)**: 17–40.

26 Giacomini KM, Giacomini JC, Gibson TP, *et al*. Propoxyphene and norpropoxyphene plasma concentrations after oral propoxyphene in cirrhotic patients with and without surgically constructed portacaval shunt. *Clin Pharmacol Ther* 1980; **28**: 417–24.

27 Gibson TP, Giacomini KM, Briggs WA, *et al*. Propoxyphene and norpropoxyphene plasma concentrations in the anephric patient. *Clin Pharmacol Ther* 1980; **27**: 665–70.

28 Bailie GR, Johnson CA. Safety of propoxyphene in dialysis patients. *Sem Dialysis* 2002; **15**: 375.

29 Beers JH, Ouslander JG, Rollingher I, *et al*. Explicit criteria for determining inappropriate medication use in nursing home residents. *Arch Intern Med* 1991; **151**: 1825–31.

30 AGS Panel on Chronic Pain in Older Persons. The management of chronic pain in older persons. *J Am Geriatr Soc* 1998; **46**: 635–651.

31 Crome P, Gain R, Ghurye R, *et al*. Pharmacokinetics of DPP and NPP in elderly hospital patients after single and repeated doses of Distalgesic. Preliminary analysis. *Hum Toxicol* 1984; **3**: 43s–48s.

32 Mercadente S, Salvaggio L, Dardanoni G, *et al*. DPP vs morphine in opioid-naïve cancer patients with pain. *J Pain Sympt Manag* 1998; **15**: 76–81.

33 Moertel CG, Ahmann DL, Taylor WF, *et al*. Relief of pain by oral medications. *J Am Med Ass* 1974; **229**: 55–9.

34 Hill CS, Jr. Oral opioid analgesics. In: Patt RB (Ed.) *Cancer Pain*. Philadelphia: JB Lippincott, 1993, p. 133.

35 Po ALW, Zhang WY. Systematic overview of co-proxamol to assess analgesic effects of addition of dextropropoxyphene to paracetamol. *Br Med J* 1997; **315**: 1565–71.

36 Miller RR, Ferrigold A, Paxinos J. Propoxyphene chloride. *J Am Med Ass* 1970; **213**: 996–1006.

37 Collins SL, Edwards JE, Moore RA, *et al*. Single dose dextropropoxyphene, alone and with paracetamol (acetaminophen), for postoperative pain. *Cochrane Database Syst Rev* 2000; **2**: CD001440.

Chapter 8

Morphine

Paul Glare

Morphine is the main pharmacologically active constituent of opium, the resin derived from the dried juice of the opium poppy, *Papaver sominferum*. Morphine was first introduced into clinical practice more than 200 years ago. Its effects are mediated by activating opioid receptors, mainly within the central nervous system (CNS). Globally morphine remains the strong opioid of choice for moderate-to-severe pain[1]. Other strong opioids are generally used when morphine is not readily available or the patient has intolerable adverse effects with morphine. The WHO has placed morphine on its Essential Drugs List[2].

Pharmacology

The chemical structure of morphine is that of a phenanthrene alkaloid, consisting of five condensed rings that are structurally rigid, and would be otherwise chemically inactive were it not for the hydroxyl groups at C3 and C6 (phenolic and alcoholic, respectively)[3]. Morphine is a weak base with a pK_a of 7.9. At a physiological pH, 76% of its molecules are ionized. The two –OH groups at C3 and C6 make it relatively water soluble and poorly lipid soluble. Morphine is available for therapeutic use as the hydrochloride, sulfate and tartrate, in a wide variety of formulations. The oral route is the preferred route of administration for chronic cancer pain. Oral morphine is available as normal-release (NR) and modified-release (MR) preparations.

Dynamics

Morphine produces it effects by being an agonist at opioid receptors in the spinal cord and elsewhere in the body. Morphine is a pure opioid agonist with primary affinity for the mu subclass of receptor, but also some affinity for the kappa and delta subclasses. The molecular pharmacology of opioids is discussed in detail elsewhere in this book. The main responses mediated by activation of the various opioid receptors include analgesia, sedation, respiratory depression, emesis, reduced gastrointestinal motility (leading to nausea and constipation) and changes in mood (euphoria, dysphoria and psychotomimetic).

While analgesia is the principal desirable effect of morphine, it has been used for other medicinal purposes throughout the ages, including as an anti-diarrheal agent and an antitussive. More recently, it has also been used for the relief of breathlessness in both cancer and non-malignant diseases.

Pharmacokinetics

Absorption

Morphine is readily absorbed by all routes of administration. After oral administration, morphine absorption occurs predominantly in the alkaline medium of the upper small bowel (morphine being a weak base), and is more or less complete. Absorption from the acid environment of the stomach is poor. Only a minor fraction of the morphine absorbed after oral administration reaches the systemic circulation, the oral bioavailability (BA) being approximately 33% (range 16–68%), but like all other pharmacokinetic parameters, BA demonstrates marked inter-individual variability[4–6]. Onset of action (oral, NR) is 20–30 min and duration of action 3–6 h. For MR morphine, the peak plasma concentration is typically achieved at 3–6 h with an attenuated peak and longer half-life, and plasma concentrations are maintained over 12–24 h[7–10].

Spinal

Morphine is relatively hydrophilic, and when administered epidurally or intrathecally, it is not rapidly absorbed into the systemic circulation. This results in a long half-life in cerebral fluid (90–120 min) and extensive rostral redistribution[11].

Elimination

Half-life

The half-life depends on the route of administration, being approximately 1.5 h for intravenous (i.v.) and 1.5–4.5 h for oral. In patients with normal renal function, the plasma half-life (2–3 h) is slightly shorter than the duration of action (4–6 h)[3].

Metabolism

After oral administration, extensive presystemic elimination of morphine occurs, about 90% of a dose being converted to metabolites. The liver is the principal site of morphine metabolism in humans[12–14]. Metabolism also occurs in other organs, notably the CNS[15,16]. Morphine metabolites have been identified in the human brain after ICV administration of morphine[17]. These extrahepatic sites may become important in man when liver function is impaired.

The main pathway for morphine metabolism is conjugation with glucuronic acid. Glucuronidation is catalysed by the enzyme UDP glucuronyl transferase (UGT), with two different isoforms of the enzyme have been identified in humans, UGT2B7 likely to be the major form[18]. The major metabolites of morphine are morphine-3-glucuronide (M3G) and morphine-6-glucuronide (M6G). M3G and M6G account for 50–60% of a dose[19]. Ethnicity affects morphine metabolism, Chinese patients reported to have increased morphine glucuronidation compared to Caucasians[20]. In a sample of Norwegian cancer patients, there was a lack of functional polymorphisms to UGT2B7, suggesting that other factors determine the variability seen in morphine : glucuronide ratios[21].

In patients on chronic morphine therapy, the ratio of M3G : morphine has been found to be in the range of 22–56 : 1 and M6G : morphine is 3.4–9 : 1[22,23]. The ratio of M3G : M6G has been determined to be 5.8–9.0[23]. While there is a relationship between morphine dose and plasma levels of morphine, M3G and M6G, there appears to no correlation between peak or trough plasma levels of these substances and clinical effect in patients with cancer-related pain[24].

Minor metabolites include morphine-3,6-diglucuronide, normorphine and normorphine-6-glucuronide, morphine ethereal sulfate and possibly codeine[23,25]. Recently, a novel metabolic pathway leading to the formation of morphine glucosides has been reported[26]. Their clinical relevance is not yet known. Unlike methadone, the pharmacokinetics of morphine remains linear with repetitive administration. There does not appear to be auto-induction or saturation of biotransformation even following large chronic doses[27].

Pharmacology of morphine glucuronides

Pharmacokinetics

M3G and M6G are highly polar compounds. Formation of metabolites takes time and the T_{max} of both M3G and M6G occurs approximately an hour later than for morphine, irrespective of route and formulation[23]. Because it is highly polar/hydrophilic, M6G would not be expected to cross a lipophilic structure, such as the BBB. Cerebrospinal fluid (CSF) : plasma ratios of M6G and M3G are low (0.1–0.2 : 1). It has been suggested that M6G is a 'molecular chameleon' that can exist in both extended and folded forms, the latter providing unexpected lipophilicity[28]. Consequently, there is believed to be substantially passage of M6G across the BBB, although this passage may be inhibited in some patients.

M3G and M6G are excreted by the kidney, the renal clearance of morphine being greater than that of its metabolites. M6G excretion by the kidney is directly related to creatinine clearance[29]. Its elimination half-life is 2–3 h in patients with normal renal function (similar to that of morphine), but becomes progressively longer with deteriorating function, resulting in significant accumulation, accounting for morphine toxicity in these patients. M3G and M6G also accumulate in the CSF in patients with renal failure[30].

Pharmacodynamics

M6G binds to opioid receptors whereas M3G does not[31]. M6G has the same affinity for mu$_1$ receptors as morphine, but much less affinity for mu$_2$ receptors (the receptor responsible for respiratory depression by opioids). It has a similar affinity to morphine for kappa and delta receptors.

M6G

This produces potent opioid effects in animals[31-33]. Even though it is widely stated that M6G contributes substantially to the analgesic effect of morphine in humans[31,34-38], the data are less consistent than in animals[39], and the exact role and contribution of M6G to morphine effects/side effects in humans remains unresolved at this time[40]. The relative potency of M6G to morphine is not yet known in humans and needs to be elucidated[23]. It can be expected that this will need to be very high or the concentrations in CSF very high for M6G to have much of a role. It is not yet clear whether M6G will have fewer side effects than morphine, although a number of small clinical studies suggest this is the case. M6G may cause emesis and respiratory depression in animals[41,42]. In humans, the evidence for an emetic effect of M6G is contradictory. Likewise, it has been suggested that M6G causes less respiratory depression due to its lower affinity for the mu$_2$ receptor.

M3G

There has been much controversy in recent years about the possible role of M3G as an opioid antagonist or as a mediator of the adverse effects of morphine. For many years it was assumed that M3G is inert, as is the case with most glucuronide metabolites[43]. Behavioral studies in rodents, however, have suggested that M3G may produce a functional antagonism of the analgesic effects of morphine and its active metabolite M6G[44,45]. There has also been some evidence in animal models that M3G may be responsible for the CNS excitatory side effects seen with morphine such as myoclonus[46,47].

It is clear that M3G does not bind to opioid receptors. Non-opioid mechanisms for any effect of M3G that have been postulated include including activation of NMDA receptors and blockade of inhibitory glycinergic pathways in the spinal cord[23]. Findings that contradict for a role of M3G include data from electrophysiological animal models, indicating no evidence of an antagonistic effect of M3G, and recent studies in human volunteers, indicating that M3G is devoid of significant activity[38,48,49]. In particular, there is no evidence of functional antagonism of morphine or M6G in humans. In conclusion, it currently appears that M3G plays no significant role in the pharmacodynamics of morphine.

Excretion

The kidney is the main site of excretion. It undergoes glomerular filtration and tubular secretion. Morphine and its metabolites accumulate in patients with renal failure (see below).

Routes of administration

Preparations are commercially available for oral, rectal, parenteral and intraspinal administration. The time to onset of effect of different morphine formulations varies, as does the time to peak drug levels[50]. NR morphine preparations have an onset of action of about 20 min and reach peak drug levels on average at 60 min. NR preparations are recommended for use in initiating therapy for severe pain and for breakthrough pain because of their rapid onset of analgesia[51]. NR preparations must be given every 4 h to maintain constant analgesic levels. When given by this regimen, these preparations will reach a steady plasma concentrations and, hence, full effect within 12–15 h. Thus, the full effect of any dose change can be assessed at this time. In practice, during titration, dose adjustments are usually made every 24 h unless the pain is more severe, when adjustments may be made sooner[1].

MR morphine preparations have a slower onset and a later peak effect. Many are twice-daily preparations with an onset of action of 1–2 h that reach peak drug levels at 4 h. The once-daily MR preparations have a slower onset and reach peak levels at 8.5 h[50]. It has been said that MR preparations generally do not allow rapid titration for patients in severe pain, due to slow onset and the long dosing intervals[51], although experimental evidence to the contrary has recently appeared[52].

Oral to parenteral relative potency of morphine

This issue has been controversial. Single dose studies of morphine in postoperative cancer patients in the 1960s demonstrated an oral to intramuscular (i.m.) potency of 1 : 6[53]. However, empirical clinical practice using chronically administered oral morphine in cancer patients has generated a different ratio of 1 : 3 or 1 : 2[54,55]. The reason for this apparent discrepancy in the relative potency of morphine derived from single dose versus chronic dosing studies is probably associated with both methodological differences and the pharmacokinetics and pharmacodynamics of M6G[54,56]. It is possible that M6G accumulation relative to morphine may be greater with oral than with parenteral administration. This would lead to an increase in the relative potency of the orally administered drug when given on a chronic basis.

The important principle for clinical practice is that there is a difference in relative analgesic potency when the route of administration is changed. Adjustment of the dose is necessary in order to avoid either under dosing or toxicity. When given regularly the oral to s.c. ratio is normally between 1 : 2 and 1 : 3[1,57]. The usual practice when converting from oral morphine to subcutaneous morphine is to divide the dose by two or three. The same ratio holds true for i.m. and i.v. injections.

Drug interactions and toxicity

Drug interactions

Drug interactions are uncommon with morphine. Drug interactions may be broadly classified into pharmacokinetic (one drug interferes with the disposition of another), pharmacodynamic (one drug interacts with the other at the site of action, either a receptor or a physiological mechanism) or pharmaceutical (one drug is physically incompatible with another)[58].

Pharmacokinetic

Morphine has few specific pharmacokinetic interactions, although any drug that impairs hepatic or renal function can reduce morphine clearance. There are no drugs that are known to interfere with the absorption of oral morphine from the gut. Other drugs influence UGT activity[23]. As morphine does not undergo significant oxidative metabolism, the concurrent use of drugs that induce the hepatic mixed function oxidase system (cytochrome P450) do not alter the disposition of morphine. Tricyclic antidepressants and oxazepam has been shown to inhibit morphine conjugation by UGT, and clomipramine and amitriptyline have been shown to increase plasma morphine levels, as measured by an increase in bioavailability and the half-life of morphine in cancer patients[59]. Ranitidine reduces the M3G : M6G ratio though the clinical significance of this is unclear[23]. A Japanese group has found that MR morphine may interfere with the efficacy of $5HT_3$ receptor antagonists in chemotherapy-induced emesis, but these findings await confirmation[60].

Pharmacodynamic

Morphine is more likely to be involved in pharmacodynamic interactions involving physiological mechanisms. The additive side effects of morphine with the toxicity of other drugs are much more of a problem than true drug interactions *per se* and these are of two types. First, there are the extra sedative effects of morphine with other CNS depressants (anxiolytics, neuroleptics, antidepressants and alcohol). Secondly, there are the additive constipating effects of morphine with anticholinergic drugs and the $5HT_3$ antagonists. Recently, it has been suggested that there is an interaction between morphine and benzodiazepines at the level of the opioid receptor, benzodiazepines antagonizing the effect of opioids[61].

Pharmaceutical

Physical compatibility can be an issue when morphine is combined with other drugs in syringe drivers in palliative care. Morphine is considered to be compatible with many commonly used drugs, including baclofen, bupivacaine, clonidine, dexamethasone, glycopyrrolate, haloperidol, hyoscine, ketamine, metoclopramide and ondansetron. It is usually, but not always, compatible with midazolam. It is considered incompatible with phenytoin and phenobarbitone[62].

Toxicity

Successful pain management with morphine requires that adequate analgesia be achieved without excessive side effects. Excessive side effects account for some of the

10–30% of patients who fail to respond to treatment. The management of excessive side effects remains a substantial clinical challenge. Multiple approaches have been tried to address this problem. However, there is a lack of studies comparing the various options which guide choice and it has become controversial[63]. Patients receiving morphine (and other strong opioids) experience predictable side effects that need to be prevented/minimized if titration of the dose is not to be limited. All strong opioids tend to cause the same range of adverse effects although to a varying degree. These are shown in Table 8.1. Sedation, respiratory depression, constipation, and nausea and vomiting are the most widely recognized, but many other adverse effects are common. The reported frequency of these symptoms is based on their incidence in pharmacological studies of new morphine.

Symptoms attributed to the adverse effects of morphine are difficult to assess in patients with advanced cancer, as they may not, in fact, be due to the drug. Other possibilities include symptoms of the cancer, side effects of anti-cancer treatment, debility, or comorbidities and/or concomitant medications. Morphine side effects are also difficult to assess because of the influence of pharmacokinetic and pharmacodynamic factors in individual patients, such as the differential development of tolerance, changes in dose, route and regimen of administration, alterations in liver and renal function, and drug interactions.

To further complicate things, the mechanisms underlying the various side effects are only partly understood. Studies comparing the adverse effects of one opioid with another, or the same opioid by different routes, are lacking. The ability to tolerate a particular dose depends on the degree of opioid responsiveness of the pain, prior exposure to opioids, and rate of titration of dose, concomitant medications and renal/hepatic function. The caveats that apply to the use of parenteral opioids for patients in acute pain with impaired ventilation, bronchospasm and raised intracranial pressure do not apply to the careful titration of oral morphine in patients with advanced cancer.

There are five possible approaches to managing symptoms that are attributed to the adverse effects of morphine[63]. These include:

- reducing the dose;
- changing the route;

Table 8.1 Common adverse effects of morphine and all other strong opioids

Common initial	Common ongoing	Occasional	Rare
N&V	Constipation	Dry mouth	Respiratory depression
Drowsiness	N&V	Sweating	Psychological dependence
Unsteadiness		Pruritus	
Delirium/confusion		Hallucinations	
		myoclonus	

+ use of opioid-sparing adjuvant drugs;
+ opioid rotation;
+ symptomatic management of the side effect.

Treatment options for symptomatic management of common side effects are shown in Table 8.2.

Table 8.2 Therapeutic options for common adverse effects of morphine. Adapted from reference 63

Common initial	Common ongoing	Occasional	Rare
N&V: Change route (PR, SC); Symptomatic: ◆ if gastric stasis, metoclopramide or cisapride; ◆ if vestibular stimulation, try promethazine, cyclizine or methotrimeprazine	*N&V:* Symptomatic: as per initial treatment Opioid switch	*Dry Mouth* Reduce dose Artificial saliva	*Respiratory depression* Reduce dose (opioid antagonist may be indicated)
Drowsiness Usually resolves	*Constipation* Symptomatic: laxatives and or enemata; opioid antagonists Consider rotation to fentanyl or methadone	*Pruritus* Oral antihistamine Opioid switch	*Psychological dependence* Referral to addiction medicine expert
Unsteadiness Usually resolves	*Drowsiness* Reduce dose; consider methylphenidate (not available some countries) Route change, drug switch may help	*Hallucinations* Reduce dose and/or prescribe haloperidol Opioid switch	
Delirium/confusion Reduce dose and/or prescribe haloperidol Opioid switch		*Myoclonus* Reduce dose; consider benzodiazepine Opioid switch	

Sedation

This is the commonest side effect limiting titration and can cause a 'pseudo- pharmacological' ceiling dose. It can occur in the first few days of regular opioids for moderate-severe pain and subsequently if the dose is increased. This effect is augmented by concomitant use of other medication with CNS depressant effects, the prescribing of which may need to be rationalized. Patients receiving strong opioid for the first time should be aware that sedation may occur and be advised of the risks for driving or using machinery.

Constipation

The majority of patients taking morphine for either mild or moderate to severe pain will develop constipation, so preventative treatment is recommended rather than waiting for constipation to develop. Recent studies have challenged the previous view that morphine-induced constipation is dose dependent[64,65]. The best prophylactic treatment for preventing opioid induced constipation is a combination of stimulant and softening laxatives[66,67].

Nausea and vomiting

In clinical practice, it appears that in opioid naïve patients, 30–60% will develop nausea and/or vomiting. Tolerance in the majority of patients usually occurs within 5–10 days. Patients commencing opioids should have access to anti-emetics. A dopamine antagonist such as metoclopramide 10 mg t.d.s. (which is also prokinetic) or low dose haloperidol (1.5 mg nocte) will also be effective. The subcutaneous route may be required for drug delivery until the patient stabilizes.

Dry mouth

This usually occurs. It has been associated with high plasma morphine levels[23]. The xerostomatic effect of morphine is augmented by concurrent medication with a similar side effect, especially anticholinergic side effects. Patients should be encouraged to take regular sips of cool water and to maintain good oral hygiene

Neurotoxicity syndrome

This can present as subtle agitation, seeing shadows at the periphery of the field of vision, vivid dreams, nightmare, visual and auditory hallucinations, confusion and myoclonic jerking. Hyperalgesia may even be part of this syndrome[68]. Agitated confusion may be misinterpreted a uncontrolled pain and further opioid given. The sedated patient may then become dehydrated with resultant renal impairment, leading to accumulation of metabolites that cause further toxicity. The presence of opioid toxicity is an indication that the dose is too high for the patient at the particular time and it may warn of developing renal dysfunction[69]. Opioid toxicity is managed by reducing the dose of opioid, ensuring adequate hydration and treating the agitation/confusion with haloperidol (1.5–3 mg/h PRN). The opioid causing the toxicity may need switching to an alternative.

Respiratory depression

Because pain is a physiological antagonist to the central depressant effects of morphine, strong opioids do not cause clinically important respiratory depression in cancer patients in pain when used correctly[70]. Furthermore, in contrast to postoperative patients, cancer patients with pain:

- generally are not opioid naïve (have already been receiving a weak opioid);
- take medication by mouth (slower absorption, less peak concentration);
- titrate the dose upward step-by-step (less likelihood of excessive dose being given).

It is therefore extremely rare to need to use the specific opioid antagonist naloxone in palliative care. Because of the possibility of an additive sedative effect, care needs to be taken when strong opioids and psychotropic drugs are used concurrently.

Other less common side effects

These include hypotension, confusion, poor concentration, gastroparesis and urinary hesitancy/retention. Itch is a more common problem with spinal administration of morphine than systemic administration.

Hypogonadism

A recent small study of cancer survivors (disease free for >1 year) exposed to chronic high-dose (>200 mg/day) oral opioid therapy revealed marked central hypogonadism [with depressed testosterone levels and no compensatory increase in luteinizing hormone (LH)/follicle stimulating hormone (FSH)] and sexual dysfunction. Testosterone replacement therapy may be indicated in some of these patients[71]. Furthermore, it has recently been suggested that chronic opioid use may result in a more generalized hormonal derangement (hypoadrenalism, hypothyroidism), although the evidence for this is less clear[72].

Tolerance

Tolerance refers to the phenomenon of decreasing response to a drug as a consequence of continued use, manifest as a shift to the right in the dose–response curve, i.e. an increased dose is need to achieve the same effect. Tolerance occurs at a variable time after initiation of the drug. It may occur to some or all of the effects, and to a greater or lesser extent in each case. Tolerance to a drug may be pharmacokinetic (e.g. due to increased metabolism of the drug) or pharmacodynamic (e.g. due to decreased receptor responsiveness to the drug).

States of poor opioid responsiveness are common in patients with advanced cancer and tolerance may not be the only explanation. The mechanisms involved are unknown or poorly understood[73]. In the case of tolerance to morphine, this is currently thought to be a pharmacodynamic phenomenon, rather than a pharmacokinetic one. At a cellular level, tolerance has been linked to uncoupling of the opioid receptor from its associated intracellular guanosine 5'-triphosphate protein due to production of protein kinase C and activation of NMDA receptors[74,75]. Other possible explanations may include shift from a nociceptive to neuropathic pain pathophysiology, imbalance in the ratio of M3G : M6G production, opioid receptor internalization, spinal/supraspinal hypersensitivity[73] and intratumoral opioid uptake[76].

Despite these molecular changes, initiated by the occupation of the opioid receptor by morphine, tolerance to the analgesic effects of strong opioids is not a practical problem/does not occur in chronic cancer pain management, as increases in dose usually coincide with disease progression[77,78]. On the other hand, tolerance develops quickly to most, but not all (in the case of constipation) adverse effects. The initiation of opioid analgesia should not be delayed by professional anxiety over pharmacological tolerance as, in clinical practice, this does not occur.

Physical and psychological dependence

Physical dependence on chronically administered opioids may occur in cancer pain patients. Sudden discontinuation may lead to a physical withdrawal syndrome, which can be treated by administering a small dose of the opioid in question[79]. Physical dependence does not prevent a reduction in the dose of a strong opioid if the patient's pain ameliorates, e.g. as the result of radiotherapy or a nerve block[80].

The fear of patients developing psychological dependence (addiction) is unfounded/ generally does not occur in cancer patients experiencing pain and initiating treatment should not be delayed due to unfounded fears. Patients should be reassured they will not become psychologically dependent on their opioid analgesia and should not limit the use of strong opioids for cancer pain. Caution, in this respect, should be reserved for patients with a present or past history of substance abuse; even then the strong opioids should be used when there is a clinical need.

Drug abusers can develop malignancies and the prescription of analgesics in such cases nearly always results in anxiety and tension on all sides. Inadequate prescription of opioids in such cases will result in drug-seeking behavior for pain relief, commonly referred to as pseudo-addiction. A common sense approach is to accept the background drug maintenance therapy, e.g. a methadone maintenance program and to titrate the most appropriate opioid analgesic along with NSAIDS and adjuvant analgesics as appropriate. Knowledge of the pharmacokinetic/pharmacodynamic effects of morphine will usually guide the prescriber on the question of opioid titration. If the pain is opioid responsive, prescription of morphine should lead to improved function and less pseudo-addiction. Less opioid-responsive pains should be dealt with in the same way as the non-drug abuser.

Dosing in special populations

Liver failure

There are discrepancies in the data reported for the effect of hepatic dysfunction on the metabolism of morphine that probably relate to differences in the severity of the liver disease[81]. In the case of cancer patients, glucuronidation is rarely impaired in liver failure[57] and morphine is well tolerated in most patients with hepatic impairment[82], although with impairment severe enough to prolong prothrombin time, the plasma half-life of morphine may be increased and the dose of morphine may need to be reduced/given less often (6- or 8-hourly). However, extra-hepatic metabolism of morphine may also play a significant role in patients with hepatic dysfunction.

Renal failure

In patients with impaired renal function, the clearance of M3G and M6G has been shown to be significantly correlated with creatinine clearance[83]. Consequently, M6G may accumulate in blood and CSF[30], and high concentrations of this metabolite have been associated with toxicity including sedation, respiratory depression and myoclonic jerking[34,84]. Although further studies are needed to clarify the clinical importance of M6G and other metabolites, the data available are sufficient to recommend caution when administering morphine to patients with renal impairment. Patients who are receiving regular morphine and develop acute renal failure in a previously stable situation (e.g. rapidly developing obstructive uropathy in a patient with a pelvic malignancy) may develop sudden onset of signs and symptoms of opioid toxicity, necessitating temporary withdrawal of the morphine, and subsequent dose reduction and or less frequent administration. In patients with impaired renal function, M6G may accumulate in the blood and CSF, and high concentrations of this metabolite have been associated with toxicity[30,34,84]. Although further studies are needed to clarify the clinical importance of M6G and other metabolites, the data available are sufficient to recommend caution when administering morphine to patients with renal impairment. Patients who are receiving regular morphine and develop acute renal failure in a previously stable situation (e.g. rapidly developing obstructive uropathy in a patient with a pelvic malignancy) may develop sudden onset of signs and symptoms of opioid toxicity, necessitating temporary withdrawal of the morphine, and subsequent dose reduction and or less frequent administration.

Elderly

It appears that the ageing process affects all phases of pharmacokinetics, especially hepatic metabolism and renal excretion[85]. As a result, the clearance of morphine is decreased. Pharmacodynamic responses may also be altered in older patients, with increased receptor sensitivity. In practice, reducing the dose or lengthening the time interval between doses for the elderly will minimize the development of serious adverse events.

Pediatrics

The maturation of morphine clearance depends on the development of UGT activity. Even preterm infants of only 24 weeks gestation are capable of metabolizing morphine. Neonates have a 5-fold reduction in morphine clearance compared with children aged >1 year. Glucuronidation reaches adult levels between 1 and 6 months of age[86].

Evidence-based use for cancer

Morphine has been used for many millennia for the management of pain and other symptoms. It has been used for cancer pain since the 1950s. Since the development of the WHO analgesic ladder in the late 1970s, a number of major groups have developed guidelines for the use of morphine[1,51,87,88]. The evidence base for many of the recommendations contained in these documents is weak, either consensus-based or taken from studies that have not been identified in a systematic way. It was only recently that a formal systematic review of oral morphine for cancer pain has finally been published[89].

Those reviewers found that the randomized trial literature for morphine was surprisingly small. No meta-analysis of the data contained in them was possible. The reviewers concluded that it was not clear if there are clinically important differences between different formulations of oral morphine or comparator drugs. These methodological problems notwithstanding, an evidence-based medicine approach to using morphine is still useful, by addressing a series of 'well-built clinical questions'[90].

'In patients with pain due to advanced cancer . . . ':

1 Is morphine better than other strong opioids?

Morphine remains the opioid of choice by virtue of its availability, familiarity to clinicians, established effectiveness, simplicity of administration and relative inexpensive cost[63]. It is not based on proven therapeutic superiority over other options. The systematic review identified 14 RCT comparing oral morphine with other various opioids, including dextropropoxyphene, transdermal fentanyl, hydromorphone, methadone, oxycodone, tramadol and Brompton's cocktail[89]. It was not clear if any of the studies were sufficiently powered to detect any real differences between the different drugs studied.

While morphine is the preferred drug, it has its limitations:

- Its systemic BA is poor, contributing to an unpredictable onset of action and great inter-individual variation in dose requirements in some patients.

- Its active metabolites may cause toxicity esp. in renal failure[91].

- Some pains do not respond entirely (e.g. neuropathic pain).

Pharmacokinetics considerations, comorbidities, previous use of opioids for moderate pain, and available formulations all need to be considered when choosing between morphine and its alternatives:

- *Pharmacokinetic considerations*: Any opioid can be selected for the opioid-naïve patient without organ impairment. A short-half-life opioid like morphine is generally preferred to a long half-life one like methadone or levorphanol.

- *Available formulations*: The range of available formulations often influences initial drug choice. Morphine is preferred in many countries because it has a short half-life, has easy to titrate NR forms, MR forms allowing 12–24 h dosing intervals and injectable forms for parenteral administration. Although some clinicians advocate the use of modified-release morphine (MRM) when initiating morphine therapy in cancer patients a normal-release morphine (NRM) preparation is generally recommended in the dose titration period[88]. Initial dose titration with MRM is difficult because of the delay in achieving peak plasma concentrations, the attenuation of peak concentrations and the long duration of action. In this situation, dose finding is performed more efficiently with NRM. For the same reasons MRM is not appropriate for the treatment of acute pain or breakthrough pain.

- Response to previous trials of opioid therapy: this is also relevant.

- *Co-existing disease*: Mild to moderate hepatic impairment has only a minor impact on morphine clearance[92], but it may be reduced in advanced disease[93]. Patients with renal impairment may accumulate M6G and particular caution is required with morphine administration to such patients[91]. Extra care should be taken initiating/titrating in patients with renal impairment. The active metabolites of morphine are cleared through the renal system. Therefore, in patients with renal impairment, morphine metabolites may accumulate and lead to toxicity. In patients with renal dysfunction, smaller doses of morphine and longer dosing intervals are required. It is good clinical practice to avoid controlled release morphine preparations in patients with renal dysfunction. Normal release morphine preparations are safer in the presence of renal impairment.

2 How should treatment with oral morphine be initiated?

When moving up from step 2 of the analgesic ladder, start the patient on NR formulation of morphine sulfate 5–10 mg orally, every 4 h[1]. Regularly scheduled 'around the clock' dosing is intended to provide continuous relief by preventing pain from recurring. Clinical vigilance is required in patients with no previous exposure to strong opioids. A double dose may be given at bedtime and the overnight dose is then unlikely to be required[94]. In patients presenting in severe pain, parenteral opioids may be superior to the oral route if rapid control of pain (within an hour) is needed[95].

3 Is there ever a place for PRN/as-needed dosing?

In some limited situations, an as needed dosing regimen alone can be recommended. This type of dosing provides additional safety during the initiation of morphine therapy in the opioid-naïve patient particularly when rapid dose escalation is needed (see below). This technique is also recommended in the very sick/frail/elderly, in patients with respiratory failure and hypercarbia, or patients with marked hepatic/renal impairment.

4 Is morphine inappropriate for some types of moderate-severe cancer pain?

All patients with pain of moderate–severe pain should be given a trial of strong opioids irrespective of the underlying pathophysiological mechanism. The suggestion that some forms of pain (e.g. neuropathic) are intrinsically refractory to opioid analgesia has been refuted by several studies that demonstrate that pain mechanisms do not accurately predict analgesic outcome from opioid therapy[96].

5 How should breakthrough analgesia be prescribed?

Every patient on regularly morphine for moderate to severe pain needs to have access to breakthrough analgesia, usually in the form of NR morphine, for pain that breaks through the regular schedule[88]. It is applicable to all routes of administration. It is established practice when using morphine for cancer pain to prescribe one-sixth of the total daily dose of morphine at any time for breakthrough pain[1]. Breakthrough pain is defined as an unexpected increase in pain to greater than moderate intensity, occurring on a baseline pain of moderate intensity or less[97]. Breakthrough analgesia should be administered at any time in addition to regular analgesia if the patient is in pain. The frequency with which the rescue dose is administered depends on the time to peak effect for the drug used and the route of administration. In the case of morphine, the breakthrough dose is the same as the regular 4-h dose (or one-sixth of the 24-h dose), offered every 60–90 or every 15–30 min for parenteral morphine. In patients with low-level baseline pain, but severe exacerbations, the rescue dose may need to be much larger than the regular dose. Following administration of the breakthrough dose, wait 30 min to assess the response. If pain persists, repeat the dose and reassess in another 30 min. If pain still persists, full reassessment of the patient is required. NRM can be used for predictable movement-related pain. Where possible, it should administered 30 min before movement.

6 How should the morphine dose be adjusted?

Each day assess the pain control, degree of side effects and total amount of morphine required, including breakthrough doses, in the previous 24 h. Divide the total required in the previous 24 h by six. Prescribe this dose every 4 h and alter the breakthrough analgesia dose accordingly (this is the same as the 4-hourly dose). Gradually increase the dose in this way until adequate analgesia is reported or dose-limiting toxicity intervenes. Increases of <33–50% are not likely to improve analgesia significantly because the analgesic response to opioid increases linearly with the logarithm of the dose. Clinical experience indicates doses of this magnitude are safe and effective. The integration of scheduled dosing with rescue doses provides a method for rational stepwise dose escalation applicable to all routes of administration.

If the patient is unable or unwilling to use breakthrough doses, but is still in pain, the dose of NRM prescribed 4-hourly should be increased. The increase depends on the individual, but is usually 30–50% increments.

In patients with very severe pain, repeated parenteral dosing every 15–30 min may be used until the pain is partially relieved, at which time an oral dosing regimen can be initiated.

The rate of titration of morphine may be limited by drowsiness and, in some patients, longer is required to become tolerant to this effect before escalation of the dose can be continued. Opioid responsiveness is a continuum and while a trial of opioids is required in all cases of moderate to severe cancer pain some pains (e.g. neuropathic) do predictably require larger doses of opioids. However, the side effect profile associated with larger doses can restrict dose titration and, hence, limit analgesia. Careful titration with opioids is necessary and, in such situations, allow time for tolerance to develop to side effects, prior to increasing the dose.

Care should be taken when calculating a new regular dose for patients who are pain free at rest, but have pain on movement. If all the analgesia for this incident pain is incorporated into the new regular morphine dose, such patients could be rendered opioid toxic. In particular, they will be rendered excessively sleepy at rest. This is because pain is a 'physiological antagonist' to the sedative and respiratory depressant side effects of opioids, although the exact mechanism by which this occurs is not well understood. In such cases, optimum analgesia is achieved by maximizing background analgesia, anticipatory analgesia for movement-related pain, maximum use of non-opioid and adjuvant analgesics, and consideration of other treatment modalities, such as RT, nerve blocks and stabilizing surgery[98].

7 Is there a ceiling dose of morphine?

The gradual escalation of the dose can lead to extremely large doses of morphine being prescribed. The actual dose remains immaterial as long as there is a favorable balance between effects and side effects. Surveys of palliative care services have indicated median doses of 60–120 mg/day being used[99,100]. However, another retrospective study of 100 patients with advanced cancer, the average daily morphine requirement (in parenteral equivalents) was 400–600 mg/day with approximately 10% patients requiring >2 g/day, with one patient on >30 g/day[101].

8 Is tolerance a problem?

The need for dose escalation is a complex phenomenon. Most patients reach a dose that is stable for prolonged periods. When dose escalation is required, one or more processes may be involved. Clinical experience indicates true pharmacological tolerance is a much less common reason for dose escalation than disease progression or, less commonly, increasing psychological distress (as most patients needing dose increases have demonstrable progressive disease or are psychologically distressed). Changes in pharmacokinetics (changes in drug clearance, drug interactions) may also be involved. The implication is that escalating dose requirements should be taken as presumptive evidence of disease progression, rather than the development of tolerance. Concern about the development of tolerance should not delay the initiation of opioid therapy.

9 What is the correct way to use modified release formulations of morphine?

The development of modified release morphine preparations has had a major impact on clinical practice as they provide a much more convenient means of administering oral morphine[102]. The same level of analgesia can be achieved by giving the total daily amount of normal release morphine as controlled-release morphine[103,104]. When pain is controlled, add up the total daily dose of NRM the patient is receiving and give this dose as a once daily MR preparation or divide the total dose by two and give twice daily. In addition to the MRM, continue to prescribe the appropriate dose of NRM as breakthrough analgesia.

When converting from NRM to MRM preparations there is no need to administer a NR formulation as the same time as the first CR dose[105]. Discontinue the regular NR morphine when the first dose of MR morphine is given.

10 Can MR morphine formulations be used to titrate the dose?

It is generally recommended that these formulations should not be used for rapid titration of the dose in patients with severe pain. Recently, an RCT comparing MR morphine with NR morphine for the initiation of morphine treatment in patients with cancer pain found a shorter time to achieving analgesia, less tiredness and no differences in QOL or satisfaction with treatment in patients treated with MR morphine[52].

11 How does one best administer morphine to patients in whom the oral route is not available?

The oral route is inappropriate for patients with impaired swallowing or GI obstruction, for patients who require a rapid onset of analgesia, and for some patients who require very high doses and for whom it is not possible to prescribe a manageable oral opioid-regimen. When patients are unable to take morphine by mouth, parenteral administration is effective. Indications for the parenteral route include inability to swallow, nausea/vomiting, gastrointestinal obstruction and any pathology limiting GIT absorption. Uncontrolled pain is not an indication for the parenteral routes if further titration by the oral route is possible. In a survey of patients with advanced cancer, more than half required two or more routes of administration and almost a quarter required three or more[101]. The subcutaneous route is effective[106,107] and avoids the need for repeated i.m. injections, which may be painful yet are still frequently given in hospitals[108,109]. If a breakthrough injection is needed, the s.c. route should also be used.

12 What is the optimal way to deliver parenteral morphine?

The technique of continuous subcutaneous infusion (CSCI) is well established/has become first choice in palliative care for the delivery of analgesics antiemetics, anxiolytics and other agents. It avoids obtaining and maintaining i.v. access, and allows the patient to keep their limbs free. These agents can be combined provided they are all non-irritant, miscible and stable in combined solution (see below). The most appropriate for patients with a pre-existing central venous access or when the morphine dose is high and a large volume is needed, may be intravenously. The needle can be steel or Silastic, and can stay in place for up to a week[110]. The delivery devices vary in complexity and cost. Simple portable battery-operated infusion pumps are widely used. The infusion devices most often used to deliver subcutaneous continuous infusion (CSCI) are portable syringe drivers. To be suitable for s.c. administration, an agent has to be soluble, well absorbed and non-irritant. Morphine meets these requirements[110–113]. Syringe drivers do have a volume restriction (usual maximum 30 ml/infusion), which can limit the amount of morphine sulfate (MS) to be delivered (1 g MS requires 16 ml of water for injection to dissolve). To maintain the comfort of a CSCI site, the infusion rate should not exceed 5 ml/h. More soluble alternatives for patients on high doses include hydromorphone (USA, Australia) and diamorphine (heroin, UK).

Use of a PCA device allows the patient to titrate the opioid dose carefully to his/her individual analgesic needs. There is relatively little experience for using this technique, used mainly for acute postoperative pain (see below), in chronic cancer pain. Long-term PCA is accomplished using an ambulatory infusion device[114].

13 Can bolus injections be used?

Intermittent bolus injections are used for breakthrough analgesia in patients requiring a non-oral route or when rapid analgesia is required. Repeated bolus injections are effective, but may be complicated by the occurrence of untoward 'bolus' effects (toxicity at peak concentration and/or pain breakthrough at the trough). Repeated boluses can be accomplished without frequent skin punctures by using an in-dwelling i.v. or s.c. infusion device. A 25–27-gauge butterfly can be left in the skin for up to a week[115]. The discomfort associated with this technique is partly related to the volume to be injected; it can be minimized by the use of concentrated formulations.

14 Is subcutaneous as effective as intravenous?

Studies suggest that dosing with s.c. administration can proceed in a manner identical to CIVI: a postoperative study comparing patients who received an identical dose of morphine by either i.v. or s.c. infusion found no difference in blood levels.[116]. One controlled study of hydromorphine (HM) calculated the bioavailability of 78% for SQ route and that analgesic outcome are identical during CIVI and CSCI, but a study of i.v. versus s.c. morphine found that the relative potency was dose related[107].

15 How does one convert from oral morphine to subcutaneous morphine?

In clinical practice, s.c. morphine is 2–3 times as potent as oral morphine. To convert from the oral to s.c. route, add up the oral morphine requirements, both regular and breakthrough, used in the previous 24 hr and divide the dose by the equipotency ratio (2 or 3). This dose may need to be adjusted prior to the administration according to the clinical situation. Prescribe the calculated amount over 24 h as a CI, or divide by 6 and deliver as regularly scheduled four-hourly injections. A subcutaneous breakthrough dose, one sixth of the total daily regular dose, should also be prescribed. If using other opioids, s.c. DM (H) is three times more potent than OM and s.c. HM is 10–20 times more potent than OM.

If the patient's pain is well controlled, start the infusion when the next oral dose was due. If the patient's pain is uncontrolled, start the infusion immediately and give a subcutaneous breakthrough dose concomitantly. As for oral morphine, the dose should be reviewed daily and adjusted if necessary.

When the patient regains the ability to take oral morphine, the dose is 2–3 times that of the subcutaneous dose. A CR preparation can be used if the dose is stable[1].

16 How does one manage postoperative pain in patients already on morphine?

The team looking after the patient postoperatively must be aware whether the patient was taking morphine preoperatively. Patients taking morphine preoperatively need a larger than normal dose of morphine postoperative patients are commonly given the standard postoperative analgesia and suffer as a result. If possible a pain specialist should be consulted. A PCA system should be used, set with a larger background and bolus than usual, based on the preoperative opioid dosage and a short lock out time. Management in a high-dependency nursing unit postoperatively is recommended.

17 Is morphine compatible with other drugs in solution for infusions?

A variety of different combinations of drugs are commonly given by CI[117]. However, the stability/compatibility of many of these combinations is not known. The compatibility of drug combinations is dependent on a number of factors, including the type of drugs, concentrations, diluent and temperature, and exposure to UV light. A database of compatible combinations is now available on the internet.[118]. Generally, infusions should contain as few as drugs as possible, preferably no more than three. The absence of precipitation within a drug mixture is not synonymous with compatibility between the drugs in the mixture.

18 Are spinal routes superior to systemic administration of morphine?

Intraspinal opioids generally provide a longer duration of analgesia at dose lower than required by systemic administration, which may decrease supraspinal-mediated adverse effects. Opioid selection for intraspinal delivery is influenced by several factors. Hydrophilic drugs like morphine have a prolonged half-life in CSF and undergo significant rostral redistribution[119].

Analgesia obtained with spinal morphine can be improved by the addition of the LA bupivacaine, without increasing toxicity[120,121]. The a$_2$ antagonist clonidine can also be added. The conversion ratio for parenteral to spinal morphine is 1 : 10 for epidural and 1 : 100 for spinal. Thus, a patient on 100 mg s.c. morphine/day would be commenced on 10 mg epidural morphine or 1 mg intrathecal morphine/day.

A recent large trial compared intrathecal morphine with comprehensive pain management with systemic morphine. Sixty of 71 patients receiving IT morphine achieved successful analgesia compared with 51 of 72 CMM patients (85% versus 71%, $P = 0.05$), with less toxicity. The IT morphine patients had improved survival at 6 months compared with CMM patients (59% versus 37%, $p = 0.06$). The authors concluded that IT morphine improved clinical success in pain control, reduced pain, significantly relieved common drug toxicities and improved survival in patients with refractory cancer pain[122].

There have been no trials comparing epidural with intrathecal morphine in cancer patients. The epidural route is usually chosen because it is technically simpler. A combined analysis of the adverse effects observed in numerous trials suggests that the risks associated with these two approaches are similar. The potential morbidity associated with these procedures emphasizes the need for well-trained staff and long-term monitoring.

Limited experience suggests intracerebroventricular administration of morphine can provide long-term analgesia in selected patients with head, upper body or diffuse pain. Schedules have include both intermittent administration and administration via an Ommaya reservoir.

19 Does topical morphine work?

There are several case series and two small RCT examining the role of topical morphine in local analgesia. The evidence points to a role in some situations, for example, cutaneous ulcers or tumours with cutaneous infiltration. Doses of 10–40 mg of morphine are used in simple gel, saline soaks or LA gel[123–126].

20 Is morphine effective for breathlessness?

Systemic morphine has been shown to be effective in controlling dyspnea in a few controlled studies. One used oral morphine as a supplementary dose of 25–50% above this stable analgesic dose[127]. A recent RCT used low dose MS Contin[128]. Three studies report the usefulness of the s.c. route at 5 mg in opioid naïve patients or 25–50% above the stable analgesic dose in opioid tolerant patients with concomitant pain[127,129,130]. There were no reports of side effects such as respiratory depression with s.c. administration, but it has been reported in studies of oral and i.v. morphine[131,132].

21 Is nebulized morphine effective?

Nebulized morphine has been tried for breathlessness in both cancer and non-cancer patients. In uncontrolled studies, it has been reported to be effective in doses up to 30–40 mg every 4 h[133–135]. In two controlled studies that have been performed, there was no significant difference from placebo[136,137]. Because the bioavailability is low (<10%) and unpredictable, it is not recommended to use this route for pain management.

22 What is the role for opioid antagonists in managing side effects?

While systemic administration of standard doses of opioid antagonists will reverse life-threatening opioid toxicity or over dosages, their use in patients with advanced cancer on chronic opioid therapy is generally discouraged because they can precipitate severe pain and/or acute withdrawal syndrome.

Despite this caveat, there has been interest for more than a decade in the oral administration of opioid antagonists for opioid-induced constipation[138]. More recently, there has been interest in the parenteral administration of ultra-low dose opioid antagonists to control other toxicity, such as sedation, nausea and pruritus[139,140]. With regard to oral naloxone for constipation, to date five small studies using various naloxone regimens have been done on patients receiving chronic opioid therapy, only one of which was a controlled study. The extent of the anti-constipating effect, the incidence of withdrawal syndromes, and the re-emergence of pain, varies from study to study, so that no firm conclusions can be made at this stage[141]. New opioid antagonists are currently being developed that may improve the results of these trials.

23 Morphine and driving?

Driving is a complex task that requires alertness, information processing from several inputs, coordination and dexterity, and drugs that affect the CNS have the potential to impair it. There have been several reviews of the effects of opioids and other CNS depressants on driving[142–4]. From these reviews it has been concluded that opioids may impair performance, but that this depends on the particular opioid, dose involved, population studied and length of use. In patients with chronic non-cancer pain, long-term (>12 months) treatment with opioids has recently been shown not to impair cognitive function, but rather to improve some aspects of cognitive functioning consequent on pain relief, and improved mood and sensation of well-being[145]. With specific regard to opioid-dependent patients on stable doses who have some degree of tolerance to the sedative effects of the drug, it has recently been concluded that there is generally consistent data that opioids do not impair driving-related skills. For patients on chronic opioid therapy who wish to drive the following recommendations have been recently suggested[145]:

- ◆ do not drive for 4–5 days after beginning opioid therapy or after a dose increase;
- ◆ do not drive if feel sedated;
- ◆ report sedation/unsteadiness to the physician so that dose can be reduced;
- ◆ do not drive and take alcohol or illicit drugs concomitant with the opioid;
- ◆ avoid other sedatives, e.g. OTC antihistamines;
- ◆ consult physician re changes to medications.

Recent data suggest that long-term opioid use does not significantly impair psychomotor function or cognitive ability after 3 and 6 months administration[146].

Doses and routes

Morphine is available in four oral formulations: an elixir, a normal-release tablet, a MR tablet or capsule (of which there are now several preparations using different sustained-release mechanisms) and sustained-release suspension. Administered as tablets or aqueous solution (immediate or 'normal release'). In the UK, NR tablets are 10, 20 and 50 mg, and solution is 10 mg/5 ml and 100 mg/5 ml.

An increasing range of MR preparations is available worldwide: tablets, capsules and suspensions, in a range of dose formulations (10–200 mg), depending on the country, allowing considerable flexibility of use[147]. There are no generic MR tablets. Because of the differing pharmacokinetic profiles, it is best to keep individual patients on the same brand. Most are given twice daily, some once daily as either an ordinary (NR) or MR preparation.

Parenteral administration

The inorganic salts of morphine (hydrochloride, sulfate) have limited solubility. Standard formulations are available up to 20 mg/ml and morphine can be constituted from lyophilized powder up to 50 mg/ml. Morphine tartrate is substantially more soluble and, in some countries, is formulated in concentrations of 80 mg/ml.

Rectal

This is a non-invasive alternative to parenteral. Suppositories containing morphine are available in some countries. Rectal administration of MRM tablets may also be effective[148]. In practice, the potency of rectal morphine is best considered equal to that of oral dosing, even though the pharmacokinetics and bioavailability are different[149].

Transdermal

Morphine does not have the appropriate physical or chemical properties to permit transdermal administration without an electric current.

Sublingual

The utility of the SL/TM routes is limited because of the lack of true SL/TM formulations of morphine, poor drug absorption and the inability to deliver high doses. Anecdotally, sublingual administration of low doses of morphine (using an injectable formulation) has been reported to be effective. Given the poor SL absorption of this drug, this efficacy may be related in part to swallowing the dose.

Nasal

The nasal route is potentially the best alternative to oral/parenteral administration because absorption is aided by the large surface area and the highly vascular epithelium, and first pass metabolism is bypassed. The nasal route may be effective for a number of opioids[150]. A pilot study of single dose intranasal morphine gluconate (40 mg) achieved plasma morphine levels considered to be in the therapeutic range and the onset of analgesia in 2–3 min. Meaningful pain relief was achieved in approximately 50% cases[151].

Because morphine is hydrophilic it is poorly absorbed nasally. To overcome this problem, morphine has been combined with chitosan, a bio-adhesive material that slows the mucociliary clearance of morphine, allowing more time for absorption. A pilot study in the UK of a commercially available morphine-chitosan formulation for breakthrough pain in patients with cancer has recently been reported[152].

Nebulized

This route has been employed for the management of breathlessness. Giving morphine via a nebulizer has the potential advantage of reducing adverse effects because of its low systemic bioavailability, varying between 5 and 35% depending on the method of administration[153,154]. Peak plasma concentrations are reached more rapidly than with the oral route[154]. Single doses up to 40 mg and repeated doses up to 30 mg every 4 h have been reported. It is generally well tolerated, though some patients find the mask claustrophobic and complain of the bitter taste. None of the studies report adverse effects such as somnolence or respiratory depression. Nor do they report bronchospasm, even though morphine produces potent histamine release.

Topical

Doses of 10–40 mg of morphine are used in simple gel, saline soaks or LA gel[123–126].

References

1 Hanks GW, Conno F, Cherny N. Morphine in cancer pain: recommendations of European Association of Palliative Care. *Br J Cancer* 2001; **84**: 587–93.

2 World Health Organisation. *Model List of Essential Drugs (EDL)*, 11th edn, Nov 1999. Available at: http://www.who.int/medicines/organization/par/edl/infed111group.html (accessed January 19, 2004).

3 **Resine T, Pasternak G.** Opioid analgesics and antagonists. In: Gilman AG, Hardman JG, Limbird LE (Eds) *Goodman & Gilman's the Pharmacological Basis of Therapeutics*, 9th edn. NewYork: McGraw-Hill, 1996, pp. 1026–38.

4 **Sawe J, Dahlstrom B, Paalzow L,** *et al.* Morphine kinetics in cancer patients. *Clin Pharmacol Ther* 1981; **30:** 629–35.

5 **Hoskin PJ, Hanks GW, Aherne GW,** *et al.* The bioavailability of and pharmacokinetics of morphine after intravenous, oral and buccal administration in health volunteers. *Br J Clin Pharmacol* 1989; **27:** 499–505.

6 **Gourlay GK, Plummer JL, Cherry DA,** *et al.* The reproducibility of bioavailability of oral morphine from solution under fed and fasted conditions. *J Pain Sympt Manag* 1991; **6:** 431–6.

7 **Vater M, Smith G, Aherene GW,** *et al.* Pharmacokinetics and analgesic effects of slow-release oral morphine sulphate in volunteers. *Br J Anaesth* 1984; **56:** 821–7.

8 **Savarese JJ, Goldenheim PD, Thomas GB,** *et al.* Steady state pharmacokinetics of controlled release oral morphine sulphate in healthy subjects. *Clin Pharmacokinet* 1986; **11:** 505–10.

9 **Poulain P, Hoskin PJ, Hanks GW.** Relative bioavailability of controlled release morphine tablets (MST) Continus in cancer patients. *Br J Anaesth* 1988; **61:** 569–74.

10 **Gourlay GK, Cherry DA, Only MM,** *et al.* Pharmacokinetics and pharmacodynamics of 24-hour Kapanol compared to 12 hourly MST Contin in the treatment of severe cancer pain. *Pain* 1997; **69:** 295–302.

11 **Max MB, Inturrisi CE, Kaiko RF,** *et al.* Epidural and intrathecal opiates: CSF and plasma profiles in patients with chronic cancer pain. *Clin Pharmacol Ther* 1985; **38:** 631–41.

12 **Sawe J, Kager L, Svensson JO,** *et al.* Oral morphine in cancer patients: in vivo kinetics and in vitro hepatic glucuronidation. *Br J Clin Pharmacol* 1985; **19:** 495–501.

13 **Benhye S.** Morphine: new aspects in the study of an ancient compound. *Life Sci* 1994; **55:** 969–79.

14 **Hasselstrom J, Eriksson S, Person A.** Morphine metabolism in patients with liver cirrhosis. *Acta Pharmacol Toxicol* 1996; **Suppl V:** abstr 101.

15 **Mazoit JX, Sandouk P, Zelataoui P,** *et al.* Phamacokinetics of unchanged morphine in normal and cirrhotic subjects *Anesth Analg* 1987; **66:** 293–8.

16 **Sandouk P, Serrie A, Schermann JM,** *et al.* Presence of morphine metabolites in human cerebrospinal fluid after intracerbroventricular injection of morphine. *Eur J Drug Metab Pharmacol* 1991; **16(Suppl 3):** 166–71.

17 **Smith MT, Wright AWE, Williams BE,** *et al.* CSF and plasma concentrations of M, M3g, and M6G in patients before and after ICV administration of morphine. *Anaesth Analg* 1999; **88:** 109–16.

18 **Coffman BL, Rios GR, King CD,** *et al.* Human UGT2B7 catalyzes morphine metabolism. *Drug Metab Disp* 1997; **25:** 1–4.

19 **McQuay HJ, Carroll D, Faura CC,** *et al.* Oral morphine in cancer pain: influences on morphine and metabolite concentration. *Clin Pharmacol Ther* 1990; **48:** 236–44.

20 **Zhou HH, Sheller JR, Nu H,** *et al.* Ethinic differences in response to morphine. *Clin Pharmacol Ther* 1993; **54:** 507–13.

21 **Holthe M, Rakvag TN, Klepstad P,** *et al.* Sequence variations in the UDP-glucuronosyltransferase 2b7 (UGT 2B7) gene: identification of 10 novel single nucleotide polymorphisms (SNP) and analysis of their relevance to morphine glucuronidation in cancer patients. *Pharmacogenom J* 2003; **3:** 17–26.

22 **Osborne R, Joel S, Trew D,** *et al.* Morphine and metabolite behavior after different routes of morphine administration: demonstration of the importance of the active metabolite M6G *Clin Pharmacol Ther* 1990; **47:** 12–19.

23 Andersen G, Christup L, Sjogren P. Relationships among morphine metabolism, pain and side effects during long-term treatment: an update. *J Pain Sympt Manag* 2003; **25:** 74–91.

24 Quigley C, Joel S, Patel N, *et al.* Plasma concentrations of morphine, M6G and M3G and their relationship with analgesia and side effects in patients with cancer related pain. *Palliat Med* 2003; **17:** 185–90.

25 Glare PA, Walsh TD, Pippenger CE. Normorphine: a neurotoxic metabolite? *Lancet* 1990; **335:** 725–6.

26 Chen XY, Zhao LM, Zhong DF. A novel metabolic pathway of morphine: formation of morphine glucosides in cancer patients. *Br J Clin Pharmacol* 2003; **55:** 570–8.

27 Sawe J, Svensson JO, Rane A. Morphine metabolites in cancer patients on increasing oral doses—no evidence for autoinduction or dose dependence. *Br J Pharmacol Ther* 1983; **16:** 85–93.

28 Carrupt PA, Testa B, Bechalany A, *et al.* M6G and M3G as molecular chameleons with unexpected lipophilicity. *J Med Chem* 1991; **34:** 1272–5.

29 Portenoy RK, Foley KM, Stulman J, *et al.* Plasma M and M6G during chronic morphine therapy for cancer pain: plasma profiles, steady state concentrations and consequences of renal failure. *Pain* 1991; **47:** 13–19.

30 D'Honneur G, Gilton A, Sandouk P, *et al.* Plasma and CSF concentrations of M and Mg's after oral M. the influence of renal failure. *Anaesthesia* 1994; **81:** 87–93.

31 Paul D, Standifer KM, Inturrisi CE, *et al.* Pharmacological characterisation of M6G, a very potent morphine metabolite. *J Pharmacol Exp Ther* 1989; **251:** 477–83.

32 Shimiomura K, Kamata O, Ueki S, *et al.* Analgesic effect of morphine glucuronides. *Tohoku J Exp Med* 1971; **105:** 45–52.

33 Pasternak GW, Bodnar RJ, Clark JA, *et al.* Morphine-6-glucuronide: a potent mu agonist. *Life Sci* 1987; **41:** 2845–9.

34 Osborne RJ, Joel SP, Slevin ML. Morphine intoxication in renal failure: the role of morphine-6-glucuronide. *Br Med J* 1986; **292:** 1548–9.

35 Osborne R, Thompson P, Joel S, *et al.* The analgesic effect of morphine-6-glucuronide. *Br J Clin Pharmacol* 1992; **34:** 130–8.

36 Portenoy RK, Thaler HT, Inturrisi CE, *et al.* The metabolite morphine-6-glucuronide contributes to the analgesia produced by morphine infusion in pain patients with normal renal function. *Clin Pharmacol Ther* 1992; **51:** 422–31.

37 Lotsch J, Weiss M, Ahne G, *et al.* Pharmacokinetic modelling of morphine-6-glucuronide formation after oral administration of morphine I healthy volunteers. *Anesthesiol* 1999; **90:** 1026–38.

38 Penson RT, Joel SP, Bakhshi K, *et al.* Randomised placebo controlled trial of the activity of the morphine glucuronides. *Clin Pharmacol Ther* 2000; **68:** 667–76.

39 Hoffman M, Xu JC, Smith C, *et al.* A pharmacodynamic study of morphine and its glucuronide metabolites after single dose morphine dosing in cancer patients. *Cancer Invest* 1997; **15:** 542–7.

40 Lotsch J, Geisslinger G. Morphine-6-glucuronide: an analgesic of the future? *Clin Pharmacokinet* 2001; **40:** 485–99.

41 Thompson PI, Bingham S, Andrews PL. Morphine-6-glucuronide: a metabolite with greater emetic potency than morphine in the ferret. *Br J Pharmacol* 1992; **106:** 3–8.

42 Osborne RJ, Joel SP, Slevin ML. Morphine intoxication in renal failure: the role of morphine-6-glucuronide. *Br Med J* 1986; **292:** 1548–9.

43 Hanks GW. Morphine pharmacokinetics and analgesia after oral administration. *Postgrad Med J* 1991; **67**(**Suppl 2**): S60–3.

44 Smith MT, Watt JA, Cramond T. Morphine-3-glucuronide—a potent antagonist of morphine analgesia. *Life Sci* 1990; **47:** 579–85.

45 Gong QL Hedner J, Bjorkman R, *et al.* M3G may functionally antagonise M6G induced antinociception and ventilatory depression in the rat. *Pain* 1992; **48:** 249–55.

46 Labella FS, Pinsky C, Havilcek V. Morphine derivatives with diminished opiate receptor potency show enhanced central excitatory activity. *Brain Res* 1979; **174:** 263–71.

47 Yaksh TL, Harty GJ. Pharmacology of the allodynia in rats evoked by high dose intrathecal morphine. *J Pharmacol Exp Ther* 1987; **244:** 501–7.

48 Hewett K, Dickenson AH, McQuay HJ. Lack of effect of M3G on the spinal anti-nociceptive action of morphine in the rat: an electrophysiological study. *Pain* 1993; **53:** 59–63.

49 Penson RT, Joel SP, Clark S, *et al.* Limited phase I study of M3G. *J Pharmaceut Sci* 2001; **90:** 1810–16.

50 McQuay H, Moore A. *Bibliography and Systematic Reviews in Cancer Pain.* A report to the NHS National Cancer Research and Development Program. Oxford, 1997.

51 Scottish Intercollegiate Guidelines Network (SIGN). *Cancer Pain Guidelines.* Edinburgh: SIGN, 2000.

52 Klepstad P, Kaasa S, Jystad A, *et al.* Immediate or sustained release morphine for dose finding during start of morphine to cancer patients: a randomised double blind trial. *Pain* 2003; **101:** 193–8.

53 Houde RW, Wallenstein S, Beaver WT. Clinical measurement of pain. In: Stevens G (Ed.) *Analgesics.* New York: Academic Press, 1965, pp. 75–122.

54 Hanks GW, Hoskin PJ, Aherne GW, *et al.* Explanation for potency of repeated oral doses of morphine? *Lancet* 1987; **ii:** 723–5.

55 Twycross RG. The therapeutic equivalence of oral and subcutaneous/im morphine in cancer patients. *J Palliat Care* 1987; **2:** 67–8.

56 Kaiko RF. Commentary: equianalgesic dose ratio of i.m./oral M, 1:6 versus 1:3. In: Foley KM, Inturrisi CE (Eds.) *Advances in Pain Therapy Research*, vol. 8. New York: Raven Press, 1986, pp. 87–93.

57 Max MB, Payne R (co-chairs). Principles of analgesic use in terminal cancer. In: Max MB, Payne R (Eds.) *Principles of Analgesic Use in the Treatment of Acute Pain and Cancer Pain.* New York: American Pain Society, 1992, p. 12.

58 Bernard S, Bruera E. Drug interactions in palliative care. *J Clin Oncol* 2000; **18:** 1780–9.

59 Ventafridda V, Ripamonti C, deConno F, *et al.* Antidepressants increase the bioavailability of morphine in cancer patients. *Lancet* 1987; **i:** 204.

60 Shoji A, Toda M, Suzuki K, *et al.* Insufficient effectiveness of 5HT-3 receptor antagonists due to oral morphine administration in patients with cisplatin-induced emesis. *J Clin Oncol* 1999; **17:** 1926–30.

61 Gear R, Miaskowski C, Heller PH, *et al.* Benzodiazepine mediated antagonism of opioid analgesia. *Pain* 1997; **71:** 25–9.

62 Therapeutic Guidelines. *Palliative Care*, version 1. North Melbourne: Therapeutic Guidelines Ltd, 2001, pp. 280–1.

63 Cherny N, Ripamonti C, Pereira J, *et al.* Strategies to manage the adverse effects of oral morphine: an evidence-based report. *J Clin Oncol* 2001; **19:** 2542–54.

64 Fallon MT, Hanks GW. Morphine, constipation sand performance status in advanced cancer patients. *Palliat Med* 1999; **13:** 159–60.

65 Bennett M, Cresswell H. Factors influencing constipation in advanced cancer patients: a prospective study of opioid dose, Dantron dose and physical functioning. *Palliat Med* 2003; **17:** 418–22.

66 Sykes NP. A volunteer model for the comparison of laxatives in opioid-related constipation. *J Pain Sympt Manag* 1996; **11:** 363–9.

67 Fallon MT, Hanks GW. Morphine constipation and performance status in advanced cancer patients. *Palliat Med* 1999; **13:** 159–60.

68 Mercadante S, Ferrara P, Villari P, *et al.* Hyperalgesia: an emerging iatrogenic syndrome. *J Pain Sympt Manag* 2003; **26:** 769–75.

69 O'Neill B, Fallon M. ABC of palliative care. Principles of palliative care and pain control. *Br Med J* 1997; **315:** 801–4.

70 Bjorgberg FM, Nielsen K, Franks J. Experimental pain stimulates respiration and attenuates morphine-induced respiratory depression: a controlled study in human volunteers. *Pain* 1996; **64:** 123–8.

71 Rajagopal A, Vassilopoulo-Sellin R, Palmer JL, *et al.* Hypogonadism and sexual dysfunction in male cancer survivors receiving chronic opioid therapy. *J Pain Sympt Manag* 2003; **26:** 1055–61.

72 Abs R, Vehrelst J, Mayaart J, *et al.* Endocrine consequences of long term intrathecal administration of opioids. *J Clin Endocrinol Metab* 2000; **85:** 2215–222.

73 Mercadante S. Portenoy RK. Opioid poorly-responsive cancer pain. Part 1: clinical considerations. *J Pain Sympt Manag* 2001; **21:** 144–50.

74 Mao J, Price DD, Mayer DJ. Mechanisms of hyperalgesia and morphine tolerance: a current view of their possible interacions. *Pain* 1995; **62:** 259–74.

75 Mayer DJ, Mao J, Holt J, *et al.* Cellular mechanisms of neuropathic pain, morphine tolerance and their interactions. *Proc Nat Acad Sci USA* 1999; **96:** 7731–6.

76 Arcuri E, Ginnobi P, Froldi R, *et al.* Preliminary *in vivo* experimental evidence of an intra-tumoral morphine uptake. Possible clinical implications in cancer pain and opioid responsiveness. *J Pain Sympt Manag* 2002; **24:** 1–3.

77 Foley KM. Pharmacological approaches to cancer pain management. In Fields HL, Dubner R, Cervero F (Eds) *Proceedings of the 4ᵗʰ World Congress on Pain*, Advances in Pain Research Therapy, vol. 9. New York: Raven Press, 1989, pp. 629–53.

78 Collin E, Poulain P, Gauvain-Piquard A, *et al.* Is disease progression the major factor in morphine 'tolerance' in cancer pain treatment? *Pain* 1993; **55:** 319–26.

79 Hunt R. Transdermal fentanyl and the opioid withdrawal syndrome. *Palliat Med* 1996; **10:** 347–8.

80 Twycross RG. *Pain Relief in Advanced Cancer*, 2nd edn. Edinburgh: Churchill Livingstone, 1994, pp. 339–42.

81 Hoyumpa AM, Scenker S. is glucuronidation truly preserved in patients with liver disease? *Hepatology* 1991; **13:** 786–95.

82 Regnard CFB, Twycross RG. Metabolism of narcotics, *Br Med J* 1984; **288:** 860.

83 Peterson GM, Randall CTC, Paterson J. Plasma levels of morphine and morphine glucuronides in the treatment of cancer pain: relationship to renal function and route of administration. *Eur J Clin Pharmacol* 1990; **38:** 121–4.

84 Lehmann KA, Zech D. M6G a pharmacologically active metabolite of M: a review of the literature. *Eur J Pharmacol* 1993; **12:** 28–35.

85 Owen JA, Sitar DS, Berger L, *et al.* Age-related morphine kinetics. *Clin Pharmacol Ther* 1983; **34:** 364–8.

86 McRorie TI, Lynn ASM, Nepesca MK, *et al.* The maturation of morphine clearance and metabolism. *Am J Dis Childh* 1992; **146:** 958–63.

87 Jacox A, Carr DB, Payne R, *et al. Management of Cancer Pain*, Clinical Practice Guideline No. 9, AHPCR Publication No. 94–0592. Rockville: AHPCR, March 1994.

88 Expert Working Group of the European Association of Palliative Care. Morphine for cancer pain: modes of administration. *Br Med J* 1996; **312**: 823–6.

89 Wiffen PJ, Edwards JE, Barden J, *et al*. Oral morphine for cancer pain (Cochrane Review). In: *The Cochrane Library*, Issue **4**, 2003. Chichester, UK: John Wiley & Sons, Ltd.

90 Richardson WS. Wilson MC, Nishikawa J, *et al*. The well-built clinical question: a key to evidence based decisions. *Am Coll Phys J Club* 1995; **123**: A-12.

91 McQuay HJ, Moore RA. Opioid problems and morphine metabolism and excretion. In: Dickenson AH, Besson JM (Eds) *Handbook of Experimental Pharmacology*. Berlin: Springer-Verlag, 1997, pp. 335–60.

92 Neal EA, Meffin PJ, Gregory PB, *et al*. Enhanced bioavailability and decreased clearance of analgesics in patients with cirrhosis *Gastroenterol* 1979; **77**: 96–102.

93 Hasselstrom J, Eriksson LS, Person A, *et al*. The metabolism and bioavailability of morphine in painters with severe liver cirrhosis. *Br J Clin Pharmacol* 1990; **29**: 289–97.

94 Regnard CF, Badger C. Opioids, sleep and the time of death. *Palliat Med* 1987; **1**: 107–10.

95 Harris JT, Kumar S, Rajagopal MR. Intravenous morphine for rapid control of severe cancer pain. *Palliat Med* 2003; **17**: 248–56.

96 Portenoy RK, Foley KM, Inturrisi CE. The nature of opioid responsiveness and its implications for neuropathic pain: new hypotheses derived from studies of opioid infusions. *Pain* 1990; **43**: 273–86.

97 Foley KM. Acute and chronic cancer pain syndromes. In: Doyle D, Hanks G, Cherny N, *et al*. (Eds) *Oxford Textbook of Palliative Medicine*, 3rd edn. Oxford: Oxford University Press, 2004, pp. 298–315.

98 Fallon MT. O'Neill WM. Spinal surgery in the treatment of metastatic back pain: three case reports. *Palliat Med* 1993; **7**: 235–8.

99 Walsh TD, Cheater FM. Use of morphine for cancer pain. *Pharmaceut J* 1983; **231**: 525–8.

100 Brooks DJ, Gamble W, Ahmedzai S. A regional survey of opioid use by patients receiving specialist palliative care. *Palliat Med* 1995; **9**: 229–38.

101 Coyle N, Adelhart J, Foley KM, *et al*. Character of terminal illness in the advanced cancer patient: pain and other symptoms during the final four weeks of life. *J Pain Sympt Manag* 1990; **5**: 83–9.

102 Hanks GW. Controlled release morphine (MST Continus): the European experience. *Cancer* 1989; **623**: 2378–82.

103 Welsh J. A DBXO study of two oral formulations of morphine. In: Harrap KR, Davis WE, Calvert AH (Eds) *Cancer Chemotherapy and Selective Drug Development*. Boston: Nighoff 1984, pp. 153–8.

104 Gilletet JF, Ferme C, Gehanno P, *et al*. DBXO clinical and pharmacokinetic comparison of oral M syrup and sustained release morphine capsules in patients with cancer related pain. *Clin Drug Investig* 1997; **Suppl**: 1–6.

105 Hoskin PJ, Poulain P, Hanks GW. Controlled release M in cancer pain. Is a loading dose required when the formulation is changed? *Anaesthesia* 1989; **44**: 897–901.

106 Moulin DE, Johnson NG, Murray Parsons N, *et al*. Subcutaneous narcotic infusions for cancer pain: treatment outcome and guidelines for use. *Canadian Medical Association Journal* 1992; **146**: 891–7.

107 Nelson KA, Glare PA, Walsh D, *et al*. A prospective within-patient crossover study of CIV and s.c. morphine for chronic cancer pain. *J Pain Sympt Manag* 1997; **13**: 262–7.

108 Urch CE, Field GB, Chamberlain JH. A comparative study of syringe driver use in community, hospice and hospital. *Palliat Med* 1996; **10**: 75.

109 **Panda M, Doshi N, Desbiens N.** Use of i.m. narcotic injections in hospitalised patients with i.v. access: causing pain to relieve pain (letter). *J Pain Sympt Manag* 2003; **25:** 297–9.

110 **Bruera E, Brenneis C, Michaud M, *et al.*** Patient controlled subcutaneous hydromorphone versus continuous subcutaneous infusion for the treatment of cancer pain. *J Nat Cancer Inst* 1988; **80:** 1152–4.

111 **Russel PSB.** Analgesia in terminal disease. *Br Med J* 1979; **I:** 1561.

112 **Oliver DJ.** The use of the syringe driver in terminal care. *Br J Clin Pharmacol* 1985; **20:** 515–16.

113 **Portenoy RK.** CIVI of opioid drugs. *Med Clin N Am* 1987; **71:** 233–41.

114 **Citron ML, Kalra JM, Seltzer VL, *et al.*** PCA for cancer pain: a long-term study of inpatient and outpatient use. *Cancer Invest* 1992; **10:** 335–41.

115 **Coyle N, Cherny NI, Portenoy RK.** Subcutaneous opioid infusions in the home. *Oncology* 1994; **8:** 21–7.

116 **Waldmann CS, Eason JR, Rambohul E, *et al.*** Serum morphine levels: a comparison between CSCI and CIVI in postoperative patients. *Anaesthesia* 1984; **39:** 768–71.

117 **O'Doherty CA, Hall EJ, Schofield L, *et al.*** Drugs and syringe drivers: a survey of adult specialists palliative care practice in the United Kingdom and Eire. *Palliat Med* 2001; **15:** 149–54.

118 Sdrivers-drug compatability database. http://www.pallmed.net. Accessed September 4, 2004.

119 **Moulin DE, Inturrisi CE, Foley KM.** Epidural and intrathecal opioids: CSF and plasma pharmacokinetics in cancer pain patients. In: Foley KM, Inturrisi CE (Eds) *Advances in Pain Research Therapy*, vol. 8. New York: Raven Press, 1986, pp. 369–84.

120 **Du Pen S, Williams AR.** Management of patients receiving combined epidural morphine and bupivacaine for the treatment of cancer pain. *J Pain Sympt Manag* 1992; **7:** 125–7.

121 **Hogan Q, Haddox JD, Abram S, *et al.*** Epidural opiates and local anaesthetics for the management of cancer pain. *Pain* 1991; **46:** 271–9.

122 **Smith TJ, Staats PS, Deer T, *et al.*** Randomized clinical trial of an implantable drug delivery system compared with comprehensive medical management for refractory cancer pain: impact on pain, drug-related toxicity, and survival. *J Clin Oncol* 2002; **20:** 4040–9.

123 **Stein C.** The control of pain in peripheral tissues by opioids. *N Engl J Med* 1995; **332:** 1685–90.

124 **Back IN, Finlay I.** Analgesic effect of topical opioids on painful skin ulcers. *J Pain Sympt Manag* 1995; **10:** 493.

125 **Kranjik M, Zylicz Z, Finlay I, *et al.*** Potential uses of topical opioids in palliative care—report of six cases. *Pain* 1999; **80:** 121–5.

126 **Zepetella G, Paul J, Ribiero MDC.** Analgesic efficacy of M applied topically to painful ulcers. *J Pain Sympt Manag* 2003; **25:** 555–8.

127 **Allard P, Lamontagne C, Bernard P.** How effective supplementary doses of opioids for dyspnoea in terminally ill cancer patients? A randomised continuous sequential clinical trial. *J Pain Sympt Manag* 1999; **17:** 256–65.

128 **Abernethy A, Currow DC, *et al.*** RCT of MST for breathlessness. *Br Med J* 2003; **327:** 523–8.

129 **Mazzocato C, Buclin T, Rapin CH.** The effects of morphine on dyspnea and ventilatory function in elderly patients with advanced cancer: an RCT. *Annl Oncol* 1999; **10:** 1511–14.

130 **Bruera E.** s.c. Morphine for dyspnoea in cancer patients. *Annl Int Med* 1993; **119:** 906–7.

131 **Cohen MH, Anderson AJ, Krasnow SH, *et al.*** CIVI M for severe dyspnoea. *Sthn Med J* 1991; **84:** 229–34.

132 **Boyd KJ, Kelly M.** Oral morphine as symptomatic treatment of dyspnoea in patients with advanced cancer. *Palliat Med* 1997; **11:** 277–81.

133 Farncombe M. The use of nebulised opioids for breathlessness: a chart review. *Palliat Med* 1994; **8**: 306–12.

134 Tanaka K, Shima Y, Kakinuma R, *et al*. Effect of nebulised morphine in cancer patients with dyspnoea: a pilot study. *Jap J Clin Oncol* 1999; **29**: 600–3.

135 Zepetella G. Nebulised morphine in palliation of dyspnoea *Palliat med* 1997; **11**:267–75

136 Peterson GM, Young RS, Dunne PF, *et al*. Pilot study of nebulised M for dyspnoea in palliative care patients. *Aust J Hosp Pharm* 1996; **26**: 545–7.

137 Davis CL, Penn K, A'Hern R, *et al*. Single dose RCT of nebulised morphine in patients with cancer-related breathlessness (abst.). *Palliat Med* 1996; **10**: 64–5.

138 Sykes NP. Oral naloxone in opioid-associated constipation. *Lancet* 1991; **337**: 145.

139 Cepeda MS, Alvarez H, Morales O, *et al*. Addition of ultralow dose naloxone to postoperative morphine PCA: unchanged analgesia and opioid requirements but decreased incidence of opioid side effects. *Pain* 2004; **107**: 41–6.

140 Mercadante S, Villari P, Ferrera P. Naloxone in treating central adverse effects during opioid titration for cancer pain (letter). *J Pain Sympt Manag* 2003; **26**: 691–3.

141 Choi YS, Billings JA. Opioid antagonists: a review of their role in palliative care, focussing on use in opioid-related constipation. *J Pain Sympt Manag* 2002; **24**: 71–90.

142 Zacny J. A review of the effects of opioids on psychomotor and cognitive functioning in humans. *Exp Clin Psychopharmacol* 1995; **3(4)**: 432–66.

143 O'Neill W. The cognitive and psychomotor effects of opioid drugs in cancer pain management. *Cancer Surv* 1994; **21**: 67–84.

144 Fishbain DA, Culter B, Rosomoff HL, *et al*. Are opioid dependent/tolerant patient impaired in driving-related skills? A structured evidence-based review. *J Pain Sympt Manag* 2003; **25**: 559–77.

145 Tassain V, Attal N, Fletcher D, *et al*. Long term effects of oral SRM on neuropsychological performance in patients with chronic non-cancer pain. *Pain* 2003; **104**: 389–400.

146 Jamison RN, Schein JR, Vallow S, *et al*. Neuropsychological effects of long term opioid use in chronic pain patients. *J Pain Sympt Manag* 2003; **26**: 913–21.

147 Forman WB, Portenoy RK, Yanagihara RH, *et al*. A novel morphine sulphate preparation: clinical trial of a controlled release morphine suspension in cancer pain. *Palliat Med* 1993; **7**: 301–6.

148 Walsh D, Tropiano PS. Long-term rectal administration of high-dose sustained release morphine tablets. *Support Care Cancer* 2002; **10**: 635–5.

149 Hanning CD. The rectal absorption of opioids. In: Benedetti C, Chapman CR, Giron G (Eds) *Advances in Pain Research Therapy*, vol. 14 New York: Raven, 1990, pp. 259–69.

150 Dale O, Hjortkjaer R, Kharasch ED. Nasal administration of opioids for pain management in adults. *Acta Anesth Scand* 2002; **46**: 759–70.

151 Fitzgibbon D, Morgan D, Dockter D, *et al*. Initial pharmacokinetic, safety and efficacy evaluation of nasal morphine gluconate for breakthrough pain in cancer patients. *Pain* 2003; **106**: 309–15.

152 Pavis H, Wilock A, Edgecombe J, *et al*. Pilot study of nasal morphine for the relief of breakthrough pain in patients with cancer. *J Pain Symptom Manage* 2002; **24**: 598–602.

153 Chrubasik J, Wust H, Friedrich G, *et al*. Absorption and bioavailability of nebulized morphine. *Br J Anaesth* 1988; **61**: 228–30.

154 Masood AR, Thomas SHL. Systemic absorption of nebulised morphine compared with oral morphine in healthy subjects. *Br J Clin Pharmacol* 1996; **41**: 250–2.

Chapter 9

Hydromorphone

Paul Glare

Hydromorphone (HM) is a semi-synthetic derivative of morphine with a long history of successful use as an opioid analgesic, having been developed in 1922 by Knoll and used for cancer pain since 1932[1]. It is almost pharmacologically identical to morphine, but has the advantages of high solubility in water and availability in a variety of dosage forms. HM is widely used in cancer pain management for opioid rotation[2].

Pharmacology

HM is a hydrogenated ketone of morphine and, like the parent compound, has the pharmacological properties of a pure mu opioid agonist. As with many of the morphine derivatives, few data exist that distinguish the effects of HM from those of morphine; in the absence of such data, it has to be assumed at this stage that the effects of HM are similar to the other.

Pharmacodynamics

HM is considered to be 5–10 times more potent than morphine. Its analgesic efficacy is very similar to morphine, peak effects being reached in 0.5–1 h after a parenteral dose and 1.5–2 h after oral, and the duration of analgesia is 4–6 h. It has been said that tolerance develops more slowly to HM than morphine[1,3].

The side effects of HM are also similar to those of morphine, but comparative data are conflicting and generally come from non-cancer populations. Old data (more than 50 years ago) suggested less vomiting, constipation and euphoria, but more respiratory depression with HM than morphine[1]. The Boston surveillance study of almost 40,000 hospitalized patients being treated with parenteral opioids reported the highest adverse event rate with HM, and reported more confusion, drowsiness and constipation, but less nausea and vomiting with HM than morphine, but HM was used uncommonly in that series (<1% cases)[4]. More recent studies suggest a less prolonged respiratory depression with HM compared to morphine[1]. Anecdotally, HM has always been said to be less addictive than other opioids. One of the four who became addicted to opioids administered for medical reasons out of some 11,000 cases was given HM[5].

Pharmacokinetics

Absorption

HM appears to be well absorbed from all routes of administration. The lipophilicity of HM is uncertain. It is generally considered to be more lipophilic than morphine, but has been reported to be less so by some and this discrepancy still awaits clarification[6,7].

Elimination

HM is excreted primarily as HM-3-glucuronide (HM3G), with HM3G:HM ratios being normally in the vicinity of 25 : 1[8]. Small amounts of the parent drug and minor amounts of the 6-hydroxy reduction metabolite are also excreted. The contribution of the 6-hydroxy metabolite to analgesia and toxicity of HM is unknown. HM3G may accumulate in renal failure and levels may be four-fold normal. Accumulation of HM3G and other potentially neurotoxic metabolites may account for the side effects occasionally reported by patients on very high doses of HM. In laboratory animals HM3G, like morphine-3-glucuronide, is devoid of analgesic activity, but can evoke a range of dose-dependent excitatory behaviors, including allodynia, myoclonus and seizures, following intracerebroventricular administration to rats. It has been suggested that when the HM3G concentration in the CSF exceeds the neuroexcitatory threshold, excitatory behaviors will be evoked in patients. In the case of neurotoxicity, rotation of the opioid from morphine/HM to a structurally dissimilar opioid, such as methadone or fentanyl, is recommended to allow clearance of HM3G (or M3G) from the patient central nervous system over hours to days, thereby producing a time-dependent resolution of the neuroexcitatory behaviors while maintaining analgesia[9].

Half-life

Elimination half-life is 2.64 ± 0.88 h and the volume of distribution is estimated at 1.22 l/kg[10].

Metabolism

HM undergoes extensive first pass metabolism, being metabolized primarily in the liver, where it undergoes glucuronidation. The major metabolite is HM3G. Single dose studies indicate an oral bio-availability (BA) of oral HM of 0.2, but with repeated oral administration this becomes more like 0.5[11]. Others have estimated BA of HM to be 0.6[10]. The dose proportionality for the 2 and 4 mg Dilaudid tablets has not yet been established for the 8-mg tablet.

Routes of administration

HM is available in several oral formulations (solution, immediate release tablets, controlled release tablets). The tablets make HM in attractive alternative to morphine in some patients, allowing titration as described for oral morphine without the nausea that morphine liquid may cause. It is also available as a suppository for rectal administration and for parenteral administration as ampoules (in regular and high-potency dosage forms). Parenteral HM can be administered by continuous subcutaneous (s.c.) and intravenous (i.v.) infusions. The increased solubility and potency of HM is particularly attractive for patients who require high-dose injections in small volumes. An implantable s.c. system has been developed[12]. Spinal HM has been mainly reported in the postoperative setting[13,14].

Drug interactions and toxicity

As with other strong opioids, HM may interact with other drugs causing central nervous system (CNS) depression, such as benzodiazepines, alcohol and central muscle relaxants. There has been a case report of respiratory depression not reversed by naloxone in a patient receiving spinal HM and droperidol[15]. HM is compatible with many other drugs in mixtures and stable for many days[16]. A comparison of cost-effectiveness and feasibility of using continuous subcutaneous ambulatory infusion of HM versus i.v. ambulatory morphine found that HM was stable for 28 days in two different dilutants and cost analysis of a HM 28-day supply resulted in substantial savings over the equivalent costs of morphine infusions[17].

Dosing in special populations

Pregnancy

HM is teratogenic in laboratory animals at high doses; the relevance to humans is unknown, so it is labeled Pregnancy Category C. HM can cause respiratory depression in the newborn so should be used with caution in labor. Low levels of opioids are detectable in human milk and as a rule should be avoided by mothers who are breast-feeding.

Pediatrics

The safety and effectiveness of HM have not been established in the pediatric population[18]. Analgesic intravenous doses of 0.015 mg/kg/dose every 4–6 h as needed have been used in pediatric patients[19]. Intramuscular analgesic doses of 1–2 mg/dose every 4–6 h as needed have been used in older children[19]. Oral analgesic doses of hydromorphone, 0.05–0.1 mg/kg/dose up to 5 mg/dose every 6 h have been used in pediatric patients[20]. Subcutaneous analgesic doses of 1–2 mg/dose every 4–6 h as needed have been used in older children[19]. A small study comparing the efficacy and side effect profile of morphine and HM, while utilizing patient-controlled analgesia for mucositis pain after bone marrow transplantation found no superiority of one drug over the other[21]. However, the data suggests that in the population of children studied, hydromorphone is less potent than what is generally documented in adult equipotency. Intravenous HM (2 mg) was approximately equipotent with i.v. morphine (10 mg).

This finding may be significant when calculating dosages in the setting of opioid switching during long-term opioid use.

Elderly

Due to greater frequency of decreased hepatic, renal or cardiac function, and of concomitant disease or other drug therapy, elderly patients should be dosed cautiously with HM, as with all strong opioids, usually starting at the low end of the dosing range.

Evidence-based use for cancer pain

HM is now included in clinical practice guidelines and recommended for the management of pain associated with malignancy[22]. HM has also been used extensively for the management of postoperative pain[13,14,23]. Despite widespread use, there appear to be gaps in our understanding of the efficacy and potency of HM[24].

A Cochrane Review published in 2000 evaluated 10 controlled clinical trials (645 subjects) involving HM[25]. The studies all had active controls and no placebo-controlled studies were found. HM was the active control in six studies using different prescribing regimes, routes and formulations. Morphine was used as the control in three studies and oxycodone the control in one study. Six studies used a 'double-dummy' design. A cross-over model was used in eight of the trials. Pain intensity, need for rescue analgesia and adverse effects were the primary outcome measures in eight studies. Two studies, by the same author, chose relative potency and equianalgesic dose ratios as the primary endpoints[11]. Eight studies assessed pain using a 10-cm or 100-mm visual analogue scale (VAS), with or without a verbal rating score (VRS). The results of the review were as follows.

Hydromorphone versus morphine

Two studies, from the same research group, compared oral controlled-release HM and oral controlled-release morphine sulfate[26,27]. These two studies included a total of 138 evaluable patients. The dose of HM was based on the assumption that HM is 7.5 times more potent than morphine. The larger study, involving 89 patients, did not find any significant difference between any of the outcome measures (pain VAS, pain VRS, nausea/sedation VAS, nausea/sedation VRS) for either group[26]. However, pain scores were generally low, with overall pain VAS less than 11 mm. Seventy-nine per cent (70 patients) did not require rescue analgesia with either treatment. Similarly, adverse effects were mild and infrequent.

The second study, involving 49 patients with cancer pain, reported significantly higher pain scores with HM[27]. In addition, significantly more doses of rescue analgesia were required by patients in the HM group. Overall pain scores were low, being less than 2/10 throughout the study. Withdrawals were higher in the HM group (16 versus two) due to either inadequate analgesia or adverse effects. Diarrhea was a significant problem in the HM group. There were no significant differences in other adverse effects between both groups.

Earlier studies compared intramuscular HM and morphine in 48 patients with cancer pain[11]. The endpoint was to determine equianalgesic doses of both drugs. It was concluded that 1.3 mg of HM was equivalent to 10 mg of morphine in terms of analgesia and adverse effects. HM appeared to be shorter acting, but demonstrated a higher peak effect. This study was not reported as blinded.

A recent Irish study has compared continuous subcutaneous infusion (CSCI) of HM and morphine in 74 terminally ill patients cared for in the palliative care setting[28]. The study found HM to be at least as effective as morphine when delivered by CSCI. Adverse effects were rare and similar in both groups. Because the patients were dying, a proxy usually completed the assessments.

HM versus oxycodone

One study compared oral sustained release oxycodone and HM[29]. There were no significant differences between pain outcomes (overall pain VAS 28 mm for oxycodone, 30.6 mm for HM), rescue analgesia and adverse effects (sedation VAS 23.6 mm for oxycodone, 18.2 mm for HM; nausea VAS 15.5 mm for oxycodone, 13.1 mm for HM). Two patients reported hallucinations with HM.

HM as active control

Two studies compared HM immediate-release formulation with controlled-release formulation[30,31]. Both formulations were reported as being equally efficacious. There were no significant differences in adverse effects. In the first study, classic opioid adverse effects, such as nausea, constipation and drowsiness were observed in an open follow-up phase[30]. No patient withdrew as a result of adverse effects.

An earlier paper by the same investigators compared patient controlled (PCA) subcutaneous (s.c.) bolus HM injections with CSCI HM[32]. Adequate analgesia was reported with both regimes, with a similar total daily dose of HM required with both continuous and bolus administration. There was no significant difference in patient preference between groups. A controlled cross-over study of eight patients similarly compared PCA HM with CSCI HM[33]. Pain intensity was similar for both groups. However, the PCA group required less HM to achieve an equivalent degree of analgesia.

A randomized, double-blind, double-dummy study compared CSCI HM with i.v. infusion of HM in 20 patients[34]. Both routes provided a significant improvement in analgesia. There was no difference between groups in terms of analgesia, side effects and rescue analgesia.

Oral and intramuscular (i.m.) HM have been compared in a randomized, double-blind, cross-over study of 96 patients with chronic cancer pain[11]. The aim of the study was to determine the potency ratio between both routes. Intramuscular HM was reported as being five times more potent than oral HM. Adverse effects, such as sleepiness and nausea, were dose-related. At equianalgesic doses more side effects were observed with i.m. administration.

The limited number of studies available suggests that there is little difference between HM and morphine in terms of analgesic efficacy, adverse effect profile and patient preference. However, as most studies involved small numbers of patients, it is difficult to determine real differences between both drugs.

The issue of equianalgesic ratios between morphine and hydromorphone was not resolved by the Cochrane review. The potency ratio for hydromorphone: morphine has been variously reported as between 3 : 1 and 7.5 : 1[26,35–38]. It has been suggested that the direction of the switch is important, HM being more potent than morphine when given second (5 : 1) than when it is given first[38].

The Scottish Cancer pain guidelines[39] recommend that HM should be considered as a useful alternative in patients if morphine is causing drowsiness or cognitive impairment despite careful titration with morphine or is otherwise poorly tolerated[2]. Furthermore, they posit that HM is approximately 7.5 times as potent as morphine and has similar pharmacokinetic properties[26].

Dose and routes

+ Instant release tablets: 2, 4 and 8 mg.
+ Oral instant release liquid: 1 mg/ml.
+ Rectal suppositories: 3 mg.
+ Ampoules for injection: 2 and 10 mg/ml, 50 mg/5 ml and 500 mg/50 ml (vial).

References

1 Steinberg SK, Kornijenko M. The role of hydromorphone in the treatment of cancer pain. *Canad Pharm J* 1988; **121**(**March**): 182–6.

2 de Stoutz ND, Bruera E, Suarez-Almazor M. Opioid rotation for toxicity reduction in terminal cancer patients. *J Pain Sympt Manag* 1995; **10**: 378–84.

3 Angst MS, Drover DR, Lotsch J *et al.* Pharmacodynamics of orally administered sustained-release hydromorphone in humans. *Anesthesiology* 2001; **94**(**1**): 63–73.

4 Miller RR. Clinical effects of parenteral narcotics in hospitalised medical patients. *J Clin Pharmacol* 1980; **20**: 165–71.

5 Porter J, Jick H. Addiction is rare in patients treated with narcotics. *N Engl J Med* 1980; **302**: 123.

6 Murphy MR, Hug CC. Pharmacokinetics of intravenous morphine in patients anaesthetized with enflurane-nitrous oxide. *Anesthesiology* 1981; **54**: 187–92.

7 Coyle DE, Parab PV, Streng WH *et al.* Is hydromorphone more lipid soluble than morphine? *Anesthesiology* 1984; **61**: A240.

8 Cone EJ, Phelps BA, Gorodetzky CW. Urinary excretion of hydromorphone and metabolites in humans, rats, dogs, guinea pigs, and rabbits. *J Pharm Sci* 1977; **66**: 1709–1713.

9 Smith MT. Neuroexcitatory effects of morphine and hydromorphone: evidence implicating the 3-glucuronide metabolites. *Clin Exp Pharmacol Physiol* 2000; **27**: 524–8.

10 Vallner JJ, Stewart JT, Kotzan JA, *et al.* Pharmacokinetics and bioavailability of hydromorphone following intravenous and oral administration to human subjects. *J Clin Pharmacol* 1981; **21:** 152–6.

11 Houde RW. Clinical analgesic studies of hydromorphone. In: Foley KM, Inturrisi CE (Eds) *Advances in Pain Research and Therapy*, Vol. 8. New York: Raven Press, 1986, pp. 129–35.

12 Lesser GJ, Grossman SA, Leong KW, *et al. In vitro* and *in vivo* studies of subcutaneous hydromorphone implants designed for the treatment of cancer pain. *Pain* 1996; **65:** 265–72.

13 Chaplan SR, Duncan SR, Brodsky JB *et al.* Morphine and hydromorphone epidural analgesia. *Anesthesiology* 1992; **77:** 1090–4.

14 Goodarzi M. Comparison of epidural morphine, hydromorphone and fentanyl for post-operative pain control in children undergoing orthopaedic surgery. *Paediat Anaesth* 1999; **9:** 419–22.

15 Cohen SE, Rothblatt AJ, Albright GA. Early respiratory depression with epidural narcotic and intravenous droperidol. *Anesthesiology* 1983; **59:** 559–60.

16 Walker SE, DeAngelis C, Iazzetta J. Stability and compatibility of combinations of hydromorphone with a second drug. Can J Hosp Pharm 1991; **44:** 289–95.

17 Fudin J, Smith HS, Toledo-Binette CS, *et al.* Use of continuous ambulatory infusions of concentrated subcutaneous (s.q.) hydromorphone versus intravenous (i.v.) morphine: cost implications for palliative care. *Am J Hospice Palliat Care* 2000; **17:** 347–53.

18 Product Information. *Dilaudid-HP, hydromorphone hydrochloride.* Mount Olive: Knoll Pharmaceuticals, revised October 1999, reviewed March 2002.

19 Siberry GK, Iannone R. *Formulary: hydromorphone HCl. The Harriet Lane Handbook.* St. Louis: Mosby Inc., 2000, pp. 735–6.

20 Koren G, Maurice L. Pediatric uses of opioids. *Pediat Clin N Am* 1989; **36:** 1141–56.

21 Collins J, Grier H, Weinstein H *et al.* Patient-controlled analgesia for mucositis pain in children: a three-period crossover study comparing morphine and hydromorphone. *J Pediat* 1996; **129:** 722–8.

22 Jacox A, Carr D, Payne R. New clinical practice guidelines for the management of pain in patients with cancer. *N Engl J Med* 1993; **330:** 651–5.

23 Hanna C, Mazuzan JE, Abajian J. An evaluation of dihydromorphinone in treating post-operative pain. *Anesth Analg* 1962; **41:** 755–61.

24 Chen ZR, Irvine RJ, Somogyi AA, *et al.* Mu-receptor binding of some commonly used opioids and their metabolites. *Life Sci* 1991; **48:** 2165–71.

25 Quigley C. *Hydromorphone for acute and chronic pain* (Cochrane Review), The Cochrane Library, Issue 4. Chichester: John Wiley & Sons Ltd, 2003.

26 Moriarty M, McDonald CJ, Miller AJ. A randomised crossover comparison of controlled release hydromorphone tablets with controlled release morphine tablets in patients with cancer pain. *J Clin Res* 1999; **2:** 1–8.

27 Napp Laboratories. *A Comparative Efficacy and Tolerability Study of Palladone Capsules and MST Continus Tablets in Patients with Cancer Pain.* Edinburgh: Royal College of Physicians.

28 Miller MG, McCarthy N, O'Boyle CA, *et al.* Continuous subcutaneous infusion of morphine vs. hydromorphone: a controlled trial. *J Pain Sympt Manag* 1999; **18:** 9–16.

29 Hagen NA, Babul N. Comparative clinical efficacy and safety of a novel controlled-release oxycodone formulation and controlled-release hydromorphone in the treatment of cancer pain. *Cancer* 1997; **79:** 1428–37.

30 Bruera E, Sloan P, Mount B, *et al.* A randomized, double-blind, double-dummy, crossover trial comparing the safety and efficacy of oral sustained-release hydromorphone with immediate-release hydromorphone in patients with cancer pain. *J Clin Oncol* 1996; **14:** 1713–17.

31 Hays H, Hagen N, Thirlwell M, *et al.* Comparative clinical efficacy and safety of immediate release and controlled release hydromorphone for chronic severe cancer pain. *Cancer* 1994; **74:** 1808–16.

32 Bruera E, Brenneis C, Michaud M, *et al.* Patient-controlled subcutaneous infusion for the treatment of cancer pain. *J Nat Cancer Inst* 1988; **80:** 1152–4.

33 Vanier MC, Labrecque G, Lepage-Savary D, *et al.* Comparison of hydromorphone continuous subcutaneous infusion and basal rate subcutaneous infusion plus PCA in cancer pain: a pilot study. *Pain* 1993; **53:** 27–32.

34 Moulin DE, Kreeft JH, Murray-Parsons N, *et al.* Comparison of continuous subcutaneous and intravenous hydromorphone infusions for management of cancer pain. *Lancet* 1991; **337:** 465–8.

35 Keeri-Szanto M. Drugs or drums: what relieves postoperative pain. *Pain* 1979; **6(2):** 217–30.

36 Dunbar PJ, Chapman CR, Gavrin JR. Clinical analgesic equivalence for morphine and hydromorphone with prolonged PCA. *Pain* 1996; **68:** 265–70.

37 Bruera E, Pereira J, Watanabe S, *et al.* Opioid rotation in patients with cancer pain. A retrospective comparison of dose ratios between methadone, hydromorphone and morphine. *Cancer* 1996; **78:** 852–7.

38 Lawlor P, Turner K, Hanson J, *et al.* Dose ratio between morphine and hydromorphone in patients with cancer pain: a retrospective study. *Pain* 1997; **72:** 79–85.

39 Scottish Intercollegiate Guideline Network. Control of Pain in Patients with Cancer, SIGN publication no. 44, June 2000. Available at: www.sign.ac.uk. Accessed 9 September, 2004.

Chapter 10

Oxycodone

Mellar P. Davis

Introduction

Oxycodone (14-hydroxy-7,8-di-hydrocodeinone) is a semisynthetic thebaine derivative that has been in clinical use since 1917. Oxycodone was originally formulated with non-steroidal anti-inflammatory agents. In 1981 oxycodone became available in the USA as a single agent and, by 1996, a sustained-release (SR) double matrix product became commercially available. The total dose of oxycodone was limited by the non-steroidal anti-inflammatory drug in the original formulation and, as a result, oxycodone classified as a step II or weak opioid. The availability of immediate release oxycodone without a non-steroidal anti-inflammatory drug lead to its use for severe pain as a potent opioid without dose limitations, and the SR added form further convenience and improved compliance[1].

Pharmacodynamics

The analgesic activity of oxycodone is mediated to a certain extent by kappa opioid receptors as demonstrated in Sprague–Dawley rats[2]. Anti-nociceptive testing in Dark Agouti rats using the tail flick latency test demonstrated the pain-relieving properties of oxycodone were mediated by a distinctively different opioid receptor subtypes than morphine[3]. Subanalgesic doses of morphine and oxycodone produce pronounced antinociceptive activity in these experimental animals with less sedation than equivalent doses of either opioid alone[4]. In the same rat model (Sprague–Dawley) nociceptive activity of oxycodone was selectively blocked by kappa receptor antagonists, which was not seen with morphine[4].

Oxycodone was originally reported to have analgesic potency close to morphine. By competitive binding assays using ^{3}H-DAMGO (a specific opioid agonist) the inhibitory constant (K_i) for oxycodone was 47.4 nmol, but only 1.2 nmol for morphine demonstrating a greater affinity to the mu opioid receptor (MOR) by morphine. This difference in *in vitro* binding affinity, and analgesia between oxycodone and morphine may be explained by:

- the kappa opioid receptor (KOR) binding activity of oxycodone;
- species specific differences in oxycodone binding of metabolism;

- difference in opioid binding affinities and receptor activation between oxycodone and morphine;

- the presences of potent MOR binding oxycodone metabolite[5].

Metabolites derived from oxycodone, noroxycodone and oxymorphone, are MOR[6]. The relative MOR potency of noroxycodone to oxycodone for MOR is 0.17 in the Sprague–Dawley rat model. Noroxycodone is also capable of inducing a neuroexcitatory response in animals that are not reversed by naloxone[7]. An unidentified metabolite of oxycodone, which is neither noroxycodone or oxymorphone has a strong affinity to MOR[8–10]. The analgesic potency of oxycodone diminishes relative to morphine when converting from oral to parenteral dosing, and this is perhaps due to the loss of oxycodone metabolism to this unidentified metabolite[8–10]. Although oxymorphone has 14 times the potency of oxycodone for MOR, it accounts for only 2% of oxycodone metabolites and thus plays little if any role in pain relief[11]. Oxycodone pain responses do not correlate with oxymorphone production; nor is it associated with oxymorphone plasma levels. The intrinsic efficacy of oxycodone (the ability of oxycodone to activate opioid receptors independent of the receptors' affinity) is essentially unknown[12].

Although some oxycodone pharmacodynamic effects (such as pupil size) correlate with oxycodone levels, pain response does not[11,13]. Most studies demonstrate wide differences in oxycodone pharmacodynamic between individuals that are not accounted for by changes in oxycodone metabolism.

Similar to most opioids, oxycodone increases prolactin levels, but oxycodone's influence on testosterone levels is unknown. In animal studies, oxycodone can induce mast cells to degranulate causing histamine release[14]. Oxycodone, unlike morphine, is devoid of immunosuppressive effects as measured by natural killer cell activity and interleukin 2 production *in vitro*[15].

Pharmacokinetics

Absorption

Immediate release oxycodone has monoexponential absorption rates and SR oxycodone is bi-exponential SR oxycodone has an initial half-life of 37 min accounting for 38% of the dose and a second half-life of 6.2 h accounting for 62% of the dose. Overall the bioavailability of immediate release oxycodone and SR oxycodone is the same[16,17,18]. Oxycodone elixirs have pharmacokinetics that are influenced by a high fat meal, whereas the SR form is not altered by diet. There is an increase in the bioavailability of oxycodone elixir by 20% as measured by the area under curve (AUC; confidence intervals 109–132%) and a reduced maximum serum concentration to 18% (confidence interval 47–91%) compared with a non-fat meal. The clinical relevance of these mild changes due to high fat meal is unknown, but should not influence the timing or dose whether given with meals or not[19]. Sustained-release oxycodone has less variability between individuals in oral bioavailability relative to SR morphine as measured by maximum and minimal values in AUC[20].

The high oral bioavailability (60–87%) of oxycodone is due to reduced first pass hepatic clearance related to the 3-methoxy group on oxycodone and not due to increased absorption[8,9,21–23]. As a result of its high oral bioavailability, the conversion ratios from oral to parenteral oxycodone is 2 : 1[10,23,24]. However, there may be diurnal variations in oxycodone bioavailability with low peak and trough levels occurring in the afternoon[17]. There is probably little clinical relevance to this minor alteration in bioavailability.

Variation in absorption has been claimed to be due to gender and age. Elderly individuals and females have a higher oxycodone bioavailability compared with younger patients and males. Oxymorphone levels are inversely related to oxycodone levels in older individuals and females, which may be due to reduced CYP2D6 activity in older individuals and females and first pass hepatic metabolism in both groups[11,25].

A buccal adhesive oxycodone disk preparation containing glycerol, sorbitol and gelatin has been developed, but is not commercially available. Absorption appears to be similar to oral immediate release oxycodone as measured by drug half-life, maximum plasma concentrations and AUC in studies of cancer patients. It is assumed that mucosal oxycodone is absorbed through the mucosal membranes, rather by swallowing[26]. It is this author's opinion that the kinetics described in this study suggest that the most likely route of absorption is by swallowing the dissolved opioid.

Sublingual oxycodone at normal mucosal pH (pH of 6.5) is not well absorbed. The absorption of oxycodone sublingual at a pH of 7.43 is only 15% (22.5% for morphine and 25% for hydromorphone)[27,28]. Theoretically, delivering oxycodone in an alkaline solution may improve absorption, since the pKa of oxycodone is 8.3. Akaline solutions would increase the percentage of unionized, thereby favoring absorption.

Nasal absorption of medication is largely independent of lipid solubility. The nasal mucosa capillaries are fenestrated and lack elastic membrane. The olfactory perineural spaces are intimately connected to subarachnoid spaces. A relatively high blood flow to volume is found within the nasal cavity, which is distinctly different to blood flow to volume ratios involving sublingual and buccal surfaces. Intranasal oxycodone is 46 ± 34% bioavailable and has a time to maximum plasma concentration of 25 min, but with large individual variability[29,30]. Rectal oxycodone bioavailability is 61%, which is similar to oral oxycodone. There is greater individual variability in absorption (+30%, range 16.4–126.8%) with a rectal route when compared with the oral route. Administration of oxycodone in a pectinate suppository produces sustained-release kinetics. Analgesia occurs in 30 min, but peak plasma concentrations are delayed to 2.8 h after administration[8]. The variability in maximum concentration is large amongst individuals (37.2–100.8 mcg/l) for the same dose, which may have more to do with route than type of preparation. In another study, the AUC for equivalent dose was the same for rectal oxycodone and morphine. The mean time to onset of analgesia is 0.52 ± 0.33 h for oral and 0.76 ± 0.47 h for rectal oxycodone[13,22].

Topical oxycodone has been reported to reduce pain when applied to skin ulcers associated sickle cell disease. No information about oxycodone plasma levels after topical application is available[31].

Intrabursal oxycodone after orthopedic surgery reduces pain similar to parenteral oxycodone, but with significantly lower plasma levels[32].

Metabolism

Oxycodone is metabolized to noroxycodone, its major metabolite, by N-demethylation, which does not involve the cytochrome enzyme CYP2D6[11,32]. Therefore, quinidine, a potent blocker of CYP2D6 activity, does not reduce noroxycodone levels[11]. Oxycodone plasma levels will normally exceed those of noroxycodone. The maximum plasma concentration of oxycodone and noroxycodone are 23.2 ± 8.6 ng/ml and 15.2 ± 4.5 ng/ml, respectively, for 20 mg of SR oxycodone. The AUC is 236 ± 102 ng/h/ml and 233 ± 102 ng/h/ml, respectively, for the same oxycodone dose. Noroxycodone production is less with parenteral administration of oxycodone indicating that the major source of noroxycodone comes from liver metabolism[21].

Oxymorphone is produced by O-demethylation (at position 3) through the cytochrome enzyme CYP2D6. Patients who are poor metabolizers (CYP2D6 4, 5 or 6) or who are receiving medications that block CYP2D6, such as quinidine, fluoxetine or paroxetine, or are female produce lower levels of oxymorphone[25,32]. Oxymorphone is produced in such small quantities that, despite its high analgesic potency it plays little role in the pain relief and side effects associated with oxycodone[8,32]. Oxymorphone's maximum concentration after 20 mg of SR oxycodone is 0.82 ± 0.85 ng/ml and the AUC is 12.3 ± 12 ng/h/ml that is less than 5% of the AUC of oxycodone. Oxymorphone once formed is glucuronidated before it is excreted.

A small portion of oxycodone undergoes a 6-keto reduction to 6-oxycodal. Oxycodone, though a weak base (pKa of 8.3), binds to albumin rather than alpha$_1$ acid glycoprotein. It has similar lipid solubility to morphine[33]. The mean partition co-efficient (reflection of lipid solubility) for oxycodone is 0.5 (octanol to water drug partition) and is 0.7 for morphine[34]. At physiological pH and temperature, the mean protein binding is 45% (+0.4%) as compared with morphine, which is 35 ± 0.2%[22]. In other studies, oxycodone protein binding was 38%[34]. It is unlikely that there will be significant change in oxycodone kinetics through competitive drug interactions at albumin protein binding sites.

Oxycodone's mean elimination half-life of 3.5 ± 1.43 h is independent of the route of administration (rectal, parenteral or oral). The volume of distribution is approximately 3 l/kg (211 ± 186 l in a 70-kg individual). Oxycodone has a plasma clearance of 48.6 ± 26.5 l/h[13,21,22]. The oxycodone pharmacokinetics in children approximates those of adults[35]. Although there does not appear to be any saturation to oxycodone clearance with dose, there are large individual variations in pharmacokinetics as seen in the volume of distribution and plasma clearance[36]. As a result, the maximum to minimum oxycodone concentration ratios (c-max to c-min) are similar to morphine[10,11,22]. Variations in the c-max to c-min ratio occur regardless of the route of administration and can range from 1.5 to 5.4. The individual differences in kinetics results in as wide a difference in plasma levels per dose as morphine has among individuals[9,37].

Renal elimination

Eight to 14% of oxycodone dose is excreted in the urine either unchanged or as a conjugated form of the parent drug. The oxymorphone metabolite is excreted predominately as a glucuronidated metabolite and noroxycodone is excreted mostly unconjugated[11,21]. Noroxycodone clearance is dependent upon renal function to a greater extent than oxycodone.

Routes of administration

The pharmacokinetics of immediate release and equal doses of SR oxycodone are the same in randomized double-blind cross-over trials involving cancer patients[18]. The pharmacokinetics of two 10-mg SRd oxycodone tablets are equivalent to one 20-mg SR tablet[38]. A double-blind cross-over trial involving normal individuals demonstrated similar pharmacokinetics for immediate release oxycodone by mouth, by oral solution and SR oxycodone, all of which were in 20 mg doses[16]. The same is true for the oral bioavailability of immediate release oxycodone in a 10-mg dose, in solution and in SR oxycodone also in a 10-mg dose in normal individuals[17].

The relative analgesic potency of epidural oxycodone compared with morphine is 1 to 8–10[39]. The loss of oxycodone analgesic potency with epidural administration may be related to the relative lack of kappa receptors in the dorsal horn for an important yet unidentified oxycodone metabolite needed for pain relief and requiring liver metabolism[10].

Equivalence with other opioids

Morphine

Oral oxycodone analgesic potency relative to morphine has been published to be 1.5 : 2[1,6,11,25]. Many of these studies have potential statistical problems due to small numbers of patients and large confidence intervals. In addition, the order of rotation influences appears to influence equivalence. The dose ratio of oxycodone to morphine is 2 : 3 if morphine is given first and 3 : 4 if oxycodone is given initially. A study by Glare found a ratio of 1 : 1 when rotating from oxycodone to morphine, but it was reported to be 1.5 in other studies[40–42]. The maximum potency ratio is 2.3 : 1 and the minimum is 1 : 1 (morphine to oxycodone) as published in the literature. Noted with each study was a large individual variation in dosing rates, wide confidence intervals and a small group size[40–42]. This is similar to postoperative patients where the potency of oxycodone relative morphine is 1.8 with confidence intervals of 1.09 to 2.42 : 1 and for peak effect 2.2 with confidence intervals of 0.9–4.59[43]. In a relatively large trial involving 100 consecutive patients the mean daily SR oxycodone dose was 101 mg (range 40–360 mg) and for SR morphine the daily dose was 140 mg (range 60 to 300 mg) with similar breakthrough dose requirement and acceptability among patients.

Gender differences in oxycodone metabolism play a minor role in the variability of equivalence between oxycodone and morphine. Women receiving oxycodone have a 41% greater AUC and a 35% greater maximum plasma concentration compared with men when controlled for body weight[11]. The overall clearance was 25% lower for women[11]. Pharmacodynamics as measured by pupil size and respiratory rate correlated with oxycodone levels[11,23]. There is little data to suggest gender differences in oxycodone analgesia as there is little correlation between pain relief and oxycodone plasma levels.

There is also a diversity of oxycodone to morphine equivalence for parenteral oxycodone. Oxycodone is reported to be more potent relative to morphine for postoperative pain. Doses for pain relief postoperatively were 13 mg of oxycodone compared with 25 mg for morphine[43]. After breast reconstructive surgery and back surgery, morphine dose of 45 mcg/kg produced the same degree of pain relief as an oxycodone dose of 30 mcg/kg[44]. However, in cancer pain, the relative parenteral to oxycodone ratio is 0.71[10,24,45]. The confidence intervals for relative parenteral potencies between oxycodone and morphine are quite wide. For total analgesic effect, the potency ratio ranges from 0.32 to 1.07, while for peak analgesic effect the potency ratio ranges from 0.12 to 2.67[24]. In a small number of cancer patients[8], Gagnon and colleagues found that 91 ± 81 mg of subcutaneous morphine was equivalent to 75 ± 39 mg of subcutaneous oxycodone for an overall ratio of 1.2 : 1[46]. The reliability of potencies in equivalent ratios, which are given in the literature, must be taken as a rough estimate in light of the small numbers of patients studied and the wide individual differences in equivalence[1].

Oral oxycodone is 7–9.5 times more potent than oral codeine and parenteral oxycodone is 10–12 times more potent than parenteral codeine[1]. Parenteral tramadol dose of 0.6 mcg/kg produces comparable analgesia to a dose of 0.04 mcg/kg of parenteral oxycodone. Oxycodone, however, produces a greater degree of respiratory depression than tramadol dose for equivalent analgesia[47]. In a group of 31 cancer patients, SR oxycodone doses of 120 ± 22 mg were equivalent to SR hydromorphone doses of 24 ± 4 mg. The final mean oxycodone dose was 124 ± 24 mg and hydromorphone dose was 30 ± 6 mg[48]. The overall potency ratio is 0.25 comparing oxycodone with hydromorphone. No comparison has been made between oxycodone and methadone, or between oxycodone and fentanyl. Equivalents for oxycodone have been established through morphine equivalents and may be inaccurate[1,49]. An oral transmucosal fentanyl dose of 10 mcg/kg was equivalent to the oral oxycodone dose of 0.2 mcg/kg in a study involving 22 pediatric patients treated in a burn unit[50].

There appears to be no major advantage of SR oxycodone over SR morphine or methadone, or significant patient preference for SR oxycodone over the other long-acting opioids. The adverse side effects were similar as found in four randomized trials. The major disadvantages of SR oxycodone are its cost and, as a result, SR morphine and/or methadone are preferred as long-acting opioids[49].

Drug interactions

There are a number of drug interactions with oxycodone, which appear to be clinically important. Quinidine, paroxetine and fluoxetine are strong inhibitors of CYP2D6 metabolism[51]. It is thought that the inhibition of CYP2D6 might lead to oxycodone toxicity, yet quinidine combined with oxycodone does not alter levels of side effects[33]. There is no difference in psychomotor responses or subjective drug effects with oxycodone related to CYP2D6 activity. Fluoxetine, like quinidine, prevents the demethylation of oxycodone to oxymorphone, but side effects do not appear to be greater with the combination of the two drugs[52]. Paradoxically, sertraline with oxycodone has been associated with hallucinations and tremor in patients receiving increasing doses of oxycodone, although sertraline does not block CYP2D6 activity[53,54].

Unlike morphine, oxycodone does not interact with amitriptyline, cirprofloxacin or levoquin[8,11,55]. Oxycodone delays the time to maximum concentrations of gatifloxacin from 1.8 ± 0.8 h to 4.3 ± 1.5 h, but does not decrease its overall bioavailability, nor does it appear to be clinically relevant[55]. Oxycodone does reduce the oral bioavailability of cyclosporin in half[56]. Ritonavir influences oxycodone kinetics perhaps through CYP2D6 metabolism. Rifampicin may increase oxycodone clearance but the documentation for this interaction is not as definite as morphine's interaction with rifampicin[57].

Adverse effects

Individuals who have the genotype CYP2D6 alleles 3, 4 and 5 are said to be more susceptible to oxycodone toxicity[58]. Side effects are similar to other opioids, and include confusion, constipation, dizziness, dry mouth, nausea, pruritus, somnolence and vomiting[1,9]. Side effects appear to be related to levels of oxycodone, but not to levels of oxymorphone[11]. As a result, there is little evidence that the CYP2D6 geneotype influences toxicity. Oxycodone neurological side effects are more cognitive than motor (myoclonus) and hallucinations are reported less frequently with oxycodone than with morphine[8,10]. Morphine is more often associated with nightmares where oxycodone is not[41]. Morphine neurotoxicity, such as delirium, resolves when rotating from morphine to oxycodone[59–61]. In normal volunteers, reaction time, vigilance, attention, body balance, and the coordination of extraocular and muscle performance diminishes to the greatest extent around the time of maximum plasma concentrations (1.5 h). Mental slowness and impairment are still present at 4.5 h after the initial dose. However, these single dose toxicity studies were performed in normal individuals and may not apply to patients on chronic oxycodone who have cancer pain[62].

Nausea and vomiting with oxycodone occurs more frequently in women[11,63]. In comparison with morphine, oxycodone is more constipating, produces less vomiting, but has similar levels of nausea[41]. In another series, there was less nausea with oxycodone than with morphine, while a further series found the frequency of gastrointestinal toxicity comparable to that of morphine[10,64]. Vomiting has been reported to be less with SR oxycodone as compared with immediate release oxycodone[65]. In another series of patients, the frequency of nausea with SR oxycodone was the same as immediate release[18]. Nausea and vomiting occurs with greater frequency using parenteral oxycodone compared with using oral oxycodone[9,22]. Nausea was found to be greater with rectal oxycodone than with oral oxycodone[9,13,22].

Bile duct pressures are increased by oxycodone as with other opioids, which can lead to colicky pain with bile duct obstruction[66].

Parenteral oxycodone produces greater respiratory depression with a dose of 0.05 mg/kg bolus and 0.275 mg/kg/h than morphine does with a dose of 0.039 mg/kg bolus and 0.215 mg/kg/h infusion[67]. There is also a greater respiratory depression with parenteral oxycodone at a dose of 0.04 mg/kg compared with parenteral tramadol (0.6 mg/kg)[47]. Oxycodone produced greater respiratory depression in children than other opioids[35]. However, this was not a randomized comparison.

Oxycodone accounts for only 3.3% of drug deaths due to drug abuse. Most drug oxycodone deaths are related to polysubstance abuse (benzodiazepines, alcohol, cocaine and other opioids, marijuana and antidepressants)[68,69]. Fatal oxycodone concentrations found at postmortem vary widely[70,71]. By case report, respiratory depression from massive doses of SR oxycodone could not be reversed by naloxone. Intravenous injections of dissolved oxycodone suppositories has been described, and produce a fibrillary glomerolopathy and chronic renal failure[72]. Oxycodone abuse during pregnancy causes a neonatal withdrawal syndromes due to transplacental absorption of oxycodone[73]. The detection of this drug and its metabolites in urine requires special procedures and a special order by the physician if abuse is suspected[73]. However, there is no data from clinical trials to suspect that oxycodone is more addicting than any other opioid[74].

Special populations

Liver failure and cirrhosis

The first pass hepatic clearance of oxycodone is less than that of morphine and, as a result, oxycodone's bioavailability will be influenced less by the reduced hepatic blood flow associated with cirrhosis than morphine. However, oxycodone elimination is significantly influenced by hepatic impairment. The maximum concentration of oxycodone is 40% higher in hepatic impairment and the AUC is 90% greater as compared with normal individuals with comparable age, weight, height, gender and race[25,75]. The half-life of oxycodone is prolonged by 2 h, peak oxymorphone levels are 15% lower and the AUC is 50% higher in hepatic impairment reflecting reduced activity of CYP2D6[25]. Patients with end stage liver disease will have the half-life of oxycodone prolonged to 14 h (prior to transplant), which can range from 4.6 to 24 h and returns to normal after transplant (range 2.6–5.1 h). Oxycodone clearance will increase from 0.26 l/min pretransplant to 1.3 l/min post-transplant. Hence, oxycodone will be associated with a significant risk for respiratory depression in the pretransplanted patient. Doses will need to be reduced in half for mild or moderate hepatic cirrhosis[75,76].

Renal failure

Despite a normally low oxycodone renal clearance, its elimination is impaired in the uremic patient. Plasma oxycodone and noroxycodone increase and renal clearance is delayed. Oxycodone concentrations, even 4.5–6 h after oral dosing, are higher in uremic patients as compared with normal individuals[77]. In uremia, the half-life, volume of distribution and the central compartment of oxycodone are all increased. The AUC of noroxycodone relative to oxycodone is also increased from the normal of 0.41–1.22 indicating that noroxycodone clearance has a greater sensitivity to renal failure than oxycodone. The recovery of unconjugated oxycodone and noroxycodone in urine is greatly reduced. The conjugated metabolites of oxycodone are not affected by renal disease[77]. Yet, oxymorphone and its conjugated metabolites are affected by renal disease, and are eliminated very poorly. Individual variations in oxycodone kinetics with renal failure are greater than in individuals with normal renal function. Oxycodone's half-life is 3.9 h, but can range from 1.8 to 26 h. In normal renal function, half-life is 2.3 h with a range of 1.3–4 h[77]. One of the causes for reduced oxycodone clearance in renal failure is uremia-induced suppression of hepatic CYP2D6 activity, although this is speculative[78].

The elderly

The bioavailability of oxycodone is increased by 15% in the elderly[79]. This increase in bioavailability is related to changes in hepatic blood flow, in the volume of distribution and in renal function, rather than the changes of CYP2D6 activity, even though there is some evidence that CYP2D6 activity gradually diminishes with age[80,81]. The changes in oxycodone kinetics with aging are such that it is unlikely to influence doses or intervals in the healthy elderly.

Oxycodone for cancer pain

Case reports and prospective cohort trials

A single case report was used to illustrate equipotency between morphine and oxycodone. A 31-year-old was converted from a SR oxycodone dose of 300 mg every 12 h and 50 mg every 2 h as needed, to a parenteral morphine dose of 15 mg/h and 15 mg each h as needed. For this patient, 3 mg of oral oxycodone was equivalent to 1 mg of parenteral morphine when pain was controlled[82].

In a prospective non-randomized study involving 944 cancer patients receiving combination analgesics (codeine 60 mg plus acetaminophen, oxycodone 5 mg plus acetaminophen, dextropropoxyphene 90 mg plus acetaminophen, buprenorphine 0.2 mg plus acetaminophen and pentazocine), 34% received an oxycodone combination analgesic[83]. The mean daily oxycodone dose in this study was 20 mg limited by acetaminophen. As a result, two-thirds of the patients required rotation to non-compounded potent opioids by week 4 of the study. One-third of the patients continued to have their pain controlled by week 4. Side effects to the combination analgesic included dry mouth (33%), drowsiness (31%), constipation (24%), sweating (20%), agitation (20%), trembling (12%) and pruritus (10%), which were related to the opioid and not to acetaminophen. There was no differences in side effects between the opioids[83].

A prospective dose finding study reported by Glare involved 24 cancer patients.[40] Twenty patients completed the study. The age range was from 26 to 78 years. Patients received immediate release oxycodone every 4 h with rescue doses of 25–50% of the four-hourly dose as needed. Pain control and total doses were reviewed every 24–48 h. Efficacy was determined by use of the visual analog scale (VAS) and verbal rating scale (VRS). Most study participants were taking compounded analgesics prior to the beginning of the study. The median starting dose was 15 mg every h with a range of 5–30 mg and, at completion of the study, the dose was 20 mg every 4 h with a range of 15–60 mg. Doses for those less than 65 years of age were 45 mg every 4 h and patients who age was greater than 65 years received doses of 20 mg every 4 h. This was not statistically significant. The median VAS pain relief was 7.6 ± 1.5 cm (the scale being 0 for no pain relief, to 10 for complete pain relief). The median number rescue doses per day were 1.8 during the titration phase and 0.7 during the stable phase. Ten patients required rotation from oxycodone to parenteral morphine and the relative potency in these patients were 1.0. Adverse effects included mild sedation, constipation in 13, and nausea and vomiting in 8. Side effects appeared to be unrelated to oxycodone dose. Three patients experienced dose limiting side effects and the rest were rotated because of their for reasons of inability to swallow. Most patients preferred oxycodone to morphine when asked[40].

Leow and colleagues performed an open-labeled prospective trial in 12 cancer patients, one being opioid naïve[13]. Patients received parenteral or rectal oxycodone and pharmacokinetics were performed. Parenteral doses were 0.11 mg/kg and rectal doses were 30 mg in a pectinate base suppository. Patients with liver function abnormalities received reduced doses. Pain was measured by VAS (0–100 with 0 indicating no pain and 100 indicating the worst pain imaginable). Pharmacokinetics included oxycodone half-life, clearance and volume of distribution, which was the same regardless of route. Not surprisingly, pain relief was quicker with parenteral oxycodone. There was a 25% reduction in the baseline VAS by 5–8 min with parenteral injection. The same degree of analgesia was experienced 1–2 h after rectal oxycodone. Analgesia lasted longer with the pectinate suppository (8 h) compared with the parenteral bolus (4 h). There was no correlation with amount of pain relief and oxycodone plasma levels. Individual variability in dose and response was as great with oxycodone as with morphine in the experience of the authors, although there this was not a randomized trial. Side effects included drowsiness, lightheadedness, sweating, vomiting and pruritus. Nausea appeared to be greater with rectal oxycodone.

Oxycodone was used as a second line opioid in a prospective study by Maddock and colleagues[59]. Thirteen patients were rotated from morphine to oxycodone for reasons of neurotoxicity or intractable nausea and vomiting. Pain scores improved and side effects resolved with the rotation.

A second trial by Leow was a prospective cohort of 12 patients with moderate to severe cancer pain, which used a single dose cross-over design to compare oral with parenteral oxycodone[9]. Pharmacokinetics were also done. Pain relief scales to determine benefits with multiple dosing and a VAS (a 10-cm horizontal line with 0 cm indicating no pain and 10 cm indicating the worst pain imaginable) were also used. The half-life, clearance and volume of distribution were not different by route of administration (oral or parenteral). There were a large individual kinetic and dose differences reflected in the maximum concentration to minimum concentration ratios at steady state. The VAS decreased by 30 min and continued to do so at 1, 2 and 4 h. Pain relief was the same for parenteral and oral route except at 30 min. There was no correlation between plasma oxycodone levels, and pain intensity or pain relief. Side effects occurred more frequently with parenteral oxycodone than with oral and with greater intensity as measured by a VRS. Side effects included drowsiness, lightheadedness, nausea, vomiting, dry mouth and pruritus. The oral to parenteral ratio is 0.7 in this group of patients with an overall oral bioavailability of 87%. In the discussion, the author makes three major points:

♦ the pharmacokinetics of oxycodone in advanced cancer differ from those of postoperative patients;

♦ the maximum concentration to minimum concentration among individuals with cancer is similar to that of morphine in their experience;

♦ oxycodone produces pain relief which does not correlate well with drug levels.

A prospective experience of the use of subcutaneous oxycodone as a second line opioid for cancer pain and opioid toxicity was reported by Gagnon[46]. Sixty-three patients were assessed daily by the Edmonton Symptom Assessment Scale. The study involved patients on either morphine or hydromorphone. Potency ratios were determined at steady state as defined as not more than 20% differences in daily dose for 2 days. The parenteral oxycodone doses varied from 4.5 to 660 mg per 24 h and the duration of treatment varied from 1 to 49 days. Forty-eight patients were rotated for reasons of delirium of these, 13 improved and 19 could be evaluated for equivalence. Eight patients were rotated from parenteral morphine to oxycodone. The mean morphine dose was 91 ± 81 mg and for oxycodone was 75 ± 39 mg with a morphine to oxycodone ratio of 1.2, and a median ratio of 1. Eleven patients were rotated from hydromorphone to oxycodone. The mean parenteral hydromorphone dose was 28 ± 26 mg, and the mean oxycodone dose was 138 ± 99 mg with a mean hydromorphone to oxycodone ratio of 5 ± 4.0 and a median of 4. Pain control was the same before and after oxycodone rotation (VAS of 56 ± 29 pre- and 53 ± 31 postrotation). A group of patients were converted from oral to subcutaneous oxycodone using a ratio of 1 : 2 (parenteral to oral). The wide confidence intervals, differences in doses and small number of patients suggests that equivalence should be taken as a general guideline but subject to individual patient variability.

A bucco-adhesive oxycodone disc was used in a study of 11 cancer patients[26]. The age range for these patients was 50–78 years. Oxycodone was combined with sorbitol and gelatin, and solidified with heat and placed into a mold. The disc measured 11 mm and was placed against the buccal surface. Ketorolac was used for a rescue dose. The reasons for oxycodone were; uncontrolled pain on NSAIDs[4], severe opioid-related side effects[3] and difficulty swallowing[4]. The mean 'resident time' on buccal surfaces was roughly 2.7 h. The plasma concentrations and oxycodone kinetics were previously discussed. Response by VAS was noted to be excellent in 27% of the patients and good in 45%. The recovery of oxycodone, in the plasma was 80% of the oral dose (79.5 ± 5.2%). Side effects included mild sedation, nausea and sweating. Oxycodone kinetics were similar to those described with oral oxycodone.

An open-labeled prospective cohort of cancer patients was reported by Citron and colleagues[84]. This same cohort had previously participated in a randomized double-blind comparison of immediate release and SR oxycodone. All patients received SR oxycodone doses of 10–20 mg every 12 h. Patients were provided with a rescue dose of immediate release (IR) oxycodone. Responses were measured by VRS. A total of 87 patients participated in this study, Seventy-nine were evaluable and 51% completed 3 months of treatment. Fifty-seven per cent of the patients studied required a higher dose and 54% required at least the rescue dose for 75% of the study days. Rescue doses were more frequent between noon and 4 p.m. The mean daily dose of oxycodone was 23.6 ± 3.7 mg. Fifteen per cent of the patients discontinued the study due to adverse side effects. Constipation occurred in 77%, nausea in 45% and somnolence in 47%. The mean daily dose seemed quite low compared with the usual experience, which may reflect patient selection in the study.

In summary, these prospective cohort trials and case reports demonstrate equivalence between morphine and oxycodone near unity. There are wide individual variations in drug requirements with regular dosing. Oxycodone reduces opioid neurotoxicity and gastrointestinal toxicity when used in rotation as the second opioid. Responses occur in advanced cancer patients equivalent to morphine and hydromorphone. Side effect profiles appear to be similar to other opioids and may be route dependent.

Comparisons between oxycodone and NSAIDS

A randomized comparison of oxycodone and zomepirac, with oxycodone and aspirin, phenacetin and caffeine (oxycodone plus APC) which involved 170 cancer patients[85]. On three separate days patients received either 100 mg of zomepirac or (APC plus oxycodone) or a placebo as a single dose–response study. Pain relief was measured at 30 min, and 1, 2, 3, 4, 5 and 6 h following analgesic dose or placebo. A VRS was used to measure pain relief. Pain intensity differences from initial pain severity and with each time point were measured. Pain intensity differences over the entire 6 h were summed and total pain relief was calculated. Patients were allowed conventional analgesics after two hour or subsequent pain was not relieved.

A second part of this trial randomized 170 patients into three separate groups. The first group of patients received doses of oxycodone plus APC with the second and third groups receiving zomepirac in either 100- or 50-mg doses. Patients were assessed for pain relief and acceptability every hour.

Thirty-seven of 40 patients finished the first trial. In the single dose trial, a dose of oxycodone of 5 mg plus APC was equivalent to a 100 mg dose of zomepirac, and both were better than placebo. The patient overall rating of analgesia was good to excellent in 73% of those on oxycodone plus APC. It was 71% of those on zomepirac and 46% of those receiving placebo, which was a significant difference.

In the multidose part of this study doses of oxycodone plus APC were superior to doses of zomepirac of 100 and 50 mg. Therapeutic responses occurred in 69% of those patients receiving oxycodone plus APC, in 49% receiving doses of 100 mg of zomepirac and in 40% of those receiving 50 mg of zomepirac. Previous exposure to opioids influenced patient preference. Adverse effects occurred in 76% of oxycodone-treated patients, in 65% of those on zomepirac 100 mg and in 40% with doses of zomepirac 50 mg. Premature discontinuation occurred in 17% of patients receiving oxycodone, in 13% with zomepirac 100 mg and in 7% with zomepirac 50 mg.

A double-blind comparison of oxycodone plus acetaminophen (5 and 325 mg, respectively) was added to either placebo or ibuprofen alone[86]. Patients received four doses of oxycodone plus acetaminophen daily. Ibuprofen doses were 600 mg given four times daily or placebo given four times daily. Pain dairies were used and analgesic consumption, pain intensity and relief were measured each afternoon. Only one rescue dose was allowed each day. Ibuprofen plus oxycodone/acetaminophen reduced the use of oxycodone alone from an average of 8.9–7.4 tablets daily. There was a 33% reduction in pain with ibuprofen plus oxycodone/acetaminophen compared with oxycodone plus acetaminophen and placebo. In the placebo arm, there was a 10% increase in oxycodone/acetaminophen consumption, which was significantly different from the ibuprofen, plus oxycodone/acetaminophen treated patients. Patients all rated improved analgesia with ibuprofen and oxycodone plus acetaminophen compared with oxycodone plus acetaminophen alone. All of these patients were required to have bone pain that may have influenced the pain responses. It appears that this subset of patients do better with the addition of NSAIDs to oxycodone plus acetaminophen.

Comparisons of immediate release oxycodone with sustained-release oxycodone

Kaplan and colleagues performed a double-blind double-dummy parallel group study comparing immediate and SR oxycodone[65]. Early in the study breakthrough (rescue) doses were not allowed and many patients dropped out of study. However, the study was amended to allow for rescue dosing. Rescue dosing with immediate release oxycodone was available for a maximum of four times daily. Pain intensity and patient acceptance were measured by VRS four times daily. A subset of 12 patients underwent pharmacokinetic studies. One-hundred-and-eighty patients enrolled and, out of this initial number, 164 were evaluable. The mean age was 59 years. Previous analgesics included combination opioids, NSAIDs and morphine. The mean daily SR morphine dose was 127 mg with a range of 40–640 mg and for IR oxycodone the mean dose was 114 mg with a range of 20–400 mg. The mean number of supplemental doses after protocol amendment was 0.6 per day for SR oxycodone and 1 for IR oxycodone, and was not significantly different. The mean baseline pain intensity was similar between groups in the mild to moderate range. Patients with neuropathic pain had slightly higher pain intensity scores. Relative analgesic effectiveness and patient acceptance were the same between IR and SR oxycodone. Discontinuation after amendment occurred in 4 and 19% of patients on SR and IR oxycodone, respectively. There was an inverse relationship between plasma levels of oxycodone and pain intensity. Sustained-release oxycodone had fewer side effects particularly gastrointestinal side effects, as compared with immediate release oxycodone. The low intensity of pain at baseline may have biased the findings of equivalence in this study. Future study design requires the provision of breakthrough doses necessary to avoid high drop out rates.

A prospective double-blind randomized double-dummy trial was performed by Parris and colleagues for patients whose pain was controlled on 6–12 tablets of a fixed opioid combination analgesic[87]. Patients received either 30 mg of SR oxycodone twice daily for 5 days or 15 mg of IR oxycodone four times daily for 5 days. Patients requiring supplemental analgesics or titration were removed from study. A VRS was used to measure pain intensity and relief. The duration of the study was five days. Diaries were kept four times daily. One-hundred-and-three of 111 patients were evaluable; however, only 59% completed the 5-day study. Mean baseline pain scores were 1.5 ± 0.1 and

1.3 ± 0.1 for SR and IR oxycodone, respectively. The VRS scoring (0 indicating no pain and 3 indicating the most severe pain imaginable) did not differ between IR and SR oxycodone. The subgroup with neuropathic pain required slightly higher dose levels, but did respond to oxycodone. Patients acceptance was the same for SR and IR oxycodone. Side effects occurred will equal frequency SR and IR oxycodone (69 and 70%, respectively) and the majority were either gastrointestinal (43%) or central nervous systems (33%). Eleven patients discontinued therapy due to side effects (10%), four in the SR oxycodone arm of the study and seven in the IR arm. This study suffers from a high drop out rate due to the lack of provision for rescue dosing and titration. The maximum daily dose allowable was 60 mg, which would predict a high (50%) drop out rate. Unlike the Kaplan study, side effects were the same between both SR and IR oxycodone, and like the Kaplan study neuropathic pain responded to oxycodone.

Salzman and colleagues reported the use of SR and IR oxycodone for patients with cancer pain also and in a group with non-malignant back pain[63]. To enter the study the pain was not adequately controlled on analgesics. Patients with cancer requiring more than 40 mg of oxycodone/day were excluded. Patients on SR oxycodone were dosed at 8 a.m. and 8 p.m. Patients on IR oxycodone was dosed four times daily. Rescue oxycodone was provided and doses adjusted based upon the around-the-clock (ATC) dose of oxycodone. Pain was rated four times daily in a dairy with a VRS (0 indicating no pain and 3 indicating the most severe pain imaginable). Titration was allowed until the VRS was 1.5. Fifty cancer patients were enrolled and 35 completed the titration. Baseline intensity was 1.8 ± 0.2 for SR oxycodone and 1.5 ± 0.2 for IR oxycodone. Pain relief did not differ between SR or IR oxycodone. Seven of the 50 did not respond and/or dropped out due to side effects. Time to stable analgesia was the same; for both groups. The mean number of dose adjustments were the same between groups. The mean daily dose was 104 ± 20 mg for SR and 113 ± 74 mg for IR oxycodone. The incidence of side effects were similar. Most side effects involved the gastrointestinal system (nausea, vomiting, and constipation) or the central nervous system (somnolence or dizziness). Nausea was more common in women. The oxycodone dose requirement per day on this trial closely matched the findings of Kaplan.

A double-blind cross-over study by Stambaugh compared SR and IR oxycodone in cancer pain[18]. The initial phase was an open label titration with IR oxycodone, which measured length of time to stable pain control (2–21 days). The next phase involved a double-blind randomized comparison of SR and IR oxycodone. Immediate release oxycodone was given four times daily and SR oxycodone was given every 12 h for 3–7 days. A numerical rating score (NRS) was used (0 indicating no pain and 10 indicating the worst pain imaginable). Pain diminished from 6.0 ± 2.2 to 2.7 ± 1.1 with IR oxycodone titrated to comfort level in the first phase of the trial. Throughout the double-blind randomized phase of the trial, pain remained 2.7 ± 1.9 for SR oxycodone and 2.8 ± 1.9 for IR oxycodone. Patient acceptance rate and the number of adverse side effects were similar between groups.

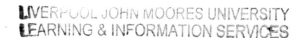

These four studies confirm that oxycodone relieves cancer pain. Three of the four studies required that pain be controlled at the time of randomization. These studies demonstrate that oxycodone can maintain pain control in cancer pain, and there is no significant difference between SR and IR oxycodone in regards to efficacy, dose, patient acceptance or side effects. The average daily dose in two of the trials ranged between 100 and 130 mg daily.

Oxycodone in comparison to other opioids

Morphine

A series of comparisons between intramuscular morphine and oxycodone were performed by Beaver and colleagues[24]. Cross-over comparisons were made using a morphine dose of 16 mg as a reference point. The mean change in pain intensity from baseline was scored hourly. Thirty-four patients started the study and 28 completed at least one round of drug comparisons. Overall, parenteral oxycodone was 0.68 (0.32–1.07) as potent as morphine, but 0.82 (0.12–2.67) as potent if measured by peak analgesic effect. Oxycodone had a shorter duration of action as compared with morphine. Side effects were said to be typical of opioids and were too infrequent to allow meaningful comparisons. The confidence intervals in this drug comparison needs to be acknowledged. Both for total effect had and peak effect confidence intervals, which were wide and overlapped with unity.

A study by Kalso and colleagues involved 10 patients with severe pain requiring potent analgesics[10]. The study required discontinuation of other opioids and the use of meperidine 1 mg/kg intramuscularly as needed for 12–24 h prior to starting patient controlled analgesia (PCA). In the next 48 h, patients used either oxycodone 3 mg or morphine by bolus with a tail dose of 2 mg/h. Lockout intervals were set at 15 min. The next phase involved converting from parenteral oxycodone or morphine to oral using a conversion ratio of 1 : 3 for morphine and a ratio of 1 : 2 for oxycodone (parenteral to oral). Pain relief was measured by VAS done 4 times daily. Pharmacokinetics were also performed. Pain relief required 30% more oxycodone parenterally than morphine and 25% less oral oxycodone than oral morphine. The mean parenteral to oral dose ratio for morphine was 0.29 (range 0.16–0.35) and the oxycodone conversion ratio was 0.51 (range 0.58–0.65). A plasma receptor assay by competitive binding with dihydromorphine demonstrated that oxycodone MOR binding affinity was 1/10th that of morphine. The analgesic potency of oxycodone appeared much greater than the binding affinity of oxycodone to MOR. This was an *in vitro* finding that was a significant part of this study (Kalso, 1990).

A double-blind cross over trial of 20 cancer patients reported by Kalso and Vainio required participants have severe pain on weak opioids before entrance to the trial[45]. The design was similar to the previous study by the same author. The pretrial opioid was stopped and a meperidine dose of 1.1 mg/kg was used as needed for 12–24 h.

A PCA device was used in the second phase of this trial and patients were self-titrated to pain relief. A conversion to an oral opioid was then performed and patients were subsequently crossed-over to the alternative opioid in a double-blind fashion. The oral bioavailability was split into two groups. Ten patients were converted and rotated based upon morphine at a projected bioavailability of 44% and a bioavailability of oxycodone of 66%. The second group of 10 patients was rotated on the basis of a morphine bioavailability of 33% and oxycodone bioavailability of 50%. Pain intensity was measured by VAS every 4 h from 8 a.m. to 8 p.m. The PCA morphine and PCA oxycodone reduced pain levels from a mean of 7.6 to 1.1. The median oxycodone consumption by PCA was 30% higher. Three patients required less than 50 mg/day of parenteral oxycodone and when crossed over to morphine, 11 required 50–100 mg/day and 5 more than 100 mg daily. The median daily oral morphine requirement in Group 1 was 168 mg compared with 130 mg for oxycodone. In the second group of patients either a median dose of 228 mg of morphine and 162 mg of oxycodone were needed. There was no difference in pain control between oxycodone and morphine. Adverse effects included sedation, nausea, vomiting, as well as visual hallucinations. Morphine was more nauseating than oxycodone. Hallucinations occurred in two patients on parenteral morphine, but was not observed on parenteral oxycodone. Hallucinations occurred in three patients on oral morphine and in none of the patients on oxycodone. Otherwise, side effects were the same. Patient's preference did not differ between oxycodone or morphine.

A study by Heiskanen compared SR oxycodone and morphine as a separate study from the pharmacokinetic trial published 2 years later by the same author[37,41]. This trial was a randomized double-blind cross over designed to compared two SR opioids. There was an initial open-labeled titration phase with either SR oxycodone or morphine for a maximum of 21 days. Opioid naïve patients were started on either 40 mg of SR oxycodone or 60 mg of SR morphine. Rescue doses were provided. Patients kept diaries for dose, adverse effects and recorded pain severity by VRS using a four-point scale (0 indicating no pain and 4 indicating severe pain recorded four times daily). Treatment acceptability by VRS was recorded twice daily. Once stable pain control was achieved patients were switched to the other SR opioid using a rotation equivalence of 2 to 3 (oxycodone to morphine). Patients remained on the alternative SR opioid for a minimum of three days. Pharmacokinetics were done at steady state. Twenty-seven of the 45 patients were evaluable. Seven had adverse side effects and five were removed from study due to poor pain control. Twelve were titrated on SR oxycodone, 15 were titrated on SR morphine. The mean daily dose of SR oxycodone at the end of the titration phase was 123 and 180 mg for SR morphine. At cross-over, pain control was maintained with SR morphine better than with SR oxycodone. More breakthrough doses were required on SR oxycodone as compared with SR morphine (mean of 1.26 for oxycodone compared with a mean of 0.79 for morphine). The mean total amount of rescue opioid in the last three days of titration was 79 mg for

SR oxycodone and 74 mg for morphine. There were directional differences in equivalence depending upon the sequence of opioids. It was 2–3 (oxycodone to morphine) if oxycodone was given second and 3–4 if oxycodone was the initial opioid. More rescue opioid was required in the afternoon for both groups. Constipation was worse with oxycodone and vomiting was worse with morphine. Nightmares occurred only with morphine. All other side effects were the same. Sustained-release morphine appeared to have better acceptance during the night despite nightmares in a few patients. Both opioids were equally acceptable to patients during the day. This particular study has influenced the literature regarding equivalents between morphine and oxycodone but had a high drop out rate and small numbers of patients (<30), which may diminish the reliability of the results. Sustained-release oxycodone may have performed better in the study used equivalence closer to unity. Pharmacokinetics within this study have previously been discussed.

The largest trial comparing SR oxycodone with SR morphine was published by Mucci LoRusso and colleagues[88]. A block randomized, prospective, double-dummy design involved using multiples of 20 mg doses of SR oxycodone compared with multiples of 30 mg doses of SR morphine. Both IR morphine and IR oxycodone were available for rescue. Initial doses were determined by equivalence to the prestudy opioid. Stable pain control by definition was less than or no more than two rescue doses per day. Pain was assessed by a four-point VRS. Medications usage, pain intensity and adverse effects were recorded daily in a diary. The acceptability of therapy was rated on a 5-point VRS. Pharmacokinetics were done during the stable phase at which time both the VAS (0–100 mm) and VRS for pain intensity were used to measure pain response. Of the 101 patients enrolled, 100 had a least one dose of study medication. The mean age was 59 (30–83) years. Neuropathic pain was evenly distributed in 10 of 48 patients with SR oxycodone and nine of 52 patients with SR morphine. Seven in the SR oxycodone group and nine in the SR morphine group dropped out of the study before stable pain control was reached. Seventy-nine patients (39 on SR oxycodone and 40 on SR morphine) reached stable pain control and 66 of these patients underwent pharmacokinetic studies. Pain relief was similar for both groups. The mean final daily SR oxycodone dose was 101 mg (range 40–360) and the dose was 140 mg for SR morphine (range 60–300). The use of rescue dose and drug acceptability were equivalent between both SR opioids. Adverse side effects occurred in 83% of patients receiving SR oxycodone and in 75% of patients receiving SR morphine. Hallucinations occurred in two patients on morphine, but in no patients on oxycodone. Otherwise, the frequency of side effects were similar. Three patients in the oxycodone group and six patients in the morphine group discontinued the study due to adverse side effects. The correlation between pharmacodynamics pain control and adverse side effects with plasma levels of opioids was poor. There was better relationship between decreased pain intensity and plasma levels of opioids with oxycodone. The potency ratio was close to unity between oxycodone and morphine with overlapping dose ranges. There were large individual differences in daily doses with oxycodone and morphine, which completely overlapped in range.

Bruera and colleagues performed a prospective, double-dummy, blinded comparison of SR oxycodone and SR morphine[42]. Patients were required to have stable pain control for 3 days prior to entering the study. Equivalents were calculated for those not on prestudy oxycodone or morphine. A 1.5–1 ratio (morphine to oxycodone) was used for rotation. Both a VAS (0–100 mm) and a VRS (5-point scale) were recorded four times daily. An Edmonton staging system was used to grade prognostic factors for pain control. Effectiveness of therapy was determined by VRS (four-point scale) on days 8 and 15. Adverse events were monitored by a checklist. Twenty-three of 30 patients completed the study with no differences in response between opioids. The mean SR oxycodone dose was 46.5 ± 57 mg every 12 h versus 72.6 ± 102 mg every 12 h for SR morphine. The equivalence ratio was 1 : 1.5 (oxycodone to morphine) with a minimum and maximum ratio of 1 and 2.3, respectively. There was no change in dose ratios with dose. Rescue doses were more frequent with SR oxycodone, and occurred more frequently between 2 and 6 a.m. Adverse events, side effects and severity of side effects were similar between oxycodone and morphine. There was no difference in patient preference at the end of trial. This is a small trial with large variations in equivalence as demonstrated by the maximum and minimum equivalence ratio. More rescue doses occurred with oxycodone as per with the Heiskanen trial. This may indicate that if dose ratios were closer to unity less breakthrough doses might be necessary for oxycodone.

None of the trials, at the time of comparison, involved patients with uncontrolled pain. Trial design required a prestudy titration to pain response prior to randomization or patients entered trial with stable pain control as a prerequisite. It appears that oxycodone is equivalent to morphine in maintaining pain relief associated with cancer[89]. The closer the ratio of oxycodone to morphine is to unity the less need for oxycodone rescue dosing. Two studies found hallucinations with morphine, otherwise, side effects were similar.

Comparisons of oxycodone with opioids

Codeine

A double-blind, double-dummy trial comparing both oral and intramuscular codeine with oxycodone was reported by Beaver and colleagues[24]. Thirty-seven patients with a mean age of 53 years entered the trial and 27 completed the study. The parenteral to oral codeine conversion ratio was 1 : 2 (parenteral to oral). Patients were allowed other analgesics and response was based upon single dose with cross-over. A VRS (4-point scale) for severity of pain and a VRS (5-point scale) was used for pain relief. The estimated oral and parenteral potency ratio of oxycodone was 1 : 2 (equivalence 2 : 1) with a confidence interval of 0.19–1.3 for overall effect. In a comparison study, 28 of 34 patients were evaluated. The estimated equivalence of parenteral codeine to parenteral oxycodone was 9.7–1 (median) with a range of 4.7–39 (for total analgesia) and a mean of 12.2–1 range 6.9–87 for peak effect. Side effects were not addressed. The conversion ratio between oral and parenteral oxycodone and oral to parenteral codeine is approximately the same. The equivalence between codeine and oxycodone is 10 : 1 with a wide confidence interval.

Hydromorphone and oxycodone

A double-blind, double-dummy comparison of SR hydromorphone with SR oxycodone was performed by Hagen and colleagues[48]. Patients were required to have stable opioid requirements before participating in the study. Each SR opioid was given every 12 h for 7 days. Rescue opioids were provided. The prestudy opioid requirements were limited to a maximum of two rescue doses per day prior to comparison. Matching IR opioids were provided for rescue doses. Cross-over occurred to the alternative opioid and doses adjusted to stable pain control levels. Pain intensity was measured four times daily by VAS (0–100 mm) and by VRS (5-point scale). Side effects were measured by VAS. Patient's preference was elicited at the end of each treatment. Thirty-one of 44 patients completed the study with a mean age of 56 ± 3 years. The mean daily SR oxycodone dose was 124 ± 22 mg and the mean daily SR hydromorphone dose was 30 ± 6 mg. The mean pain intensity was not different (28 ± 4 mm for SR oxycodone 31 ± 4 mm for SR hydromorphone. There was no difference in VRS. The greatest amount of pain experienced by patients, regardless of the opioid, occurred between 12 and 4 p.m. Daily rescue doses were the same. There was no difference in preference for either opioid. Side effects were similar except drowsiness, which was more frequently experienced with SR oxycodone. Hallucinations were seen with only SR hydromorphone. Patients with neuropathic pain required slightly higher oxycodone doses (136 ± 36 mg daily) than patients with nociceptive pain (114 ± 26 mg).

This study establishes an oxycodone to hydromorphone equivalence of 4 : 1. Both were equally effective. Neuropathic pain required higher doses of opioid. Hallucinations were seen only with SR hydromorphone.

Dose and routes

Immediate release oxycodone comes in 5, 10 and 20 mg tablets in the USA and in an oral solution of 1 mg/ml concentration. Sustained-release oxycodone is available in 10-, 20-, 40- and 80-mg tablets. Thirty milligram oxycodone pectinate suppositories are available in the UK.

In the USA oxycodone tablets come in 5 and 20 mg IR. An oral oxycodone concentrate of 20 mg/ml is available, as well as SR oxycodone in increments of 10, 20, 40 and 80 mg. Oxycodone is available in combination with acetaminophen and aspirin in various dose sizes. Some countries will have a parenteral oxycodone formulation.

Sustained-release oxycodone should not be crushed since it will lose its time release characteristics. Oxycodone IR and SR have been given per rectum with pain relief, but formal prospective studies are lacking. Topical oxycodone has only been reported anecdotally.

References

1 **Anon.** Oxycodone and Oxycontin. *Med Lett* 2001; **43(1113):** 80–1.

2 **Ross FB, Smith MT.** The intrinsic antinociceptive effects of oxycodone appear to be kappa-opioid receptor mediated. *Pain* 1997; **73(2):** 151–7.

3 **Nielsen CK, Ross FB, Smith MT.** Incomplete, asymmetric, and route-dependent cross-tolerance between oxycodone and morphine in the dark agouti rat. *J Pharm Exp Ther* 2000; **295:** 91–9.

4 **Ross FB, Wallis SC, Smith MT.** Co-administration of sub-antiociceptive doses of oxycodone and morphine produces marked antinociceptive synergy with reduced CNS side-effects in rats. *Pain* 2000; **84:** 421–8.

5 **Chen ZR, Irvine RJ, Somogyi AA, et al.** Mu receptor binding of some commonly used opioids and their metabolites. *Life Sci* 1991; **48:** 2165–71.

6 **Kalso E, Poyhia R, Onnela P, et al.** Intravenous morphine and oxycodone for pain after abdominal surgery. *Acta Anaesth Scand* 1991; **35(7):** 642–6.

7 **Leow KP, Smith MT.** The antinociceptive potencies of oxycodone, noroxycodone and morphine after intracerebroventricular administration to rats. *Life Sci* 1994; **54(17):** 1229–36.

8 **Poyhia R, Vainio A, Kalso E.** A review of oxycodone's clinical pharmacokinetics and pharmacodynamics. *J Pain Symptom Manage* 1993; **8(2):** 63–7.

9 **Leow KP, Smith MT, Williams B, et al.** Single-dose and steady-state pharmacokinetics and pharmacodynamics of oxycodone in patients with cancer. *Clin Pharm Ther* 1992; **52:** 487–95.

10 **Kalso E, Vainio A.** Morphine and oxycodone hydrochloride in the management of cancer pain. *Clin Pharm Ther* 1990; **47(5):** 639–46.

11 **Kaiko RF, Benziger DP, Fitzmartin RD, et al.** Pharmacokinetic-pharmacodynamic relationships of controlled-release oxycodone. *Clin Pharm Ther* 1996; **59(1):** 52–61.

12 **Duttaroy A, Yoburn BC.** The effect of intrinsic efficacy on opioid tolerance. *Anesthesiology* 1995; **82(5):** 1226–36.

13 **Leow KP, Cramond T, Smith MT.** Pharmacokinetics and pharmacodynamics of oxycodone when given intravenously and rectally to adult patients with cancer pain. *Anesth Analg* 1995; **80(2):** 296–302.

14 **Ennis M, Schneider C, Nehring E, et al.** Histamine release induced by opioid analgesics: a comparative study using procine mast cells. *Agents Actions* 1991; **33(1–2):** 20–2.

15 **Sacerdote P, Manfedi B, Mantegazza P, et al.** Antinociceptive and immunosuppressive effects of opiate drugs: a structure-related activity study. *Br J Clin Pharm* 1997; **121(4):** 834–40.

16 **Mandema JW, Kaiko RF, Oshlack B, et al.** Characterization and validation of a pharmacokinetic model for controlled-release oxycodone. *Br J Clin Pharm* 1996; **42(6):** 747–56.

17 **Reder RF, Oshlack B, Miotto JB, et al.** Steady-state bioavailability of controlled-release oxycodone in normal subjects. *Clin Ther* 1996; **18(1):** 95–105.

18 **Stambaugh JE, Reder JF, Stambaugh MD, et al.** Double-blind, randomized comparison of the analgesic and pharmacokinetic profiles of controlled and immediate-release oral oxycodone in cancer pain patients. *J Clin Pharm* 2001; **41(5):** 500–6.

19 Benziger DP, Kaiko RF, Miotto JB, *et al.* Differential effects of food on the bioavailability of controlled-release oxycodone tablets and immediate-release oxycodone solution. *J Pharm Sci* 1996; **85(4):** 407–10.

20 Colucci RD, Swanton RE, Thomas GB, *et al.* Relative variability in bioavailability of oral controlled-release formulations of oxycodone and morphine. *Am J Ther* 2001; **8(4):** 231–6.

21 Poyhia R, Olkkola KT, Seppala T, *et al.* The pharmacokinetics of oxycodone after intravenous injection in adults. *Br J Clin Pharm* 1991; **32(4):** 516–18.

22 Leow KP, Smith MT, Watt JA, *et al.* Comparative oxycodone pharmacokinetics in humans after intravenous, oral, and rectal administration. *Ther Drug Mon* 1992; **14(6):** 479–84.

23 Beaver WT, Wallenstein SL, Rogers A, *et al.* Analgesic studies of codeine and oxycodone in patients with cancer. I Comparisons of oral with intramuscular codeine and of oral with intramuscular oxycodone. *J Pharm Exp Ther* 1978; **207(1):** 92–100.

24 Beaver WT, Wallenstein SL, Rogers A, *et al.* Analgesic studies of codeine and oxycodone in patients with cancer. II Comparisons of oral with intramuscular codeine and of oral with intramuscular oxycodone. *J Pharm Exp Ther* 1978; **207(1):** 101–8.

25 Kaiko RF. Pharmacokinetics and pharmacodynamics of controlled-release opioids. *Acta Anaesth Scan* 1997; **41:** 166–74.

26 Parodi B, Russo E, Caviglioli G, *et al.* Buccoadhesive oxycodone hydrochloride disks: plasma pharmacokinetics in healthy volunteers and clinical study. *Eur J Pharm Biol* 1997; **44:** 137–42.

27 Gong L, Middleton RK. Sublingual administration of opioids. *Annl Pharmacother* 1992; **26(12):** 1525–7.

28 Weinberg DS, Inturrisi CE, Reidenberg B, *et al.* Sublingual absorption of selected opioid analgesics. *Clin Pharm Ther* 1988; **44(3):** 335–42.

29 Takala A, Kaasalainen V, Seppala T, *et al.* Pharmacokinetic comparison of intravenous and intranasal administration of oxycodone. *Acta Anaesth Scand* 1997; **41(2):** 309–12.

30 Dale O, Hjortkjaer R, Kharasch ED. Nasal administration of opioids for pain management in adults. *Acta Anaesth Scand* 2002; **46:** 759–70.

31 Ballas SK. Letter to the editor: Treatment of painful sickle cell leg ulcers with topical opioids. *Blood* 2002; **99(3):** 1096.

32 Heiskanen T, Olkkola KT, Kalso E. Effects of blocking CYP2D6 on the pharmacokinetics and pharmacodynamics of oxycodone. *Clin Pharm Ther* 1998; **64(6):** 603–11.

33 Leow KP, Wright AW, Cramond T, *et al.* Determination of the serum protein binding of oxycodone and morphine using ultrafiltration. *Ther Drug Mon* 1993; **15(5):** 440–7.

34 Poyhia R, Seppala T. Liposolubility and protein binding of oxycodone *in vitro*. *Pharm Tox* 1994; **74(1):** 23–7.

35 Olkkola KT, Hamunen K, Seppala T, *et al.* Pharmacokinetics and ventilatory effects of intravenous oxycodone in postoperative children. *Br J Clin Pharm* 1994; **38(1):** 71–6.

36 Gammaitoni AR, Galer BS, Bulloch S, *et al.* Randomized, double-blind, placebo-controlled comparison of the analgesic efficacy of oxycodone 10 mg/acetaminophen 325 mg versus controlled-release oxycodone 20 mg in postsurgical pain. *Clin Pharm* 2003; **43(3):** 296–304.

37 Heiskanen TE, Ruismaki PM, Seppala TA, *et al.* Morphine or oxycodone in cancer pain? *Acta Oncol* 2000; **39(8):** 941–7.

38 Benziger DP, Miotto J, Grandy RP, *et al.* A pharmacokinetic/pharmacodynamic study of controlled-release oxycodone. *J Pain Symptom Manage* 1997; **13(2):** 75–82.

39 Backlund M, Lindgren L, Kajimoto Y, *et al.* Comparison of epidural morphine and oxycodone for pain after abdominal surgery. *J Clin Anesth* 1997; **9:** 30–5.

40 Glare PA, Walsh D. Dose-ranging study of oxycodone for chronic pain in advanced cancer. *J Clin Oncol* 1993; **11(5)**: 973–8.

41 Heiskanen T, Kalso E. Controlled-release oxycodone and morphine in cancer related pain. *Pain* 1997; **73**: 37–45.

42 Bruera E, Belzile M, Pituskin E, *et al.* Randomized, double-blind, cross-over trial comparing safety and efficacy of oral controlled-release oxycodone with controlled-release morphine in patients with cancer pain. *J Clin Oncol* 1998; **16(10)**: 3222–9.

43 Curtis GB, Johnson GH, Clark P, *et al.* Relative potency of controlled-release oxycodone and controlled-release morphine in a postoperative pain model. *Eur J Clin Pharm* 1999; **55(6)**: 425–9.

44 Silvasti M, Rosenberg P, Seppala T, *et al.* Comparison of analgesic efficacy of oxycodone and morphine in postoperative intravenous patient-controlled analgesia. *Acta Anaesthesiol Scand* 1998; **42(5)**: 576–80.

45 Kalso E, Vainio A, Mattila MJ, *et al.* Morphine and oxycodone in the management of cancer pain: plasma levels determined by chemical and radioreceptor assays. *Pharm Toxicol* 1990; **67(4)**: 322–8.

46 Gagnon B, Bielech M, Watanabe S, *et al.* The use of intermittent subcutaneous injections of oxycodone for opioid rotation in patients with cancer pain. *Support Care Cancer* 1999; **7**: 265–70.

47 Tarkkila P, Tuominen M, Lindgren L. Comparison of respiratory effects of tramadol and oxycodone. *J Clin Anesth* 1997; **9**: 582–5.

48 Hagen NA, Babul N. Comparative clinical efficacy and safety of a novel controlled-release oxycodone formulation and controlled-release hydromorphone in the treatment of cancer pain. *Cancer* 1997; **79**: 1428–37.

49 Rischitelli DG, Karbowicz SH. Safety and efficacy of controlled-release oxycodone: a systematic literature review. *Pharmacotherapy* 2002; **22(7)**: 898–904.

50 Sharar SR, Carrougher GJ, Selzer K, *et al.* A comparison of oral transmucosal fentanyl citrate and oral oxycodone for pediatric outpatient wound care. *J Burn Care Rehabil* 2002; **23(1)**: 27–31.

51 Lurcott G. The effects of the genetic absence and inhibition of CYP2D6 on the metabolism of codeine and its derivatives, hydrocodone and oxycodone. *Anesth Prog* 1999; **45**: 154–6.

52 Otton SV, Wu D, Joffe RT, *et al.* Inhibition by fluoxetine of cytochrome P450 2D6 activity. *Clin Pharm Ther* 1993; **53(4)**: 401–9.

53 Rosebraugh CJ, Flockhart DA, Yasuda SU, *et al.* Visual hallucination and tremor induced by sertaline and oxycodone in a bone marrow transplant patient. *J Clin Pharm* 2001; **41(2)**: 224–7.

54 Lam YW, Gaedigk A, Ereshefsky L, *et al.* CYP2D6 inhibition by selective serotonin reuptake inhibitors: analysis of achievable steady-state plasma concentrations and the effect of ultrarapid metabolism at CYP2D6. *Pharmacotherapy* 2002; **22(8)**: 1001–6.

55 Grant EM, Nicolau DR, Nightingale C, *et al.* Minimal interaction between gatifloxacin and oxycodone. *J Clin Pharm* 2002; **42(8)**: 928–32.

56 Lill J, Bauer LA, Horn JR, *et al.* Cyclosporine-drug interactions and the influence of patient age. *Am J Health Syst Pharm* 2000; **57(17)**: 1579–84.

57 Davis MP, Wilcock A. Modified-release opioids. *Eur J Palliat Care* 2001; **8(4)**: 142–6.

58 Jannetto PJ, Wong SH, Gock SB, *et al.* Pharmacogenomics as molecular autopsy for postmortem forensic toxicology: genotyping cytochrome P450 2D6 for oxycodone cases. *J Anal Toxicol* 2002; **26(7)**: 438–47.

59 Maddocks I, Somogyi A, Abbott F, *et al.* Attenuation of morphine-induced delirium in palliative care by substitution with infusion of oxycodone. *J Pain Symptom Manage* 1996; **12(3)**: 182–9.

60 Hanks GW, Conno F De, Cherny N, *et al.* Morphine and alternative opioids in cancer pain: the EAPC recommendations. *Br J Cancer* 2001; **84(5)**: 587–93.

61 Kalso E, Vainio A. Hallucinations during morphine but not during oxycodone treatment. *Lancet* 1988; 2(8616): 912.

62 Saarialho-Kere U, Mattila MJ, Seppala T. Psychomotor, respiratory and neuroendocrinological effects of a mu-opioid receptor agonist (oxycodone) in healthy volunteers. *Pharm Toxicol* 1989; 65(4): 252–7.

63 Salzman RT, Roberts MS, Wild J, *et al.* Can a controlled-release oral dose form of oxycodone be used as readily as an immediate-release form for the purpose of titrating to stable pain control? *J Pain Symptom Manage* 1999; 18(4): 271–9.

64 Campora E, Merlini L, Pace M, *et al.* The incidence of narcotic-induced emesis. *J Pain Symptom Manage* 1991; 6(7): 428–30.

65 Kaplan R, Winston C, Parris V, *et al.* Comparison of controlled-release and immediate-release oxycodone tablets in patients with cancer pain. *J Clin Oncol* 1998; 16(10): 3230–7.

66 Tigerstedt I, Turunen M, Tammisto T, *et al.* The effect of buprenorphine and oxycodone on the intracholedochal passage pressure. *Acta Anaesth Scand* 1981; 25(2): 99–102.

67 Leino K, Mildh L, Lertola K, *et al.* Time course of changes in breathing pattern in morphine- and oxycodone-induced respiratory depression. *Anaesthesia* 1999; 54(9): 835–40.

68 Cone EJ, Fant RV, Rohay JM, *et al.* Oxycodone involvement in drug abuse deaths: a DAWN-based classification scheme applied to an oxycodone postmortem database containing over 1000 cases. *Anal Toxicol* 2003; 27(2): 57–67.

69 Drummer OH, Syrjanen ML, Phelan M, *et al.* A study of deaths involving oxycodone. *J Forens Sci* 1994; 39(4): 1069–75.

70 Anderson DT, Fritz KL, Muto JJ. Oxycontin: the concept of a 'ghost pill' and the postmortem tissue distribution of oxycodone in 36 cases. *J Anal Toxicol* 2002; 26(7): 448–59.

71 Spiller HA. Postmortem oxycodone and hyrdrocodone blood concentrations. *J Forens Sci* 2003; 48(2): 429–31.

72 Hill P, Dwyer K, Kay T, *et al.* Severe chronic renal failure in association with oxycodone addiction: a new form of fibrillary glomerulopathy. *Hum Pathol* 2002; 33(8): 783–7.

73 Rao R, Desai NS. Oxycontin and neonatal abstinence syndrome. *J Perinatol* 2002; 22(4): 324–5.

74 Davis MP, Varga J, Dickerson D, *et al.* Normal-release and controlled-release oxycodone: pharmacokinetics, pharmacodynamics, and controversy. *Supportive Care in Cancer* 2003; 11: 84–92.

75 Kaiko R, Grandy R, Hou Y, *et al.* Controlled release oxycodone pharmacokinetics/-pharmacodynamics in hepatic cirrhosis. *Proc 14th Ann Meet Am Pain Soc* 1995, Abstract#A-146.

76 Tallgren M, Olkkola KT, Seppala T, *et al.* Pharmacokinetics and ventilatory effects of oxycodone before and after liver transplantation. *Clin Pharm Ther* 1997, 61(6): 655–61.

77 Kirvela M, Lindgren L, Seppala T, *et al.* The pharmacokinetics of oxycodone in uremic patients undergoing renal transplantation. *J Clin Anesth* 1996; 8(1): 13–18.

78 Kevorkian JP, Hofmann MC, Jacqz-Aigrain E, *et al.* Assessment of individual CYP2D6 activity in extensive metabolizers with renal failure: comparison of sparteine and dextromethorphan. *Clin Pharm Ther* 1996; 59(5): 538–92.

79 Levy MH. Advancement of opioid analgesia with controlled-release oxycodone. *Eur J Pain* 2001; 5(Suppl A): 113–16.

80 Shulman RW, Ozdemir V. Psychotropic medications and cytochrome P450 2D6: pharmacokinetic considerations in the elderly. *Can J Psychol* 1997; 42(Supp 1): 4S–9S.

81 Tanaka E. *In vivo* age-related changes in hepatic drug-oxidizing capacity in humans. *Clin Pharm Ther* 1998; 23(4): 247–55.

82 Zhukovsky DS, Walsh D, Doona M. The relative potency between high dose oral oxycodone and intravenous morphine: a case illustration. *J Pain Symptom Manage* 1999, **18(1)**: 53–5.

83 De Conno F, Ripamonti C, Sbanotto A, *et al.* A clinical study on the use of codeine, oxycodone, dextropoxyphene, buprenorphine, and pentazocine in cancer pain. *J Pain Symptom Manage* 1991; **6(7)**: 423–7.

84 Citron ML, Kaplan R, Parris WCV, *et al.* Long-term administration of controlled-release oxycodone tablets for the treatment of cancer pain. *Cancer Invest* 1998; **16(8)**: 562–71.

85 Stambaugh JE Jr, Tejada F, Trudnowski RJ. Double-blind comparisons of zomepirac and oxycodone with APC in cancer pain. *J Clin Pharm* 1980; **20(4 Pt 2)**: 261–70.

86 Stambaugh JE Jr, Drew J. The combination of iburprofen and oxycodone/acetaminophen in the management of chronic cancer pain. *Clin Pharm Ther* 1988; **44**: 665–9.

87 Parris WCV, Johnson BW Jr, Croghan MK, *et al.* The use of controlled-release oxycodone for the treatment of chronic cancer pain: a randomized, double-blind study. *J Pain Symptom Manage* 1998; **16(4)**: 205–11.

88 Mucci-LoRusso P, Berman BS, Silberstein PT, *et al.* Controlled-release oxycodone compared with controlled-release morphine in the treatment of cancer pain: a randomized, double-blind, parallel-group study. *Eur J Pain* 1998; **2(2)**: 239–49.

89 Anon. Oral oxycodone: new preparation. No better than morphine. *Prescrire Int* 2003; **12(65)**: 83–4.

Chapter 11

The lipophilic opioids: fentanyl, alfentanil, sufentanil and remifentanil

Tony Hall and Janet R. Hardy

Introduction

Fentanyl, alfentanil, sufentanil and remifentanil are synthetic opioid analgesics with high affinity for the mu opioid receptor. They have been widely adopted into anesthetic practice for various surgical procedures, for example, in cardiac surgery, and for long-term analgesia and sedation.

As anesthetic agents they are generally administered by the intravenous route, although other routes of administration (epidural, intrathecal, transdermal, transmucosal, sublingual and subcutaneous) are used widely.

Important pharmacokinetic differences have been described between these analgesics. While remifentanil has the most rapid onset of analgesia, shortest time to peak effect and shortest distribution and elimination half-life, alfentanil has the smallest volume of distribution and total body clearance.

The pharmacokinetic profile of each is affected by many factors including patient age, plasma protein content, acid-base balance status, cardio-pulmonary bypass, changes in hepatic blood flow and the co-administration of other drugs which compete for plasma protein carriers and metabolic pathways. Their profile is not affected significantly by renal insufficiency or compensated hepatic dysfunction however, and this has major implications clinically.

Basic characterization

Fentanyl, alfentanil, sufentanil and remifentanil are all 4-anilidopiperidine derivatives and have similar chemical structures. Fentanyl is a 4-anilodopiperidine derivative of propanamide, alfentanil is a 4-piperidinyl analogue, sufentanil is a thienyl analogue and remifentanil a 4-phenylamino derivative (see Fig. 11.1).

Some of the physicochemical properties specific to this group of analgesics have direct effects on their pharmacokinetics. In common with most opioid analgesics, fentanyl and its congeners are tertiary amines, and with the exception of alfentanil,

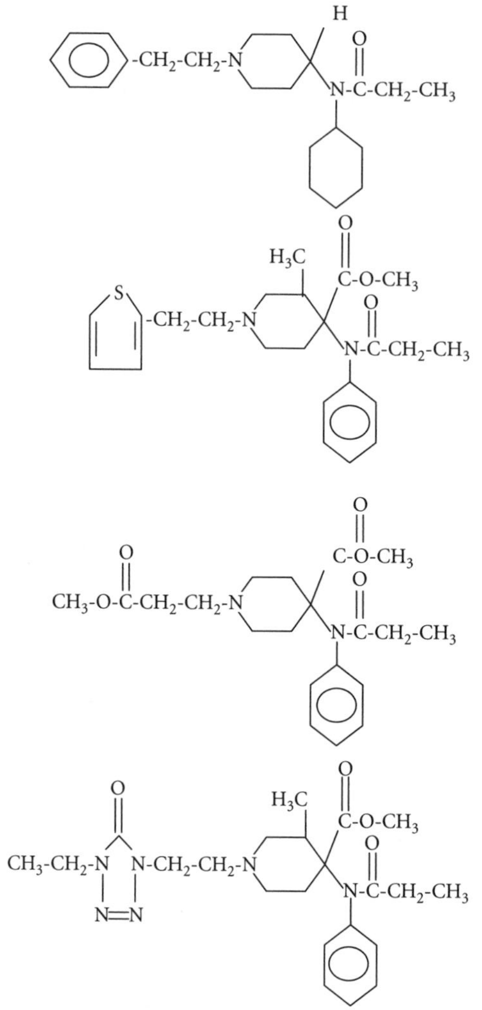

Fig. 11.1 Structural formulae for fentanyl and derivatives.

have pK$_a$ values in excess of physiological pH. Thus, alfentanil is the only derivative in which the un-ionized form predominates at physiological pH (7.4). This, together with the lower lipid solubility of alfentanil free base, imparts unusual distribution and binding characteristics. Sufentanil, in comparison, has extremely high lipid solubility and high affinity for the mu receptor[1].

The 'fentanyls' are more potent analgesics than morphine. Much of this difference in potency can be explained in terms of access to central opioid receptors. Fentanyl is reputed to be 75–100 times more potent than morphine[2,3], although potency ratios of 150:1 are recommended by the manufacturer. Direct comparison in animal studies (Table 11.1) suggests that fentanyl is almost 300 times more potent than morphine[4].

Table 11.1 Physicochemical properties and pharmacokinetics after bolus administration

Parameter	Alfentanil	Fentanyl	Sufentanil	Remifentanil	Morphine
Lipid solubility (octanol/water distribution coefficient)	129	816	1727	17.9	1.4
Non-ionized fraction at pH 7.4 (%)	89	8.5	20	NK	23
Red blood cell/plasma ratio					
Plasma binding at pH7.4 (%)	92.1	84.4	92.5	92	30
Analgesic onset (min)	0.75	1.5	1	1	7.5
Time to peak effect (%)	1.5	4.5	2.5	NK	25
Volume of distribution (l/kg)	0.75	4.0	2.9	1.0	3.2
Distribution $t\frac{1}{2}$ (min)	0.4	1.7	1.4	1.0	1.65
Elimination $t\frac{1}{2}$ (min)	94	219	164	10	177
Total body clearance (l/h/kg)	0.4	0.78	0.702	2.4	0.9

NK, not known.

Variability of parameters is not included in this table.

Adapted from Scholz (1996)[9].

When overall CNS concentrations are examined (by brain/plasma distribution coefficient), it is apparent that fentanyl has greater access to the brain (and, presumably, to central opioid receptors) than morphine. Direct delivery of opioids into the CNS, should result in unbiased potency equivalence calculations. Intraventricular fentanyl is only 12 times more potent than morphine. Alfentanil appears to be 10 times more potent than diamorphine (given subcutaneously) and one-quarter as potent as fentanyl[5]. Remifentanil is considered to be 20–40 times more potent than alfentanil.

It has been has suggested that analgesic tolerance to alfentanil develops quickly[6], but this has also been refuted for both alfentanil and sufentanil infusions[7].

Metabolism

Alfentanil is predominantly, although not exclusively, metabolized by the cytochrome P450 system via CYP3A3 and CYP3A4[8]; hence, concurrent use with inhibitors of these enzymes such as fluconazole, ketoconazole, ritonavir, erythromycin, diltiazem and cimetidine (known CYP3A4 inhibitors) will increase plasma concentrations. Fentanyl undergoes phase I metabolism predominantly by oxidative N-dealkylation and sufentanil by N-dealkylation at the piperidine and amide nitrogen atoms, as well as by O-demethylation and aromatic hydroxylation. The principal metabolites include phenylacetic acid, norfentanyl and small quantities of the pharmacologically active p-OH (phenethyl) fentanyl. Remifentanil is structurally related to alfentanil, but is rapidly metabolized by non-specific blood and tissue esterases and, to a minor extent, by N-dealkylation. A carboxylic acid derivative, remifentanil acid, is the major metabolite that is 4600 times less potent on the mu-receptor than intravenous (i.v.) remifentanil itself. Ninety per cent of a remifentanil dose appears in urine as this metabolite. Comparative animal pharmacological data are shown in Table 11.2.

Table 11.2 Physiochemical properties and pharmacokinetics after bolus administration

Opiate	Analgesic potency (rat tail flick test 55°C)			MLD$_{50}$ (mg/kg) (rat i.v. bolus)	MLD$_{50}$ / MED50	Anesthetic potency (dog intubation)		Safety margin in dog
	MED$_{50}$ (mg/kg)	TMED$_{50}$ (h)	Potency ratio			MED$_{50}$ (mg/kg)	Potency ratio	
Fentanyl	0.011	0.093	292	3.5	323	0.0012	125	160
Alfentanil	0.044	0.03	73	47.5	1080	0.005	30	50
Sufentanil	0.00071	0.14	4521	17.9	25211	0.00025	625	800
Morphine sulfate	3.21	0.31	1	223	69	0.15	1	33

From Mather (1983)[4].

Pharmacokinetics/dynamics

The physiochemical properties of the four drugs after bolus administration are shown in Table 11.2[9]. Alfentanil has a very rapid activity onset time and short time to peak effect because of its extremely high non-ionized fraction that can more easily cross the blood–brain barrier. The highest lipid solubility (defined as an octanol/water coefficient), has been found for sufentanil. Alfentanil has the smallest volume of distribution (Vd), distribution half-life ($t\frac{1}{2}\,\alpha$) and elimination half-life ($t\frac{1}{2}\,\beta$) with these parameters for sufentanil being between those of fentanyl and alfentanil. It has been suggested that the lower Vd of sufentanil, compared with fentanyl, is responsible for its higher hepatic metabolism resulting in the reduced $t\frac{1}{2}\,\beta$[10]. The plasma clearance of fentanyl and sufentanil are similar and faster than that of alfentanil.

Remifentanil is an ultrafast-acting opioid. Its duration of analgesic activity is not dependant upon the rate or duration of infusion. Cessation of administration reverses activity faster than receptor antagonism with naloxone. The elimination half-life of remifentanil after i.v. infusion is 3–10 min, but this is dose dependant and, whilst not affected by renal function, the excretion of the weakly active carboxylic acid metabolite is reduced and may culminate in severe renal impairment. There is, therefore, a theoretical risk of significant opioid activity after long-term administration in patients with severe renal impairment[11].

The pharmacokinetics of sufentanil after i.v. bolus followed by continuous i.v. infusion has been described in brain-injured patients[12]. A rapid and slow $t\frac{1}{2}\,\alpha$ (0.65 and 19 min, respectively) after the initial bolus and a clearance of 72.9 l/h (1215 ml/min) were similar to those documented for other patients. The elimination half-life ($t\frac{1}{2}\,\beta$) of 16 h was longer than that reported after bolus administration[13,14], and the Vd of 10 l/kg was higher. The long $t\frac{1}{2}\,\beta$ documented in intensive care patients[15] suggests that recovery from prolonged administration may take longer than would have been predicted from earlier pharmacokinetic data based upon i.v. bolus administration. Similar findings have also been reported for alfentanil[16] and fentanyl[10]. The prolonged $t\frac{1}{2}\,\beta$ and the different apparent volume of distribution (Vd) of the lipid soluble opioids following continuous i.v. infusion appears to be a function of the duration of administration. This characteristic is illustrated by clinical observations of prolonged effect following cessation of continuous infusions of these drugs[17].

Variation in pharmacokinetic parameters by mode of administration

Opioid analgesics are most commonly given by i.v. bolus and continuous i.v. infusion. However, other modes of administration—intraspinal (epidural and intrathecal), subcutaneous, transdermal, transmucosal and intranasal—are also used and deserve address.

Intraspinal route

Pharmacokinetic data following i.v. and epidural injection have been compared[18]. The onset of analgesia after epidural administration was 3–5-fold slower than after i.v. injection, but the duration was 3–6-fold longer. Thoracic epidural delivery was associated with a faster onset and reduced dose requirements, compared with delivery via the lumbar epidural route[19]. Lumbar epidurals were associated with a significantly higher incidence of severe respiratory depression however. The reason for this is unclear.

Baxter *et al.* (1991) compared fentanyl 1 mcg/kg/h administered either as a lumbar epidural or i.v. infusion after thoracotomy[20]. Pain scores and plasma concentrations in both groups were similar from 2 h postoperatively onwards. Several studies using epidural fentanyl have demonstrated minimal effective plasma concentrations suggesting rapid absorption of fentanyl from the epidural space into the CNS.

Epidural alfentanil has been shown to be no more effective than i.v. alfentanil as postoperative analgesia[21,22]. In a comparative single bolus dose study, sufentanil 150 mcg given i.v. resulted in a lower plasma concentration (0.58 versus 3.08 mcg/l) than the same dose given by epidural administration after 2 min, whereas plasma concentrations were comparable at later time points (up to 180 min)[23]. Transfer of sufentanil from the epidural space into CSF was slower and showed greater interindividual variation than transfer into plasma.

After major abdominal surgery, administration of epidural or i.v. sufentanil as a 15-mcg bolus followed by a 5-mcg/h infusion produced comparable levels of analgesia[24]. Within 5 min, a median serum concentration of 0.15 mcg/l was achieved following the i.v. sufentanil loading dose as compared with a medium serum concentration of 0.02 mcg/l after the epidural dose. Serum concentrations of sufentanil were significantly higher after i.v. than epidural administration during the first 3 h of treatment, whereas later, no significant differences were observed. The equianalgesic dose of epidural sufentanil was found to be approximately ¼ that of the epidural fentanyl dose.

In labor pain, similar analgesic potential was observed after epidural and i.v. administration of 10 mcg sufentanil, whereas an intrathecal injection of the same dose had a greater and a 3-fold longer analgesic effect[25].

Controversy surrounds the relative contribution of supraspinal effects secondary to the redistribution of epidural lipophilic opioids such as fentanyl, sufentanil and alfentanil. Several studies have attempted to determine whether the primary efficacy of fentanyl analogues is mediated spinally or supraspinally. A double-blind/placebo cross-over study of epidural fentanyl, sufentanil and alfentanil bolus dose administration compared plasma concentrations, adverse effects and analgesic potency[26]. Minimal effective analgesic plasma concentrations were much lower with small doses of epidural fentanyl 30 mcg, sufentanil 3 mcg or alfentanil 300 mcg, whereas larger doses (epidural fentanyl 100 mcg, sufentanil 10 mcg or alfentanil

1000 mcg) resulted in plasma concentrations of approximately one-half minimal effective analgesic concentrations. In addition, analgesia was more profound in the toe than the finger, indicating a localized spinal site of action. Upper extremity analgesia was present and attributable to either rostal spread or systemic redistribution. The authors suggest that low plasma opioid concentrations occurring after small epidural opioid doses indicate a spinal site of action, whilst larger doses result in systemic absorption, which also contributed to supraspinal analgesia and adverse effects.

Subcutaneous infusion

Subcutaneous infusions of fentanyl, sufentanil and alfentanil have been used primarily within palliative care settings. Mercadante (1997) documented the use of fentanyl in a continuous subcutaneous infusion (CSI) at a rate of 25 mcg/h in conjunction with bolus doses of 12.5 mcg during the last 2 days of a patient's life[27]. In another case history, fentanyl was used at an initial dose of 500 mcg/h and was titrated up to 4250 mcg/h over 20 days with good pain control being achieved[28]. Subcutaneous continuous infusion fentanyl has been compared with CSI morphine in hospice cancer patients[29]. There were no significant differences in the pain scores between the two drugs in this small randomized, double-blind cross-over study, although patients had more frequent bowel movements during days 4–6 whilst on the fentanyl arm. An analgesic equivalence of 150 mcg fentanyl : 10 mg morphine was suggested.

The conclusion from a retrospective study of 22 patients was that CSI fentanyl allowed for more rapid pain control than transdermal fentanyl and was better than i.v. delivery, being simpler and more comfortable in advanced cancer patients[30]. A dose ratio equivalency (morphine to fentanyl) of 100 : 1 was used and no local toxicity was noted following CSI. Paix has described the use of sufentanil in two patients using a fentanyl : sufentanil dose equivalence ratios of 24 : 1 and 16 : 1[31]. A series of 48 patients who received alfentanil by CSI at a dose equivalence of 10 mg diamorphine to 1 mg alfentanil has been reported by Urch and colleagues[17].

Continuous subcutaneous infusion alfentanil has been used in postoperative pain. A 1-mg loading dose was followed by a 0.2 mg/h continuous infusion with 0.2 mg bolus doses on demand in 12 patients after abdominal surgery[32]. Significantly smaller doses of alfentanil given by the epidural route appeared to produce better quality analgesia with fewer side effects. Plasma concentrations of fentanyl during CSI have been measured in a small number of palliative care patients[33]. There was a significant correlation between infusion rates, and both total and unbound plasma concentrations of fentanyl, but marked interpatient variation in steady state fentanyl plasma concentrations. Even with a standardization for dose, there was an 8-fold variation in total plasma concentrations and a 3.5-fold variation in unbound plasma concentrations. This emphasizes the need for careful dose individualization and titration based upon clinical response.

The major problem encountered in the use of fentanyl and alfentanil by CSI is the limited dose/volume preparations available at 50 mcg/ml and 500 mcg/ml, respectively, limiting the amount that can be delivered by many standard subcutaneous infusion systems.

Transdermal administration

The low molecular weight, high potency and lipid solubility of fentanyl make it ideal for delivery via the transdermal route and a transdermal therapeutic system (TTS) formulation 'Durogesic' has been developed[34].

The ability of this drug to penetrate the lipophilic stratum corneum before the more aqueous tissue of the epidermis and dermis, makes this system possible. The system is designed to release drug at a constant rate of from 25–100 mcg/h through a rate-limiting membrane (25 mcg/10 cm^2) using an absorption enhancer (ethanol) that increases skin flux up to 500-fold. Absorption is dependant upon the surface area of the TTS applied to the skin but is independent of the site of application[35]. The fentanyl TTS is composed of four layers, plus a removable protective lining. The drug is dissolved in ethanol and gelled with hydroxy ethyl-cellulose, and held in a reservoir between a clear occluding polyester/ethylene backing layer and an ethylene-vinyl acetate copolymer rate-controlling membrane. An adhesive silicone base allows free diffusion of the drug and also provides an initial loading dose of fentanyl upon application to the skin (Durogesic, Janssen-Cilag).

Following the application of a fentanyl TTS 'patch', a depot accumulates within skin and subcutaneous tissue resulting in a delay of between 17 and 48 h before maximal steady state plasma concentrations are achieved. The TTS is designed to deliver a constant rate for a 72-h period. Under normal physiological conditions skin temperature and peripheral blood flow have no significant effect on the absorption rate from the patch, although a rise in body temperature to 40°C may increase absorption by 33%[36]. A mean bioavailability of 92% (57–146%) has been reported, although marked interindividual variability is seen[37]. This high bioavailability suggests that there is no significant degradation by skin flora or cutaneous metabolism.

Mean maximal plasma concentrations (C_{max}) of from 0.69 to 2.6 mcg/l have been obtained from doses of 25 and 100 mcg/h, respectively[38]. Once steady state plasma concentrations (Cp_{ss}) have been obtained, these persist for the duration of the patch application (usually 72 h), although in several trials Cp_{ss} was not achieved until the application of the second patch[39]. A disadvantage of the transdermal delivery system is therefore the slow titration process. Although faster titration has been suggested, this practice is not generally recommended. The manufacturer recommends that patients are initiated on 25 mcg/h patches and that adequate rescue medication, such as immediate-release short-acting oral morphine should be available during the dose titration period.

Considerable inter- and intrapatient variation has been noted with respect to the expected and actual rate of fentanyl delivery from the transdermal system over the range 25–125 mcg/h[39]. In the first of two studies from the same center, the mean actual delivery rates were close to the expected rates; 25 mcg/h (range 13–41), 52.8 mcg/h (range 10–77) and 67.8 mcg/h (range 31–88), respectively, for the 25, 50 and 75 mcg/h systems[39]. In the second study[40], however, the 50 mcg/h patch was the most accurate with a mean actual rate of delivery of 49 mcg/h (range 29–76 mcg/h). The 75 mcg patch was the most unpredictable with a mean delivery rate of 95 mcg/h (range 48–213 mcg/h).

Elimination of fentanyl following transdermal delivery has been shown to be prolonged when compared with i.v. administration, with an elimination half-life of 13–25 h, three times longer than after i.v. administration. Whilst age did not affect absorption, the elimination half-life after removal of the patch was significantly greater in the elderly than in younger patients (43.1 compared with 20 h. $p < 0.05$)[41].

Much controversy attends the conversion from chronic oral morphine therapy to fentanyl TTS. In pooled non-blinded studies, cancer patients receiving a mean dosage of 160–257 mg morphine/day could be converted to fentanyl TTS 25–50 mcg/h (median 120 mg morphine/day converted to 63–66 mcg/h fentanyl)[34]. The manufacturers of fentanyl TTS have produced dose conversion tables. The quoted range of morphine dose equivalents for each patch size is wide, but the table is a good guide for every-day clinical practice. It has been suggested that opioid-naive patients can be started on fentanyl TTS 25 mcg/h safely and that this has the advantage of reducing any delays in achieving adequate analgesia. We would recommend caution however, as 90 mg morphine/day (the median morphine equivalent of a 25 mcg/h patch) is too high a starting dose for some patients.

A number of studies have reported the successful use of fentanyl TTS in patients with acute postoperative pain[42–46]. The US Federal Drugs Agency (FDA) does not endorse the use of fentanyl TTS in these circumstances, however, as the therapeutic benefits are thought to be outweighed by the risk of respiratory depression. Of 50 deaths reported to the FDA during 1994 in patients bearing fentanyl patches, 34 were cancer patients, where death was related to their underlying disease. Four of the remaining 16 non-cancer-related deaths were related to unlicensed use of the patches in patients with postoperative pain[34]. In general, fentanyl-associated respiratory suppression occurs within 24 h after patch application[44,47–50], but can occur up to 36 h and as late as the second night after patch application[43,44,48]. This supports the argument against the use of fentanyl patches in opioid-naive patients.

Continuous fentanyl administration by epidural, intravenous and transdermal routes has been assessed in a randomized, open single dose prospective study in postoperative patients[51]. At identical doses, all three routes, produced almost equivalent degrees of analgesia. Continuous epidural administration produced a steady rise in systemic fentanyl concentrations into the ventilatory depressant range however.

Transmucosal administration

Another unique formulation of fentanyl utilizing the lipophilic properties of the drug is 'oral transmucosal fentanyl citrate' (OTFC). This 'lozenge on a stick' utilizes the ability of fentanyl to be absorbed rapidly across the oral mucosal membranes. It has a rapid onset of analgesia (43% of patients experience analgesia within 3 min), short duration of effect, is non-invasive, convenient and, the manufacturers claim, 'easy to use'. This is facilitated by the pharmacodynamic characteristics of the drug as illustrated by the plasma concentration curve of fentanyl after buccal administration, i.e. rapid absorption, rapid redistribution, hepatic metabolism, absence of active metabolites and rapid renal excretion of metabolites[52].

The buccal cavity has a number of advantages with respect to drug absorption; it is well vascularized, with a large surface area, uniform temperature and high permeability. The buccal absorption of fentanyl is transcellular because of its lipophilicity and un-ionized state, whereas morphine is absorbed via a paracellular route because it is hydrophilic and ionized state. Fifty-one per cent of a buccal fentanyl dose is absorbed (compared with 20% for morphine and 25% for hydromorphone) and 60% of maximal absorption is achieved within 2½ min[53]. An oral transmucosal bioavailability of 25% has been reported by the manufacturer and active drug is said to cross the blood brain barrier within 3–5 min of absorption.

The product was first developed as an anesthetic premedication for pediatric patients[54]. It was subsequently developed for postoperative use as was the transdermal preparation. Both products are now marketed for primary use in chronic pain and palliative care settings. The primary indication for OFTC is for incident or 'breakthrough' pain.

Fixed doses of 200, 400, 600, 800, 1200 and 1600 mcg are available as individually packed, hard candy lozenges with a citrus flavoring on the end of a short plastic handle. Patients are instructed to place the OTFC unit between cheek and gums, and to move the unit around the mouth frequently 'painting the inside of the cheeks and gums'. Patients are advised not to chew or bite the lozenge. It takes approximately 15 min for the unit to dissolve completely. Saliva production should be sufficient for drug dissolution and patients with dry mouths can have difficulty in achieving this. It is not advised for patients with mucositis or buccal ulceration. The full analgesic effect should be expected within 30 min and may last for up to 2 h. Low pH foods or drinks can affect absorption, as can the concurrent administration of hot food or drinks. In our experience, patients with impaired cognitive ability find it difficult to utilize the OTFC units effectively.

In a multicenter, randomized, double-blind, placebo-controlled cross-over study in 130 subjects, long acting oral morphine 60–1000 mg/day or 50–300 mcg/h fentanyl TTS were used as base treatment. Eligible patients were those with 1–4 breakthrough pain episodes each day. OTFC 200–1600 mcg doses was used for the management of breakthrough pain in two phases; an initial titration phase (where the dose of OTFC that provided adequate analgesia with acceptable side effects was determined), followed by an efficacy study[55]. Although OFTC was shown to be an effective treatment for breakthrough pain, the study failed to show any correlation between the effective dose of OTFC needed for breakthrough pain and the dose of concurrent long-acting opioid. The manufacturers therefore advise starting all patients at the lowest OFTC dose (200 mcg), and titrating upwards according to response and need.

A 100 : 1 dose ratio between OTFC and i.v. morphine has been proposed, i.e. 100 mcg OTFC = 1 mg i.v. morphine = 3 mg oral morphine[56,57].

Intranasal administration

Both fentanyl, alfentanil and sufentanil have been used for intranasal administration. Once again, the lipophilic nature of these opioids predispose to high bioavailability after intranasal administration. This results primarily from the passage of venous blood flow from the nasal mucosa directly into the systemic circulation, thus avoiding first pass metabolism by the hepatic portal circulation.

The use of intranasal demand-adapted titration of fentanyl in postoperative pain management following lumbar intervertebral disk surgery has been studied[58]. In a randomized blinded study, 27 mcg fentanyl was given by intranasal or intravenous routes to postoperative patients experiencing intense pain. Doses were repeated every 5 min until patients were free of pain or refused further analgesia. Intranasal fentanyl was well tolerated by all patients. No nasal discomfort was noted and only one patient (in the i.v. group), showed a decrease in PaO_2.

In a larger unselected postoperative population, the same author demonstrated that the analgesic potential of intranasal demand-adaptive titration with fentanyl was as effective as an intravenous titration method[59]. Time to effective analgesia was significantly longer in the intranansal group (10.8 versus 16.0 min, $p < 0.05$) despite the rapid onset of action following intranasal administration.

O'Neil (1997) first reported the use of a patient-controlled intranasal analgesia device (PCINA), now called a 'GO pump', using either fentanyl or pethidine[60]. The GO pump has a reservoir volume of 0.18 ml that requires 4 min to refill. On activation of the pump, this volume is delivered as a nasal spray of approximately 80-μ particle size. Thus, a dose of either 9.5 mcg fentanyl or 9.5 mg pethidine could be delivered every 4 min (or a maximum of 142.5 mcg/h fentanyl or 142.5 mg/h pethidine). Its use in a small number of palliative care, postoperative and burns patients has been reported[60]. In another small series[61], 20 mcg intranasal fentanyl was used in cancer patients requiring immediate release morphine for breakthrough pain on an average of two occasions each day. Eight of 12 patients reported improved pain control, whilst receiving the intranasal fentanyl. Most patients reported the intranasal application simple, controllable, safe and patient-friendly. The greatest criticism raised is the small dose of fentanyl that can be administered by this method.

More potent fentanyl derivatives may be better in this regard, for example sufentanil that has been used as a nasal spray for preoperative sedation[62]. Sufentanil was chosen because of its high potency : volume ratio. In a study in two parts, sufentanil was administered as a nasal spray of 5 mcg/dose or as a nose drop of 2.5 mcg/drop. After

5, 10 or 20 mcg given intranasally, a median onset of sedation was achieved within 10 min with an average duration of 40.8 min. The 5 mcg dose was ineffective and all doses were well tolerated. In the second part of the study 1 drop (2.5 mcg)/10 kg body weight up to a maximum of eight drops was administered. Intranasal sufentanil appeared to be free of the usual opioid side effects, a short period of dizziness being the only major side effect with high patient acceptance. This formulation has also been used in pediatric patients in whom 1.5–4.5 mcg/kg intranasal sufentanil was used for pre-induction[63]. Ventilatory complications during anesthetic induction were reduced by 25%, and patients moved or coughed less during intubation. During recovery, patients given sufentanil cried less and required less analgesia, whilst recovery time remained the same. However, there was a higher incidence of vomiting in patients receiving 4.5 mcg/kg in the recovery room and during the first postoperative day.

Bioavailability studies have been carried out in patients following intranasal sufentanil[64]. At 5 and 10 min postdose, intranasal administration resulted in lower peak sufentanil concentrations—36 and 56% of that following intravenous administration. From 30 min onwards, plasma concentrations were virtually identical. The AUC during the first 120 min postintranasal administration was 78% of the AUC after intravenous administration. Peri-operative sedation of rapid onset and limited duration was seen for both routes. Onset of sedation was more rapid after i.v. administration. Intranasal dosing induced no clinically significant changes in PaO_2, whereas this was observed at 5 min after i.v. administration. Similar findings have been shown in a small group of children given sufentanil 2 mcg/kg administered via intranasal drops[65]. Onset of sedation was rapid even though peak plasma concentrations of sufentanil were not achieved until 30 min after administration.

The pharmacokinetics of intranasal and intravenous alfentanil have been compared[66]. A rapid rise in plasma concentrations and a high systemic bioavailability after intranasal administration was demonstrated.

Adverse reactions

In general, there is little variation in the side effect profile of the lipophilic opioids in comparison to morphine and other opioids. They have no active metabolites, however, and a pharmacokinetic profile that is not affected significantly by renal insufficiency or hepatic dysfunction. They are, therefore, less likely than morphine to cause toxicity in patients with renal impairment. The authors have noted unexpected toxicity when stopping fentanyl derivative infusions when converting to alternative opioids using standard dose conversions[17]. We suspect this to be related to a delayed release of the lipophilic drugs from fat stores and advise caution.

Alfentanil may cause muscle rigidity with rapid i.v. administration[67] that can be avoided by slow i.v. injection or premedication with a benzodiazepine or muscle relaxant[68]. Alfentanil may also predispose to bradycardia or hypotension due to cardiac depression or increased vagal tone, particularly when used in combination with beta-blockers and anesthetic agents.

The most frequent adverse drug reactions experienced by patients on fentanyl TTS are classic opioid side effects occurring within 24 h of patch application. When delivered by this route, fentanyl has been associated with a reduced potential for constipation. The incidence was significantly less (50.8 versus 28.6%, $p < 0.001$) than that in a comparative group receiving sustained-release morphine in one trial[69], although the incidence of diarrhea was greater for fentanyl recipients. A 66% reduction in the incidence of constipation has been reported in a group of patients previously treated with morphine, along with a 23% reduction in nausea and vomiting[70]. A number of other generally small and uncontrolled studies have suggested that at equianalgesic doses, fentanyl is less constipating than morphine[71]. Once again, this is likely due to the lipophilic nature of the drug, its rapid blood–brain barrier penetration and the resultant lower analgesic/antidiarrheal dose ratio.

Other effects on quality of life for patients with terminal cancer have been examined. A significant improvement of about 10% in both quality of sleep and morning vigilance was shown in a group of 40 cancer patients during fentanyl TTS therapy compared with morphine[69,72]. The same group also reported a significant ($p < 0.05$) reduction in vomiting and nausea compared with oral morphine.

Conclusion

Fentanyl and its derivatives alfentanil, sufentanil and remifentanil offer a number of advantages and disadvantages with respect to opioid analgesia. They have different physiochemical and pharmacological properties than morphine because of the striking difference in lipophilic profile. The octanol/water partition coefficient of fentanyl is over 1000 times higher than that of morphine. This results in rapid blood–brain penetration and high potency. This lipid solubility has also allowed for the delivery of a number of unique delivery systems (e.g. transdermal and submucousal) that have added greatly to our current analgesic armamentarium.

References

1 Wuster M, Schiltz R, Nerz A. The direction of opioid antagonists towards μ,δ and σ receptors in the vas deferens of the mouse and rat. *Life Sci* 1980; **27**: 163–70.

2 Donner B, Zenz M. Transdermal fentanyl: a new step on the therapeutic ladder. *Anticancer Drugs* 1995; **6(Suppl 3)**: 39–43.

3 Roy S, Flynn G. Transdermal delivery of narcotic analgesics—pH, anatomical and subject influences on cutaneous permeability of fentanyl and sufentanil. *Pharm Res* 1990; **7**: 842–7.

4 Mather LE. Clinical pharmacokinetics of fentanyl and its newer derivatives. *Clin Pharmacokinet* 1983; **8(5)**: 422–46.

5 Dickman A, Littlewood C, Varga J. *The Syringe Driver. Continuous Subcutaneous Infusions in Palliative Care*. Oxford: Oxford University Press, 2000.

6 Hill HF, Coda BA, Mackie AM, *et al.* Patient-controlled analgesic infusions: alfentanil versus morphine. *Pain* 1992; **49:** 301–10.

7 Schraag S, Checketts MR, Kenny GNC. Lack of rapid development of opioid tolerance during alfentanil and remifentanil infusions for postoperative pain. *Anesth Analg* 1999; **89:** 753–7.

8 Yun CH, Wood M, Wood AJ, *et al.* Identification of the pharmacogenetic determinants of alfentanil metabolism: cytochrome P-450 3A4. An explanation of the variable elimination clearance. *Anesthesiol* 1992; **77:** 467–74.

9 Scholz J, Steinfath M, Schulz M. Clinical pharmacokinetics of alfentanil, fentanyl and sufentanil. An update. *Clin Pharmacokinet* 1996; **31:** 275–92.

10 Monk JP, Beresford R, Ward A. Sufentanil. A review of its pharmacological properties and therapeutic use. *Drugs* 1988; **36(3):** 286–313.

11 Pitsiu M, Wilmer A, Bodenham A, *et al.* Pharmacokinetics of remifentanil and its major metabolite, remifentanil acid, in ICU patients with renal impairment. *Br J Anaesth* 2004; **92(4):** 493–503.

12 Scholtz J, Bause H, Schulz M, *et al.* Pharmacokinetics and effects on intracranial pressure of sufentanil in head trauma patients. *Br J Clin Pharmacol* 1994; **38:** 369–72.

13 Bovill JG, Sebel PS, Blackburn CL, *et al.* The pharmacokinetics of sufentanil in surgical patients. *Anesthesiol* 1984; **61(5):** 502–6.

14 Davis PJ, Cook DR, Stiller RL, *et al.* Pharmacodynamics and pharmacokinetics of high-dose sufentanil in infants and children undergoing cardiac surgery. *Anesth Analg* 1987; **66(3):** 203–8.

15 Alazia M, Albanese J, Martin C, *et al.* Pharmacokinetics of long term sufentanil infusion (72 h) used for sedation in ICU patients (abstract). *Anesthesiol* 1992; **77:** A364.

16 Bodenham A, Park GR. Alfentanil infusions in patients requiring intensive care. *Clin Pharmacokinet* 1988; **15(Oct):** 216–26.

17 Urch CE, Carr S, Minton O. The use of alfentanil in a palliative care setting. *Palliat Med* 2004; **18(6):** 516–9.

18 Willens JS, Myslinski NR. Pharmacodynamics, pharmacokinetics, and clinical uses of fentanyl, sufentanil, and alfentanil. *Heart Lung* 1993; **22(3):** 239–51.

19 Sawchuk CW, Ong B, Unruh HW, *et al.* Thoracic versus lumbar epidural fentanyl for post thoracotomy pain. *Annl Thorac Surg* 1993; **55(6):** 1472–6.

20 Baxter AD, Laganiere S, Samson B, *et al.* A comparison of lumbar, epidural and intravenous fentanyl infusions for post-thoracotomy analgesia. *Can J Anaesth* 1994; **41(3):** 184–91.

21 Camu F, Debucquoy F. Alfentanil infusion for postoperative pain: a comparison of epidural and intravenous routes. *Anesthesiol* 1991; **75(2):** 171–8.

22 Chauvin M, Hongnat JM, Mourgeon E, *et al.* Equivalence of postoperative analgesia with patient-controlled intravenous or epidural alfentanil. *Anesth Analg* 1993; **76(6):** 1251–8.

23 Taverne RH, Ionescu TI, Nuyten ST. Comparative absorption and distribution pharmacokinetics of intravenous and epidural sufentanil for major abdominal surgery. *Clin Pharmacokinet* 1992; **23(3):** 231–7.

24 Geller E, Chrubasik J, Graf R, *et al.* A randomized double-blind comparison of epidural sufentanil versus intravenous sufentanil or epidural fentanyl analgesia after major abdominal surgery. *Anesth Analg* 1993; **76(6):** 1243–50.

25 Camann WR, Denney RA, Holby FD, *et al.* A comparison of intrathecal, epidural, and intravenous sufentanil for labor analgesia. *Anesthesiol* 1992; **77:** 884–7.

26 Coda BA, Brown MC, Schaffer R, *et al.* Pharmacology of epidural fentanyl, alfentanil, and sufentanil in volunteers. *Anesthesiol* 1994; **81(5):** 1149–61.

27 Mercadante S, Caligara M, Sapio M, *et al.* Subcutaneous Fentanyl Infusion in a patient with Bowel Obstruction and Renal Failure. *J Pain Sympt Manag* 1997; **13**: 241–4.

28 Lenz K, Dunlap D. Continuous fentanyl infusion: use in severe cancer pain. *Annl Pharmacother* 1998; **32(6)**: 308–14.

29 Hunt R, Fazekas B, Thorne D, *et al.* A comparison of subcutaneous morphine and fentanyl in hospice cancer patients. *J Pain Sympt Manag* 1999; **18**: 111–19.

30 Watanabe S, Pereira J, Hanson J, *et al.* Fentanyl by continuous subcutaneous infusion for the management of cancer pain. A retrospective study. *J Pain Sympt Manag* 1998; **16**: 323–6.

31 Paix A, Coleman A, Lees J, *et al.* Subcutaneous fentanyl and sufentanil infusion substitution for morphine intolerance in cancer pain management. *Pain* 1995; **63**: 263–9.

32 Chrubasik J, Chrubasik S, Ren Y, *et al.* Epidural versus subcutaneous administration of Alfentanil for the management of postoperative pain. *Anesth Analg* 1994; **78**: 1114–18.

33 Miller RS, Peterson GM, Abbott F, *et al.* Plasma concentrations of fentanyl with subcutaneous infusion in palliative care patients. *Br J Clin Pharmacol* 1995; **40**: 553–6.

34 Jeal W, Benfield P. Transdermal fentanyl: a review of its pharmacological properties and therapeutic efficacy in pain control. *Drugs* 1997; **53(1)**: 109–38.

35 Roy S, Flynn G. Transdermal delivery of narcotic analgesics: Comparative permeabilities of narcotic analgesics through human cadaver skin. *Pharm Res* 1989; **6(10)**: 825–32.

36 Southam MA. Transdermal fentanyl therapy: system design, pharmacokinetics and efficacy. *Anticancer Drugs* 1995; **6(Suppl 3)**: 29–34.

37 Varvel JR, Shafer SL, Hwang SS, *et al.* Absorption characteristics of transdermally administered fentanyl. *Anesthesiology* 1989; **70**: 928–34.

38 Broome I, Wright B, Bower S, *et al.* Postoperative analgesia with transdermal fentanyl following lower abdominal surgery. *Anaesthesia* 1995; **50**: 300–3.

39 Gourlay GK, Kowalski SR, Plummer JL, *et al.* The transdermal administration of fentanyl in the treatment of postoperative pain: pharmacokinetics and pharmacodynamic effects. *Pain* 1989; **37**: 193–202.

40 Gourlay GK, Kowalski SR, Plummer JL, *et al.* The efficacy of transdermal fentanyl in the treatment of postoperative pain: a double-blind comparison of fentanyl and placebo systems. *Pain* 1990; **40**: 21–8.

41 Esteve M, Levron J, Flaisler B, *et al.* Does aging modify pharmacokinetics of transdermal fentanyl? *Anesthesiology* 1993; **75(Suppl)**: A705 (abstract).

42 Rung G, Graf G, Riemondy S, *et al.* Transdermal fentanyl for analgesia after upper abdominal surgery. *Anesth Analg* 1993; **76(Suppl.)**: 362 (abstract).

43 Sandler AN, Baxter AD, Norman P, *et al.* A double-blind, placebo-controlled trial of transdermal fentanyl for post-hysterectomy analgesia (abstract). *Anesth Analg* 1991; **72(Suppl.)**: 223.

44 Sandler AN, Baxter AD, Katz J, *et al.* A double-blind, placebo-controlled trial of transdermal fentanyl after abdominal hysterectomy: analgesic, respiratory, and pharmacokinetic effects. *Anesthesiol* 1994; **811**: 1169–80.

45 Paut O, Camboulives J, Tillant D, *et al.* Pharmacokinetics and tolerance of transdermal fentanyl in young children. *Anesthesiol* 1992; **77(Suppl.)**: A1203 (abstract).

46 Boerner TF, Bartowski RR, Torjman M, *et al.* Sympathoadrenal stress response is modified by transdermal fentanyl (abstract). *Anesthesiol* 1992; **77(Suppl.)**: A888.

47 Sevarino FB, Naulty JS, Sinatra, *et al.* Transdermal fentanyl for postoperative pain management in patients recovering from abdominal gynaecologic surgery. *Anesthesiol* 1992; **77**: 463–6.

48 Sandler AN, Baxter AD, Norman P, *et al.* A double-blind, placebo-controlled trial of transdermal fentanyl for post-hysterectomy pain relief. II. Respiratory effects. *Can J Anaesth* 1991; **38:** A114 (abstract).

49 Caplan RA, Ready LB, Oden RV, *et al.* Transdermal fentanyl for postoperative pain management. A double-blind placebo study. *J Am Med Ass* 1989; **261:** 1036–9.

50 Bulow HH, Linnemann M, Berg H, *et al.* Respiratory changes during treatment of postoperative pain with high dose transdermal fentanyl. *Acta Anesthesiol Scand* 1995; **39:** 835–9.

51 van Lersberghe C, Camu F, de Keersmaecker E, *et al.* Continuous administration of fentanyl for postoperative pain: a comparison of the epidural, intravenous, and transdermal routes. *J Clin Anesth* 1994; **6(4):** 308–14.

52 Streisand JB, Varvel JR, Stanski DR, *et al.* Absorption and bioavailability of oral transmucosal fentanyl citrate. *Anaesthesiol* 1991; **75:** 223–9.

53 Weinberg DS, Inturrisi CE, Reidenberg B, *et al.* Sublingual absorption of selected opioid analgesics. *Clin Pharm Ther* 1988; **44:** 337.

54 Dsida RM, Wheeler M, Birmingham PK, *et al.* Premedication of pediatric tonsillectomy patients with oral transmucosal fentanyl citrate. *Anesth Analg* 1998; **86:** 66–70.

55 Farrar J, Cleary J, Rauck R, *et al.* Oral transmucosal fentanyl citrate: randomised, double-blind, placebo controlled trial for treatment of breakthrough pain in cancer patients. *J Nat Cancer Inst* 1998; **908:** 611–16.

56 Lichtor J, Sevarino F, Joshi GP, *et al.* The relative potency of oral transmucosal fentanyl citrate compared with intravenous morphine in the treatment of severe postoperative pain. *Anesth Analg* 1999; **89(3):** 732–8.

57 Jacox A, Carr D, Payne R, *et al. Management of Cancer Pain*, Clinical Practice Guideline No. 9, AHCPR Publication No. 94–0592. Rockville: US Department of Health and Human Services, Public Health Service, 1994.

58 Stiebel HW, Koenigs D, Kramer J. Postoperative pain management by intranasal demand-adapted Fentanyl titration. *Anesthesiol* 1992; **77:** 281–5.

59 Stiebel HW, Pommerening J, Rieger A. Intranasal fentanyl titration for postoperative pain management in an unselected population. *Anesthesia* 1993; **48:** 753–7.

60 O'Neil G, Paech M, Wood F. Preliminary clinical use of a Patient-Controlled Intranasal Analgesia (PCINA) Device. *Anaesth Intens Care* 1997; **25:** 408–12.

61 Zeppetella G. An assessment of the safety, efficacy and acceptability of intranasal fentanyl citrate in the management of cancer-related breakthrough pain: a pilot study. *J Pain Sympt Manag* 2000; **20:** 253–8.

62 Vercauteren M, Boeckx G, Hanegreefs G, *et al.* Intranasal sufentanil for pre-operative sedation. *Anaesthesia* 1988; **43:** 270–3.

63 Henderson JM, Brodsky DA, Fisher DM, *et al.* Pre-induction of anesthesia in pediatric patients with nasally administered Sufentanil. *Anesthesiol* 1988; **68:** 671–5.

64 Helmers JHJH, Noorduin H, Van Peer A, *et al.* Comparison of intravenous and intranasal Sufentanil absorption and sedation. *Can J Anaesth* 1989; **36:** 494–7.

65 Haynes G, Brahen N, Hill H. Plasma Sufentanil concentration after intranasal administration to paediatric outpatients. *Can J Anesth* 1993; **40:** 286.

66 Schwagmeier R, Boerger N, Meissner W, *et al.* Pharmacokinetics of intranasal alfentanil. *J Clin Anesth* 1995; **72:** 109–13.

67 Bethuysen JL, Smith NT, Sanford TJ, *et al.* Physiology of alfentanil-induced rigidity. *Anesthesiol* 1986; **64(4):** 440–6.

68 Sanford TJ Jr, Weinger MB, Smith NT, *et al.* Pretreatment with sedative-hypnotics, but not with nondepolarizing muscle relaxants, attenuates alfentanil-induced muscle rigidity. *J Clin Anesth* 1994; **6(6):** 473–80.

69 Ahmedzai S, Brooks D. Transdermal fentanyl versus sustained release oral morphine in cancer pain: preference, efficacy and quality of life. The TTS-fentanyl comparative trial group. *J Pain Sympt Manag* 1998; **16(3):** 141–4.

70 Slappendel R, Lako S, Crul B. Gastrointestinal side effects diminish after switch over from morphine to transdermal fentanyl. *Annl Oncol* 1994; **5(Suppl. 8):** 200 (abstract P1004).

71 Haazen L, Noorduin H, Megens A, *et al.* The constipating-inducing potential of morphine and transdermal fentanyl. *Eur J Pain* 1999; **3:** 9–15.

72 Ahmedzai S, Allan E, Fallon M, *et al.* Transdermal fentanyl in cancer pain. *J Drug Dev* 1994; **6:** 93–7.

Chapter 12

Methadone

Mellar P. Davis

Introduction

Methadone is a synthetic opioid agonist that was developed over 50 years ago. It is a biphenyl propylamine synthetic potent mu and delta agonist[1]. The chemical structure is distinctly different from other opioid alkaloids or theobaine derivatives[2]. Methadone's physicochemical properties, pharmacodynamics and kinetics are unique compared with hydrophilic opioids. In addition methadone is not a pure mu opioid receptor (MOR) agonist, which adds complexity to the determination of opioid equianalgesia. Finally, as evidenced by clinical experience, there is a large interindividual difference in methadone pharmacology, which necessitates guidelines for safe use that are distinctly different than those used for morphine.

Pharmacodynamics

Methadone is a racemate of R(L) and S(D) methadone[3]. Its enantiomers bind to the mu agonist with an affinity (km) of 3.5 nM compared with 1.4 nM for morphine[4]. The R methadone has a 10-fold higher affinity for MOR and delta opioid receptor (DOR) receptors, and has as much as a five times greater analgesic ability as compared with S methadone (Table 12.1)[3,5,6]. R methadone displaces naloxone from its mu binding site, whereas S methadone is 30-fold weaker. Additional evidence for binding differences between morphine and methadone relates to intrinsic efficacy, that is, the activation of the receptor. Synergy between methadone and morphine, morphine 6 glucuronide, codeine and 6-acetyl morphine (heroin) suggests unique receptor binding compared with oxymorphone, oxycodone and lipophilic opioids, which are only additive in animal studies[7,8,9].

Table 12.1 Methadone enantiomers and opioid receptor binding

Ligand	MOR$_1$	MOR$_2$	DOR	KOR
R methadone	3.01	6.94	371	1332
S methadone	26.4	87.5	9532	2137
Morphine	2.55	6.59	365	213

Km = IC$_{50}$ (nM)

MOR = mu opioid receptor; DOR = delta opioid receptor; KOR = kappa opioid receptor

Source: Kristensen (1995).

Table 12.2 NMDA affinity (*Km*, mM)

S methadone	R methadone	Dextromethorphan
7.4	3.4	5.0

Source: Gorman (1997).

Both S and R methadone bind to N-methyl-D-aspirate receptors (NMDA) and methadone's affinity for the NMDA receptor is similar to dextromethorphan and ketamine.[6,10–12] Affinities to the NMDA receptor may differ depending upon the location of the NMDA receptor (spinal cord, forebrain, cortical). Both R and S methadone displace the potent NMDA blocker MK801[10]. This inhibition is non-competitive and long lasting[11]. Although methadone has a slightly reduced affinitive for the MOR compared with morphine, its intrinsic efficacy is twice that of morphine indicating different G-protein and receptor interactions[3]. Interactions with MOR differ from morphine, as certain MOR mutations shift the dose response curves of morphine, but not those of methadone (Table 12.2)[8,9].

Methadone is a strong inhibitor of serotonin and norepinephrine reuptake. The *Km* for R and S methadone is 0.014 and 0.992 mM/l, respectively. The *Km* for norepinephrine reuptake is 0.702, and for R and S methadone, it is 12.7 mM/I[6,13]. There is no relationship between opioid receptor interactions, and serotonin or norepinephrine reuptake inhibition. Methadone competes with desipramine at serotonin reuptake sites. In high doses, methadone blocks potassium channels required for rapid cardiac muscle repolarization, which may explain the risk of developing Torsades de Pointe with high doses[6].

Methadone blocks morphine tolerance as measured by rebound cyclic AMP upon morphine withdrawal (superactivation of adenylyl cyclase)[4,7]. However delta receptors are desensitized by chronic methadone through the uncoupling of G proteins[7,14]. S methadone, which does not bind to MOR prevents morphine analgesic tolerance in mice and suggests that reduced tolerance is not related to MOR interactions[15,16]. S methadone toxicity is also independent of opioid binding[5]. Adrenalectomy increases methadone potency without altering its binding characteristics to either MOR or DOR[17,18].

Methadone does not suppress the function of natural killer cells and actually improves abnormal immune response in i.v. heroin users[19,20]. HIV infections reduce delta opioid receptors in white cells, which are increased 31-fold in lymphocytes, 62-fold in monocytes and 42-fold in granulocytes by methadone[21]. Methadone increases the CCR-5 co-receptors on white cells, which are the entrance receptors for HIV invasion of lymphocytes. Methadone treated lymphocytes release more HIV than unexposed lymphocytes *in vitro*[22]. This HIV replication is promoted by methadone maintenance[23].

Lung cancer cells, dependent upon bombesin will undergo apoptosis with methadone resulting from methadone inactivation of mitogen-activated protein kinase and reduction in BCL-2[24].

Pharmacokinetics

Absorption

Methadone absorption is rapid, probably due to its lipophilic characteristic. Initial drug levels are measurable within 30 min, although peak plasma concentrations occur at 2.5 h for solutions and 3 h for tablets[3,6,25,26]. Oral bioavailability ranges between 41 and 97%, and is independent of fractional bound methadone, liver enzyme levels and liver perfusion.[3,6,27–32]. Bioavailability does not differ between enantomers[3]. Methadone is a substrate for both intestinal CYP3A4 metabolism and efflux through P glycoprotein, which may account for the variability in absorption[5,33]. Intestinal transport of methadone is increased by P glycoprotein inhibitors, such as verapramil and quinidine[33]. Plasma concentrations of methadone increase by 0.263 mg/l for every 1 mg/kg of methadone given[34]. Methadone clearance is much more variable than its absorption and absorption is not a major factor in determining the wide variations in methadone kinetics. Methadone is a highly basic drug (pKa of 9.2) and a low pH environment will keep methadone in an ionized state. Omeprazole reduces gastric acidity, and triples the maximum methadone concentrations (C-max) and the area under the curve (AUC) in experimental animals and humans[35,36]. Omeprazole does not influence methadone liver metabolism nor its clearance. Methadone absorption in advanced cancer can be delayed due to gastroparesis[6]. Methadone absorption is non-saturable and is not dose limiting[6]. However, the bioavailability of methadone decreases from 95 to 81% with time due to the induction of intestinal CYP3A4[6]. For patients with significant P glycoprotein activity and/or CYP3A4 within the gastrointestinal mucosa, parenteral methadone may lead to an unexpected increase in blood concentrations, since methadone has low hepatic extraction[33]. The average intestinal extraction of methadone by CYP3A4 is 21%[37–39]. Diets that are high in carbohydrates or fats do not alter methadone absorption.

Rectal methadone is readily absorbed. Microenemas produce analgesia within 30 min with the time to maximum concentration of 75 min. Maximum rectal methadone concentrations compared with oral methadone for the same dose (C-max of 345.5 ng/ml + 172.5 for 10 mg) are equivalent[40]. Methadone suppositories in a hydrogenated oil base delays absorption due to retention of the drug within the lipid compound[41,42].

Intranasal methadone is rapidly absorbed as maximum plasma concentrations occur within 7 min, analgesia occurs within 30 min. The duration of action can be as long as 10 h[43].

The sublinqual absorption of methadone is 34% compared with 51% for fentanyl and 18% for morphine at a same pH (6.5). Buffering the oral pH to 8.5 doubles methadone absorption to 75%. Methadone absorption by sublingual route will also depends upon the contact time with the mucosa[44].

Protein binding

Methadone's volume of distribution is much larger than physiological volume due to extensive tissue binding (brain, gut, kidney, liver, muscle and lung). The estimation of methadone's volume of distribution ranges between 2 and 5 l/kg, indicating a greater binding to extravascular tissues than circulating proteins[6]. Both the volume of distribution and the extent of plasma protein binding influences methadone clearance and half-life[45–49].

The R enantimer has a larger volume of distribution that the S enantamer (497 + 117 versus 289 + 78 l) due to the different tissue binding characteristics between R and S methadone. Alpha$_1$ acid glycoprotein (AAG) binds R methadone less well, which allows it to extrude better than S methadone, which is 86% protein bound in vascular spaces[6].

Methadone binds predominantly to alpha$_1$ glycoprotein (AAG) due to its basic properties[49]. AAG increases with inflammation and advanced cancer, and as a result the amount of unbound methadone decreases, delaying its onset to action[50,51]. However, once at steady state, the free fraction of methadone will be unchanged. There will be more bound drug with high levels of AAG delaying methadone clearance, but limited volume of distribution[3]. Increased plasma protein binding also decreases hepatic extraction, such that an unpredictable influence is added to individual patient variation due to reactive increases in AAG. Cancer patients will have greater variability (4-fold) in amounts of free and unbound methadone than the normal individuals, and less predictable drug kinetics compared with non-cancer patients[6,50].

There are two sites on AAG which binds methadone. AAG is also coded by two separate genes with different affinities for methadone. The A isoform derived from the gene ORM$_2$ binds to the R enantiomer more avidly, and influences methadone kinetics to a greater extent than the F and SL isoforms derived from the alternate structural gene[6].

Hepatic metabolism

Methadone's bi-exponential kinetics are, to some extent, related to its absorption and tissue binding, and, to a greater extent, to its hepatic metabolism. Methadone has a low hepatic extraction ratio (0.16–0.08). Drug clearance is not dependent upon hepatic blood flow nor hepatic clearance through cytochrome enzyme activity[3,47–49]. Drug dose alone accounts for only 47% of the variability in methadone concentrations at steady state[52].

This variability is due to the complexity of methadone metabolism (Table 12.3). Methadone is demethylated by CYP3A4 to 2-ethylidene 1–5-dimethyl-3–3-dephenyl pyrrolidine (EDDP), which is a non-stereospecific metabolite[53,54]. There is a 5–20-fold variation in CYP3A4 activity between individuals in the general population and at least a 5-fold difference between individuals in the excretion of EDDP. Not only are there baseline variations found in CYP3A4 activity, but there is also a time-dependent stimulation of CYP3A4 by methadone (auto-induction), which shortens the elimination half-life and increases the percentage recovery of EDDP in urine at study state from 2.45 to 16%[3,6,27,55]. Chronic dosing increases drug clearance as much as 3.5-fold[27,56]. Autoinduction reduces the elimination half-life from 120 h by single dose studies to 48 h at study state[57]. Variations in terminal half-life at steady state can range from 15 to 60 h[6,28,58]. Methadone mildly inhibits CYP3A4, which further complicates its pharmacokinetics[53,55,59]. Methadone's low affinity for CYP3A4 means that its metabolism is easily inhibited by other medications[6]. Other cytochromes also play a minor role in methadone metabolism, and are CYP2D6, CYP1A2, CYP2C9 and CYP2C19. Methadone demethylation by CYP2D6 is four times slower than by CYP3A4[6]. Unlike CYP3A4, which has a high capacity despite low affinity, CYP2D6 has a high affinity and low capacity for methadone[60]. CYP2D6 appears to be subject to stereospecific for R methadone, while other cytochromes are not limited to either enantiomer selection[61]. CYP2D6 is a contributing factor to the wide individual differences between methadone clearance. Ultra rapid metabolizers (more than two active genes for CYP2D6) will have half the methadone serum concentrations per dose at steady state compared with poor metabolizers[6]. The CYP2D6 genotype (and phenotype) influences methadone levels and R : S enantiomer ratios[6]. In addition, methadone is known to inhibit CYP2D6[6,62–64]. CYP1A2, CYP2C9 and CYPC19 isoforms play a role in methadone metabolism and drug half-life. CYP1A2 is inducible by cigarette smoking, which reduces methadone's half-life[52,54]. The final result is that methadone clearance can vary between individuals with advanced cancer by as much as 100-fold (0.023–2.1 l/min)[47–49,65]. Single dose studies in healthy populations cannot accurately reflect methadone kinetics in cancer pain[66].

The biliary excretion of EDDP and other metabolites greatly exceeds methadone biliary excretion and for this reason enterohepatic circulation appears not to be a significant factor to the highly individual differences in kinetics[67].

Table 12.3 Causes of interindividual differences in methadone pharmacokinetics

P glycoprotein polymorphism
CYP3A4 basal activity
CYP2D6 metabolizer status
Isoforms of CYP1A2, CYP2C9, CYP2C19
Genotype of alpha$_1$ acid glycoprotein
Co-medications
Urine pH

Table 12.4 Urine pH and methadone clearance

	Urine pH 5.2	Urine pH 7.8
Clearance	134 ml/min + 21	92 ml/min + 9
t½	19 + 3.6 h	42 + 8.8 h
Volume	3.51 + 0.4 l/kg	5.24 + 6.83 l/kg
% Methadone elimination in urine	35	1

Renal clearance

Methadone's renal clearance inversely relates to urine pH. A urinary pH of greater than 6 results in a methadone urinary clearance of 4%, whereas a urine pH of less than 6 will lead to 30% urinary excretion[3,68]. Urine pH can account for as much as 27% of individual variability in methadone serum levels. Methadone plasma half-life is 42 h when oral bicarbonate is used to alkalinize the urine and 19.5 h when urine is acidified by oral ammonia chloride (Table 12.4)[30,31]. However, bicarbonate use will also increase methadone's volume of distribution independent of plasma clearance and, therefore, will indirectly influence its renal elimination[6]. Under normal conditions, despite the influence of urine pH on methadone clearance, renal function plays little role in the overall drug half-life and clearance[66].

Cerebrospinal fluid methadone levels

Drug plasma levels alone cannot account for methadone analgesia. To produce analgesia methadone must first bind to central nervous system (CNS) MOR. It usually takes extra time to distribute methadone to CNS opioid receptors. This delay (or progressive analgesia with multiple doses of methadone) may reflect variability and time dependence in developing effective concentrations at central opioid receptor sites, which may involve redistribution from central compartments. Therefore, there is a wide range of methadone plasma concentrations at the time of pain relief. Steady state plasma concentrations for a 50% maximum of pain relief range from 0.04 to 1.13 µg/ml (mean 0.29 µg/ml)[28,47,48,59]. CNS methadone levels vary from 2 to 73% of corresponding serum levels for the same dose in humans[69-71].

Routes of administration

Methadone can be given via oral, intranasal, sublingual, rectal, subcutaneous, intravenous and epidural routes[26,34,43,47-49,70,72]. The safe conversion ratio from oral to parenteral methadone is reported to be 2 : 1. Sublingual bioavailability as previously mentioned is less than fentanyl, but greater than morphine. Intranasal absorption is rapid and the drug kinetics resemble oral dosing. The usual oral to rectal dosing ratio is 1 : 1. Methadone microenemas are better absorbed than within fatty suppositories. There is little advantage to spinal methadone due to its rapid systemic redistribution from epidural and subarachnoid spaces. Subcutaneous methadone is associated with local skin reactions[73,74]. However, diluting methadone, changing subcutaneous needles frequently, giving small doses of dexamethasone in the infusion or at the injection site, or using subcutaneous hyaluronidase reduces the risk for a subcutaneous inflammatory reaction[75].

Drug interactions

Co-medications produce a greater individual variability in serum concentrations per dose compared with patients on methadone alone (41- versus 17-fold, respectively)[60]. Neither age nor gender plays a major role in determining drug interactions. A significant number of deaths related to methadone use, particularly at steady state are due either to drug interactions from interfering medications or to illicit drug used to reinforce psychological dependence[76]. The severity of drug interactions depends upon competing drug plasma concentrations, enzyme affinity of the competing drug (K_i) and the type of inhibition, which is either competitive/non-competitive[53]. Methadone's metabolism, because it is dependent upon multiple type I cytochrome isoenzymes, poses a greater risk for drug interactions than morphine. Even though methadone is highly protein bound, competing drugs require higher than usual drug concentrations to displace methadone from its binding site such that few interactions are a result of competitive protein binding[50]. The antiretroviral agents are competitive inhibitors to methadone metabolism. Clinical significance drug interactions with antiretrovirals are influenced by the inhibitory constant on the antiviral, which in descending order is ritonavir, indinavir, saquinavir (Table 12.5). Combinations of antivirals may increase methadone clearance despite competitive interactions at the metabolizing enzyme site[77]. Combinations of ambrenavir and saquinavir actually increase methadone clearance, although there is an initial competitive inhibition to methadone clearance that adds complexity to the highly active antiretroviral therapy (HAART) interaction. There is displacement of protein binding and stimulation of intestinal CYP3A4 by the antiretrovials, which further complicates methadone pharmacokinetics[78]. Nelfinavir is a strong inhibitor to CYP3A4 and ritonavir stimulates P-glycoprotein enzyme, which has an overall effect of decreasing or increasing methadone clearance[6].

The combinations of fluoxetine and methadone leads to prolonged inhibition of methadone clearance. Fluoxetine's metabolite norfluoxetine has a greater inhibitory effect on CYP3A4 than fluoxetine alone. Norfluoxetine takes several weeks to clear and thus inhibits methadone metabolism for a long period of time[79].

Ethanol acutely reduces methadone N-demethylation, and increases methadone brain and liver levels. Chronic ingestion increases methadone N-demethylation and decreases methadone levels[80].

Medications which do not interact with methadone are rifambutin, famotidine, mirtazapine, haloperidol, olanzapine, valproic acid and gabapentin, and the newer antiseizure medications.

Table 12.5 Drug interactions with methadone

Drug	Effect	Cause	Clinical significance
Anti-ulcer			
Cimetidine	Delayed clearance	Inhibition CYP3A4	+
Omeprazole	Increased rate of absorption	Increased gastric pH	±
Antibiotic			
Rifampin	Increased clearance	Induces CYP3A4 and Pgp	+
Ciprofloxacin	Decreased clearance	Inhibits CYP1A2 and CYP3A4	+
Isoniazid	Increased clearance	Increased CYP3A4 activity	+
Fluconazole and ketoconazole	Reduced clearance	Inhibitor CYP3A4	+
Fusidic acid	Increased clearance	Increases CYP3A4 activity	+
Antiretroviral inhibitors			
Amprenavir	Increases clearance	Induces CYP3A4 activity	–
Indinavir	Reduces clearance	Inhibits CYP3A4 activity	
Lopinavir	Increases clearance	Induces CYP3A4 activity	+
Nelfinavir	Increases clearance	Induces CYP3A4 activity	Rarely significant
Ritonavir	Increases clearance	Induces CYP3A4, CYP2C9 and CYP2C19	+
Saquinavir	Increases or decreases clearance	Induces CYP3A4 and inhibits activity	+
Nucleoside reverse troxscritase inhibitor			
Stavudine (d4T)	Decreases D4T methadone	Cytochrome inhibition	–
Zidovudine A2T	Methadone decreases clearance	Inhibits cytochrome metabolism of A2T	+
Didanosine	Methadone decreases clearance	Inhibits cytochrome metabolism	–
Abacavir	Increases clearance	Induces CYP3A4 activity	+
Non-nucleoside reverse transcriptase inhibitor			
Efavirenz	Increases methadone clearance	Induces CYP3A4 activity	+
Nevirapine	Increases methadone clearance	Induces CYP3A4 activity	+
Antidepressants			
Amitriptyline	Decreases methadone clearance	Competitive inhibition of CYP1A2, CYP2C9, CYP2C19, CYP2D6, CYP3A4	±
Desipramine	Desipramine clearance is reduced	Methadone inhibits CYP2D6	±
Mactobemide	Reduces methadone clearance	Inhibition of CYP1A2 and CYP2D6	+
Fluoxetine	Reduces methadone clearance	Inhibition of CYP1A2, CYP2C19, CYP2C9, CYP3A4	+
Paroxetine	Reduces methadone clearance	Inhibition of CYP2D6	+

Table 12.5 (continued)

Drug	Effect	Cause	Clinical significance
Sertraline	Reduces methadone clearance	Inhibition of CYP2D6, CYP3A4, CYP1A2, CYP2C9 and moderate inhibitor CYP2C19	±
Antiseizure medications			
Carbamazepine	Increases methadone clearance	Induces CYP3A4 activity	+
Phenobarbital	Increases methadone clearance	Induces CYP3A4	+
Phenytoin	Increases methadone clearance	Induces CYP3A4	+
Antipsychotics Resperidone	Increases methadone clearance	Induces cytochrome enzymes	+
Benzodiazepines Alprazolam	Increases methadone respiratory depression	Pharmacodynamic interaction	+
Diazepam	Minor competitive interaction, but major pharmacodynamic effect	Competitive inhibition CYP3A4 and synergy for respiratory depression	+
Alcohol	Acutely decreases, chronically increases methadone	Inhibitor of CYP3A4 activity, stimulants CYP3A4 inhibition	+
Diuretics Spironolactone	Decreases methadone	Stimulate CYP3A4 activity	±
Opioids Dextromethorpton Codeine Tramadol	Decreases conversion to active metabolite (codeine tramadol)	Inhibits CYP2D6 activity	−
Cigarette smoke	Increases methadone clearance	Stimulates CYP1A2 activity	±

Toxicity

Methadone's side effects are similar to other opioids. These include constipation, dysphoria, dizziness, headaches, mental clouding, nausea, pruritus, respiratory depression, urinary retention and vomiting[6]. Dry mouth has been reported to be less, but nausea worse with methadone[81]. Less nausea and visual hallucinations were noted in one series of patients who received psychotropics plus methadone compared with those receiving methadone alone[82]. In this series, 20% of patients still developed nausea and vomiting despite receiving antiemetics. Improved constipation and reduced laxative requirements have been reported when rotating to methadone from other opioids[83,84].

Torsades de Pointes has been reported with high methadone dose combined with medications known to increase QTc intervals[85]. At risk for Torsades de Pointe are those with familial cardiac conduction defects or those with a history of cardiac disease[6]. Methadone in high doses blocks the potassium membrane transport necessary for rapid myocardial repolarization[6]. In a series of patients reported to have Torsades de Pointes on methadone, the mean daily dose was 397 + 283 mg and the mean QTc interval was 615 + 72 ms. Fourteen of the 17 patients had additional risk factors[85]. Methadone is reported to be a potential cause of ventricular arrhythmia if:

- given in high doses;

- given with medications that prolong the QTc interval;

- in individuals with congenital or acquired prolong QTc intervals[6].

General recommendations are:

- obtain an ECG if there is a history of prolongation of the QTc interval;

- repeat an ECG if methadone plasma levels greater than 800 mg/l;

- alternatively obtain an ECG when doses are 500 mg or more per day;

- draw methadone levels 4 h after the initial dose[6].

Cancer pain may require high doses of methadone for which there are few alternatives. Benefits of methadone may outweigh the risks in predisposed individuals. Therapeutic recommendations should include a risk/benefit discussion with patients.

Though the clinical response to methadone is more important than blood levels of methadone, low blood levels at high doses indicate that methadone is either rapidly cleared or that there is a lack of compliance. Doses can be safely increased once compliance has been confirmed. This may be particularly helpful for patients receiving medications that influence methadone clearance[6].

Visual hallucinations and myoclonus occur with methadone despite the absence of known neuroactive metabolites[86,87]. Euphoria and choreoathetoid movements with rapid dose adjustments have been reported accidentally[88]. Psychomotor skills are mildly impaired, but at steady state the impairment is not enough to prevent most patients from driving. There is no correlation between reduced psychomotor skills, daily dose or age[89].

Patients on chronic methadone develop a significant tolerance to morphine analgesia and there is diminished pain tolerance while on methadone maintenance[90,91]. Attempted rotations from methadone to morphine or other opioids frequently fails[92]. Equianalgesic doses from methadone to other opioids may not be the same as those used when converting to methadone. Attempted rotations to alternative opioids while on methadone maintenance not infrequently leads to pain relapse in cancer patients[93].

Deaths from methadone are more common at initiation of methadone, rather than at steady state, and are related to delated clearance from initial drug titration and interfering medications[94]. Many equianalgesic tables contain morphine to methadone ratios that are near unity, but inappropriate for chronic dosing. If these tables are followed they will predictably lead to delayed toxicity and respiratory depression.

In the psychologically-dependent population, polysubstance abuse is common. Additional drugs such as cocaine, benzodiazepines, alcohol and cannabis will either increase methadone levels (diazepam or alcohol) or enhance its psychologically reinforcing effects (cocaine, cannabis and other opioids) both will synergistically depress respiration[6]. Methadone tablets and syrups have been converted to injectable to boost doses and this can sometimes lead to respiratory depression[38]. Therefore, even though methadone is the opioid of choice for those with a history of addiction and cancer pain, its use should be monitored with caution and close observation.

Dosing in special populations

Liver disease

Methadone has a longer elimination half-life in severe compared with mild or moderate liver disease[95,96]. This is compensated for by increased elimination of methadone with chronic alcohol use such that doses are similar with patients with alcoholic liver disease and those with little to no liver disease[95–97]. Doses of methadone for patients with liver disease who are on methadone maintenance can be continued without risking undo toxicity. Hepatitis C induces CYP3A4 and increases methadone clearance[6,98]. Therefore, methadone dose reductions for patients with liver disease are necessary only for those with severe disease and dose reductions will be further dependent upon the cause of the liver disease.

Renal disease

Normally, methadone urinary elimination is only a small fraction of the total methadone dose[6]. As renal function declines the fecal excretion of methadone increases[95]. Methadone clearance is not altered either by age (which is associated with reduced renal function) or by intrinsic renal disease[99]. Recommendations for a 50% dose reduction with end-stage renal failure are not founded upon clinical evidence[59]. Methadone is not removed by dialysis, therefore dialysis would be ineffective in the management of methadone overdose[6,59,100].

Pregnancy

Cancer rarely occurs in pregnancy. However, it may occasionally be necessary to use methadone during pregnancy. Pregnancy increases methadone clearance, particularly in the third trimester, and will reduce methadone absorption overall[95,101]. As a result, the pregnant cancer patient may require higher than usual doses.

Neonates of methadone-treated mothers experience opioid withdrawal postpartum if not put on tapering opioid doses. Breast-feeding is relatively safe while on methadone. The infant will receive approximately 2.8% of the maternal dose. However, the absolute dose will depend upon the maternal dose[102]. Methadone absorption through breast-feeding is not enough to prevent opioid withdrawal in the infant who was exposed to methadone *in utero*[103].

Methadone in advanced cancer pain

Introduction

Because of its unique pharmacology, methadone has been a difficult opioid to use for cancer pain. It's bioexponential pharmacokinetics, large individual differences in drug clearance, time-dependent clearance and different intrinsic efficacy compared with morphine, makes it impossible to accurately predict equianalgesia to other opioids[92,104,105]. Most studies involving the use of methadone in cancer pain center around pain that is poorly responsive to other opioids so methadone is used in sequence in rotation rather than in parallel. The reputation for delayed toxicity and respiratory death discourages most physicians from considering methadone as an alternative first line opioid or a second line analgesic for those failing to respond to morphine. However, dosing strategies are published in retrospective and prospective trials, and if followed as a guideline provide a basis for safe prescribing.

The manufacturer's initial recommendation of 2.5–10 mg every 3–4 h in opioid-naïve patients is excessive. Overdoses will be experienced if physicians follow this initial recommendation[106]. Methadone potency is much greater than previously published in older equianalgesic tables dating from in the 1980s and early 1990s. Recent studies have found methadone's relative potency increases with the dose of morphine at the time of rotation. This is also true for hydromorphone[107]. Hence, opioid ratios will change with total opioid dose prior to methadone rotation[105,107].

Case reports

The experience with methadone by case reports illustrates the relevant issues regarding potency, particularly at high doses. Vigano reported rotating from parenteral hydromorphone to methadone for severe pain due to spinal cord compression. Analgesia was obtained at 1/30th of the expected equivalence[108]. Hunt described a patient who developed respiratory depression when rotating from 84 mg of parenteral hydromorphone to 30 mg of oral methadone every 8 h[109]. Manfredi reported rotations from morphine or hydromorphone to methadone, which resulted in pain relief at 3% of the calculated equianalgesic dose as determined by older equivalent tables[110]. Thomas and colleagues reported a methadone response with rotation from hydromorphone 200 mg/h to 800 mg methadone/6 h[111]. Fitzgibbon reported a successful switch from 1920 mg parenteral hydromorphone/day to 440 mg oral methadone/day[112]. Davis reported a response from 60 mg parenteral hydromorphone/h to 40 mg oral methadone twice a day[113].

A stop-start dosing strategy was reported by Crews which used an 'as needed' methadone dosing strategy[114]. Paalzow performed pharmacokinetics on a small series of patients using initial dose intervals of 0, 6, 12 and 24 h, then daily with successful resolution of pain[115]. These patients were opioid naïve. This loading dose strategy was chosen due to methadone's slow clearance exponential kinetics[115]. Ayonrinde and colleagues described the clinical use of a conversion ladder ratio in a small series of patients based upon previous published experience. The methadone dose was chosen by using a ratio of 3 : 1 (morphine to methadone) for daily morphine equivalents of less than 100 mg, 5 : 1 for 101–300 mg, 10 : 1 if 301–600 mg, 12 : 1 for 601–800 mg, 15 : 1 for 801–1000 mg and 20 : 1 for over 1000 mg daily. Pain relief occurred in the 11 cancer patients. Maintenance doses were reached in 3 days. This strategy also used a 'stop-start' method. Initial dosing intervals were every 6 h, then extended to 8–12 h at steady state. Morphine or oxycodone was used for rescue in this series. Final dose morphine to methadone ratios in these 11 patients ranged from 28 : 1 to 2 : 1[116].

Pharmacokinetics of rectal methadone by microenema were performed in six patients. Rectal pharmacokinetics were the same as oral[107].

Methadone has been reported in several small series of patients with neuropathic pain who responded. Morphine refractory pain and pain from bowel obstruction has been reported to improve with methadone use[117–120]. Special populations, such as children and cancer patients on methadone maintenance, will respond to methadone titration with pain relief[93,121].

There are directional differences in analgesia between morphine and methadone[105]. A small series of patients reported by Moryl and colleagues suggests that converting from methadone to different opioids frequently fails due to directional differences based upon opioid sequence that are non-reciprocal[92].

In summary, individual case reports and small retrospective cohort patient series have shown:

- the benefits of methadone in cancer pain;
- the wide range in dose equivalents;
- ratios dependent upon dose;
- improvement with neuropathic pain and morphine facilitated refractory hyperalgesia;
- benefits in special populations;
- the non-reciprocal nature of dose ratios;
- strategies that include loading dose, progressive intervals and 'stop-start' non-overlap dosing.

Retrospective studies

The earliest retrospective study was published in 1982. This series consisted of 111 patients treated with methadone and acetaminophen. A subset of 56 patients received psychotropics (haloperidol, methotrimeprazine, amitriptyline and diazepam). Initial daily doses were 37 mg (range 20–90). Dosing intervals were every 4 h, which were eventually extended to every 6 h. A subset of patients who survived 7 months were on a mean daily dose of 113 mg of methadone. Patients on psychotropics required the same daily methadone dose, but experienced less nausea, confusion and hallucinations. Cocaine was used in 12% because of sedation. Pain relief was good in 80% of patients and fair in 16%. Interestingly, 67% of patients who did not receive pyschotropics had acceptable pain relief and 33% of these patients failed to continue methadone due to side effects[81].

Fifty patients were switched either from hydromorphone to methadone or methadone to hydromorphone in a study reported by Watanabe[122]. Methadone was given either in a custom-made capsule or suppository, and hydromorphone was given parenterally. A 3-day overlapping rotation was done by reducing hydromorphone doses by 30–50% daily for 3 days, while a graduated dose escalation of methadone was started every 8 h. Equivalents were route dependent. Oral methadone to hydromorphone ratio was 1.07 + 0.9 and for hydromorphone to rectal methadone 1.88 + 1.27. Methadone suppositories were in a fatty base that differed from the microenemas reported by Ripomanti, which may have influenced bioavailability and equivalence. Constipation, sedation and nausea improved with methadone, but six of the 50 patients on study developed respiratory depression from methadone. Costs of methadone were 116.77 + 157.17 Canadian dollars for oral and 105.34 + 146.35 Canadian dollars for suppositories. The monthly parenteral hydromorphone cost was 3450.51 to 5908.58 Canadian dollars[122].

The largest methadone trial in advanced cancer is a retrospective study from Milan. Opioid-naïve patients were started on 3 mg of methadone every 8 h. Non-opioid-naïve patients on less than 60 mg of oral morphine daily before rotation received 5 mg of methadone every 8 h. For patients on 70–90 mg of morphine a ratio of 1 : 4 (methadone to morphine) was utilized and for those patients on a greater than 100 mg oral morphine/day a ratio of 1 : 6 was used. The mean age was 59 years and 62% of the patients were male. The rotation strategy was 'stop-start'. The mean methadone dose at day 7 was 14 mg and at 3 months was 24 mg. Dose levels were not associated with age or tumor type. Approximately half of the patients had a persistent reduction in pain. Twelve per cent of patients discontinued methadone for lack of efficacy, and 7% discontinued because of constipation or drowsiness. Respiratory depression or methadone related deaths were not observed with this strategy[123].

Lawlor reported 20 rotations from morphine to methadone in 19 patients. The median oral morphine dose at rotation was 1165 mg/day (range 85–24,027). A 3-day overlap schedule was used for rotation. The final equivalent ratio was 5.42 (morphine to methadone). However, those on less than 1165 mg/day had a ratio of 5 (range 2.95–9.09) and those on greater than 1165 mg a ratio of 17 (range 12.25–87.95). Both directional and dose level changes in ratios were noted with rotation from morphine to methadone and methadone to morphine. The wide ranges in doses, retrospective design and small numbers influence the conclusions about equivalents from this study[105].

A retrospective study combines the experience of clinicians from Edmonton and Milan in order to determine equianalgesic ratios between methadone and other potent opioids. A total of 88 patients were reported in this study, 37 from Edmonton and 51 from Milan. Dose ratios for parenteral hydromorphone to methadone were 1.47 (range 0.81–2.47) for Edmonton and 0.25 (range 0.17–0.44) for Milan. The final combined ratio was 0.51. Dose-related ratios were noted and different patient populations appear to have influenced the ratios from each institution. In Edmonton the mean dose of parenteral hydromorphone is 236 mg/day (36–1080) and in Milan the mean dose was 3 mg/day (range 1–60 mg). Methadone potency were 5–15 times greater than previously reported from Edmonton and 1–5 times greater than from Milan[107].

Hagen and colleagues reported their experiences with 29 patients treated with methadone over a period of 8 years using a slow overlapping rotation strategy. Median prerotation oral morphine was 1024 mg (30–2800). Rotation was performed over 25 days starting with methadone doses of 27 mg. The mean methadone dose after titration was 208 mg (range 12–1520 mg). Twenty of 29 patients reported toxicity from methadone, 12 of 20 were drowsy and nausea was present in six of 29 patients. Severe toxicity occurred in five patients. Sweating, headache and confusion were also noted[124].

Prospective studies

The earliest prospective study was reported by Sawe using 10-mg doses 'as needed' for pain for the purpose of dose finding. Pharmacokinetics were done. The first day methadone requirements ranged from 30–100 mg/day. Dosing intervals increased from 3 to 7 h on the first day to 10 h by the seventh day. The mean daily dose decreased with time by day 7. Individual dose requirements varied from 10 to 15 mg as a single dose and total daily doses ranged from 10 to 40 mg. Plasma concentrations were stable by 2–3 days. Plasma concentrations at the time of pain relief ranged from 7.4 to 54.2 mg/dl. A 7-fold difference in dose requirements occurred between individuals. Eleven of 14 patients experienced near complete pain relief[125].

A prospective trial by Hansen used 'as needed' dosing the first 3–5 days as a means of dose finding based upon pain severity and response. The first day methadone requirements were on average 44 mg and by day 7 the average dose was 22 mg. Three of 15 patients did not complete the trial, either due to nausea or lack of response. Methadone provided long-term pain relief in this small group of patients[126].

A prospective, randomized trial involving 18 patients compared the pharmacokinetics and pain response of morphine to methadone. Methadone half-life was 30.4 + 16.3 h, while that for morphine was 2.7 + 1.2 h and drug clearance was

0.19 + 0.14 l/min for methadone and 1.16 + 0.47 l/min for morphine. Methadone oral bioavailability was 79 + 11.7% compared with 26 + 13% for morphine. The coefficient of variation for oral bioavailability was 15% for methadone and 50% for morphine. Morphine doses ranged from 15 mg every 4 h to 150 mg every 3 h in the nine patients on morphine. Methadone doses ranged from 15 mg every other day to 20 mg twice a day. Adequate pain control was experienced by both groups[127].

Ventafridda randomized 27 patients between morphine and methadone. The minimum morphine dose was 4 mg and the maximum dose was 24 mg every 4 h. Total methadone daily doses ranged between 8 and 24 mg, were divided into four and given every 6 h for 3 days then every 8 h for the rest of the study. The duration of the study was 14 days and all patients were treated at home. Diclofenac and haloperdol were used as adjuvants. Initial doses were chosen based upon pain intensity and the type of opioid used prior to methadone. Pain responses were determined by an integrated pain score that took into account the daily pain duration and pain intensity. Responses occurred, on average, within 2 days. The morphine daily dose at steady state was 120 + 79.1 mg and methadone dose 18 mg at steady state. Nausea and vomiting occurred in 20% of patients. Sleep, performance score and quality of life improved on both morphine and methadone. Dry mouth was more common with morphine and headaches more frequent with methadone. Constipation, nausea, pruritus, restlessness, tremors and vomiting were the same in both groups. Methadone doses remained stable over the 14 days of the study, while patients on morphine required higher doses over time. The authors concluded that methadone dosing strategies need to be different than those for morphine[82].

Grochow and colleagues performed a double-blind, randomized trial of parenteral morphine versus methadone for cancer pain[128]. Twenty-three patients were randomized, five withdrew leaving 10 on the parenteral morphine and eight on parenteral methadone. All received their opioid through a computer-activated drug dose (CADD) pump with patient controlled analgesia as a strategy. Oral morphine dose requirements at the time of the study were 128 mg (range 24–456) and methadone doses were 344 mg (range 16–980). There was a great deal of variability in dose requirement between patients and, as a result, this aspect of the study was not statistically significant. The mean parenteral morphine dose requirement was 24 and 64 mg for oral methadone. Dose intervals and increments were not different between the opioids. All 18 patients studied had greater than a 50% reduction in pain. Sedation occurred in 11 of 18 patients. Nausea, dry mouth and constipation were noted. This small study has relatively limited applicability as a comparison between groups in opioid requirements[128].

Plummer and colleagues reported a prospective study involving 25 patients. Methadone was delivered at a dose of 0.5 mg/min until analgesia or side effects occurred. The combined experience of 162 patients was reported. Pharmacokinetics were obtained in a subset of patients. Methadone clearance was 0.186 l/min. The daily methadone requirement ranged from 8 to 67 mg[65].

The pharmacokinetics reported in the prospective part of the studies with methadone were distinctly different from those studies using morphine. These studies demonstrated the benefits of the 'as needed' dosing. Methadone dose differences in morphine equivalents were confirmed by these studies. Most if not all prospective studies are small in size (less than 40) and are subject to patient heterogeneity[65].

Prospective trials from the 1990's to the present

A prospective trial was reported by Bruera and colleagues involving 219 patients screened and 37 eligible patients. Patients were rotated to methadone over 3 days from hydromorphone. Prior to rotation, patients had poorly responsive pain to hydromorphone. Sixteen received methadone suppositories and 21 were on oral methadone. An Edmonton pain staging system was used. Methadone was given every 8 h. Comparisons with parenteral hydromorphone were made. Plasma levels of methadone were obtained in those receiving rectal methadone. The hydromorphone to methadone ratio was 1.2 (+1.3) and for methadone suppositories 3 (+2). There was a significant difference between the oral and rectal methadone dose requirements, but values overlapped in range within these differences[41].

A prospective trial sponsored by the Pain Research Institute of Liverpool used methadone dosing guidelines based upon 'as needed' for a collaborative experience involving 32 hospices and 146 patients. Rotations were from diamorphine to methadone or morphine to methadone. The mean patient age was 55.8 years and the median daily oral morphine dose was 750 mg (range 150–4500). The guidelines suggested the use of a fixed dose of 1/10th of the calculated or actual 24-h oral morphine or equivalents with a maximum single methadone dose of 30 mg. Dosing was 'as needed' every 3 h based upon pain severity. At day 6 the total daily methadone dose based upon on days 4 and 5 was divided by four and given every 12 h with a provision for methadone breakthrough doses. The previous opioid was discontinued consistent with a 'stop-start' strategy when methadone was started. Methadone requirements diminished after 2–3 days and a steady dose occurred by days 3–4. Pain control occurred in most patients. Respiratory depression was not seen in this large trial[129].

A prospective trial by Mercadante and colleagues included both opioid naïve and previously treated patients. Naive-naïve patients received 3–5 mg of methadone three times a day. Morphine treated patients were started on 50% of the calculated methadone equivalents per day divided into three doses and taken every 8 h. Breakthrough doses and dose adjustments were made if more than four rescue doses per day were required. Nineteen opioid-naïve and eight opioid-treated patients were studied. There was no correlation between methadone dose and plasma levels. Patients who were 70 or older required 11 mg of methadone (range per day. Their dose requirements gradually increased to 21 mg daily (range 14–30) by the time of death. Opioid-treated patients required 33 mg of methadone daily (range 15–60) and 56.8 mg (range 24–80) at the time of death. Side effects included constipation in 12, dry mouth in eight, drowsiness in five, nausea and vomiting in five[130].

A prospective trial involved patients on either oral or parenteral morphine that was subsequently converted to either oral or parenteral methadone. A 3-day overlap strategy was used for conversion. Morphine doses were reduced by 30–50% on the first day and again on the second. Methadone doses were gradually added based upon the prerotation morphine dose. If the daily morphine doses prior to rotation were 30–90 mg, a morphine to methadone ratio of 4 : 1 was used for 90–300 mg of daily morphine, and a ratio of 6 : 1 and greater than 300 mg, 8 : 1. Forty-nine patients were included, 11 patients were excluded and 17 patients were males. The mean age was 60.5 years (55–66). Twenty-eight patients were converted from oral morphine and 10 patients were converted from parenteral morphine. The median daily oral morphine dose or equivalent was 145 mg (range 30–800). The median daily methadone dose was 21 mg daily (range 9–60) and the median morphine to methadone dose ratio was 7.75 (range 2.5–14.3). A strong linear dose ratio was observed. Dose ratios increased dramatically from lower to high morphine doses. The actual dose ratios at the end of the study were 3.7 (for morphine 30–90 mg daily) 7.5 (for morphine 90–300 mg daily) and 12.25 (for morphine >300 mg daily)[131].

Gagnon reported a prospective trial that involved 34 of 120 patients who were evaluable. A 3-day overlap rotation strategy was utilized. Twenty-two had neuropathic pain and 18 had nociceptive pain. The morphine to methadone ratio was 3.4 + 2.5 (mean) and 7.8 + 5.9 (median) for neuropathic pain, and 4.5 + 0.5 (mean) and 6.13 + 2.3 (median) for nociceptive pain. This study involves a small number of patients, but a large difference in dose requirements among patients[132].

A prospective single-arm trial of 45 patients reported by Mercadante and colleagues involved the use of a 1% solution of methadone, which was given two or three times daily. Patients on study were opioid naïve. The mean age was 60.6 + 11.9 years and 24 patients were female. Dose requirements did not correlate with age, gender or type of pain. Starting doses were 14.4 + 5.5 mg/day with a maximum daily dose of 27.2 + 17.9 mg. Side effects included confusion in three patients, constipation in 17 patients, dry mouth in 10 patients, drowsiness in nine patients, sweating in seven patients, and nausea and vomiting in 10[133].

A second trial by the same group involved methadone in a rotation involving 24 patients. Morphine to methadone rotation used 20% of the daily morphine dose as the total daily methadone dose. Methadone was divided by 3 and administered three times daily. The indications for rotation were side effects and pain[134]. Fourteen patients were on less than 90 mg morphine/day. The mean morphine dose prior to rotation was 125 mg. The maximum daily methadone dose at the end of study was 32 mg. Methadone dose reductions were required in six patients who were on higher doses of morphine prior to rotation. Increased methadone doses were required in seven patients who were on lower morphine doses prior to rotation. Neuropathic pain required higher methadone doses[134].

A prospective single-arm trial involved patients with uncontrolled pain and opioid side effects as reported by Scholes and colleagues. Rotation to methadone was done by using a 'stop-start' strategy. Single methadone doses were 10% of the total daily morphine dose available every 3 h as needed with a single allowable maximum dose of 40 mg of methadone. Thirty-three patients with a mean age of 61 (34–91 years) and 20 females entered this trial. Neuropathic pain was present in 11 patients and a mixed neuropathic nociceptive pain was present in 19 patients. Rotation for purposes of poorly controlled pain was done in 26 patients and for side effects in seven patients. Prior to rotation patients were receiving diamorphine in 12, morphine in 19 and fentanyl in two. The median morphine or equivalent dose was 480 mg (range 20–1200). Response occurred in 78% of patients (26). Twelve per cent of patients (four) withdrew during titration because of terminal illness and one due to failure to respond. Stable doses occurred by day 3 (range 2–18 days). Nearly half of the patients required dose adjustments[135].

Mankin reported rotation from morphine to methadone in 43 patients, 18 of whom were terminally ill. The median morphine dose prior to rotation was 372 mg (range 40–4200) and median methadone dose was 76 mg (range 10–200). The mean age was 56.5 years (range 22–78). Seventy-six per cent (33) had neuropathic pain. Eight-six per cent (37) responded by day 7. Six patients had intolerable side effects. Twelve of 18 terminally ill patients were successfully converted to subcutaneous methadone from oral using a parenteral to oral conversion ratio of 1 : 2. No local cutaneous irritation was noted in this subset of patients. The author suggested using isotonic solution and hyaluronidase reduced subcutaneous toxicity from methadone[136].

Another prospective trial was reported by Mercadante and colleagues in 2001. Fifty-two patients were treated with a 'stop-start' strategy, and dose ratios were based upon the baseline morphine or equivalent morphine dose. A methadone : morphine dose ratio of 1 : 4 was used with less than 90 mg of daily morphine or equivalents, 1 : 8 for 90–300 mg of daily morphine or equivalents daily, and 1 : 12 for greater than 300 mg morphine/day. Oral doses were divided into three and given every 8 h. The mean age was 60.7 years (range 57–63) and 24 of the patients were female. Responses occurred in 80% of patients. Steady state occurred by day 3–4. Most opioid-related side effects improved with rotation. Half of the patients required a dose adjustment. Patients rotating for pain required a higher dose of methadone (by 20–33%) compared with those rotated for purposes of opioid side effects. No difference in response was noted between neuropathic and nociceptive pain, nor was response related to age or gender[137].

A small prospective trial involved patients on fentanyl who were rotated to methadone. Eighteen patients were included in this trial. The mean age was 57.6 years (23–79). Four had neuropathic pain and four had mixed neuropathic and nociceptive pain. The median fentanyl dose was 375 μg/h (50–2500 μg). The total fentanyl dose per hour when breakthrough doses were added was 483 μg (range 91.6–2706 μg). The median methadone dose per hour was 2.25 mg (range 0.4–15.4). The authors estimated that 25 mg fentanyl/h equaled a 0.1-mg dose of methadone[138].

Summary of recent prospective trials

Three rotation strategies have been reported in prospective and retrospective trials. A 3-day overlap rotation schedule utilizes a morphine or morphine equivalent reduced by 30–50% per day, while simultaneously adding methadone and has been used in a minority of groups. Respiratory depression was reported in two trials utilizing this strategy. Another rotation strategy includes a 'stop-start' method with every 8 h dosing using a linear dose ratio based upon prerotation morphine doses or an every 3 h 'as needed' dose strategy in which initial methadone doses are 1/10th of the total daily morphine or equivalent dose. Responses with these dosing methods are seen in 80% of the patients. Dose requirements do not appear to be related to age, gender or type of pain (except in one small trial). A minority of trials involved opiod-naïve patients, with most trials consisting of opiod-treated patients who are not responding well. Opiod-naïve patients on average required 10–20 mg every other day to 30–40 mg methadone/day. Side effects are similar to other opioids. One trial reported a significant cost savings with methadone compared with parenteral hydromorphone.

Dose and routes

Methadone is available in 5-, 10- and 40-mg tablets in the USA. Available oral solutions contain 5 and 10 mg/5 ml, and 10 mg/ml. Injectable methadone comes in ampuoles of 10 mg/ml. Some countries will have a 20-mg/ml oral concentrate.

References

1 Nicholson A, Davies A, Reid C. Methadone for cancer pain protocol. *Cochrane Database System Rev* 2004; 2: CD003971.

2 Bruera E, Sweeney C. Methadone use in cancer patients with pain: a review. *J Pallat Med* 2002; **5(1):** 127.

3 Garrido MJ, Troconiz IF. Methadone: a review of its pharmacokinetic/pharmacodynamic properties. *J Pharmacol Toxicol* 1999; **42:** 61–6.

4 Blake AD, Bot G, Freeman, *et al*. Differential opioid agonist regulation of the mouse mu opioid receptor. *J Biol Chem* 1997; **10:** 782–90.

5 Kristensen K, Christensen CB, Christup LL. The mu_1, mu_2, delta, kappa opioid receptor binding profiles of methadone stereoisomers and morphine. *Life Sci* 1995; **56(2):** 45–50.

6 Eap CB, Buclin T, Baumann P. Interindividual variability of the clinical pharmacokinetics of methadone. *Clin Pharmacol* 2002; **41(14):** 1153–93.

7 Yu Y, Zhang L, Yin X, *et al*. Mu opioid receptor phosphorylation, desensitization, and ligand efficacy. *J Biol Chem* 1997; **272(46):** 28869–74.

8 Bolan EA, Tallarida RJ, Pasternak GW. Synergy between mu opioid ligands: evidence for functional interactions among mu opioid receptor subtypes. *J Pharmacol Exp Ther* 2002; **303(2):** 557–62.

9 Ivarson M, Neil A. Differences in efficacies between morphine and methadone demonstrated in the guinea pig ileum: a possible explanation for previous observations on incomplete opioid cross-tolerance. *Pharmacol Toxicol* 1989; **65:** 368–71.

10 Ebert B, Thorkildsen C, Andersen S, *et al.* Opioid analgesics as noncompetitive N-methyl-D-aspartate (NMDA) antagonists. *Biochem Pharmacol* 1998; **56:** 553–9.

11 Gorman AL, Elliott KJ, Inturrisi CE. The d- and l-isomers of methadone bind to the non-competitive site on the N-methyl-D-asparate (NMDA) receptor in rat forebrain and spinal cord. *Neurol Lett* 1997; **223:** 5–8.

12 Ebert B, Andersen S, Krogsgaard-Larsen P. Ketobemidone, methadone and pethidine are non-competitive N-methyl-D-aspartate (NMDA) antagonists in the rat cortex and spinal cord. *Neurol Lett* 1995; 165–8.

13 Codd EE, Shank RP, Schupsky JJ, *et al.* Serotonin and norepinephrine uptake inhibiting activity of centrally acting analgesics: structural determinants and role in antinociception. *J Pharmacol Exp Ther* 1995; **274(3):** 1263–70.

14 Liu JG, Liao XP, Gong ZH, *et al.* The difference between methadone and morphine in regulation of delta-opioid receptors underlies the antagonistic effect of methadone on morphine-mediated cellular actions. *Eur J Pharmacol* 1999; **373(2–3):** 233–9.

15 Davis AM, Inturrisi CE. d-Methadone blocks morphine tolerance and N-methyl-D-asparate-induced hyperalgesia. *J Pharmacol Exp Ther* 1999; **289(2):** 1048–53.

16 Elliott K, Kest B, Man A, *et al.* N-methyl-D-asparate (NMDA) receptors, mu and kappa opioid tolerance, and perspectives on new analgesic drug development. *Neuophychopharmacol* 1995; **13(4):** 347–56.

17 Candido J, Lutfy K, Billings B. Effect of adrenal and sex hormones on opioid analgesia and opioid receptor regulation. *Pharmacol Biol Behav* 1992; **42(4):** 685–92.

18 Rodriguez M, Carolos MA, Ortega I, *et al.* Sex specificity in methadone analgesia in the rat: a population pharmacokinetic and pharmacodynamic approach. *Pharmacol Res* 2002; **19(6):** 858.

19 Ochshorn M, Novick DM, Kreek MJ. *In vitro* studies of the effect of methadone on natural killer cell activity. *Israel J Med Sci* 1990; **26(8):** 421–5.

20 Novick DM, Kreek MJ. Methadone and immune function. *Am J Med* 1992; **92(1):** 113–15.

21 Beck M, Mirmohammadsadegh A, Franz B, *et al.* Opioid receptors on white blood cells: effect of HIV infection and methadone treatment. *Pain* 2002; **98(1–2):** 187–94.

22 Suzuki S, Carlos MP, Chuang LF, *et al.* Methadone induces CCR5 and promotes AIDS virus infection. *FEBS Lett* 2002; **519(1–3):** 173–7.

23 Douglas SD. Methadone may promote HIV replication: study. *AIDS Alert* 2001; **16(9):** 120.

24 Heusch WL, Maneckjee R. Effects of bombesin on methadone-induced apoptosis of human lung cancer cells. *Cancer Lett* 1999; **136(2):** 177–85.

25 Wolff K, Hay AW, Raistrick D, *et al.* Steady-state pharmacokinetics of methadone in opioid addicts. *Eur J Clin Pharmacol* 1993; **44(2):** 189–94.

26 Nilsson MI, Anggard E, Holmstrand J, *et al.* Pharmacokinetics of methadone during maintenance treatment: adaptive changes during the induction phase. *Eur J Clin Pharmacol* 1982; **22(4):** 343–9.

27 Rostami-Hodjegan A, Wolff K, Hay AW, *et al.* Population pharmacokinetics of methadone in opiate users: characterization of time-dependent changes. *Br J Clin Pharmacol* 1999; **48(1):** 43–52.

28 Inturrisi CE, Colburn WA, Kaiko RF, *et al.* Pharmacokinetics and pharmacodynamics of methadone in patients with chronic pain. *Clin Pharmacol Ther* 1987; **41(4):** 392–401.

29 Wolff K, Rostami-Hodjegan A, Shires S, *et al.* The pharmacokinetics of methadone in healthy subjects and opiate users. *Br J Clin Pharmacol* 1997; **44(4):** 325–34.

30 Nilsson MI, Widerlov E, Meresaar U, *et al.* Effect of urinary pH on the disposition of methadone in man. *Eur J Clin Pharmacol* 1982; **22(4):** 337–42.

31 Nilsson MI, Meresaar U, Anggard E. Clinical pharmacokinetics of methdone. *Acta Anaesth Scand* 1982; **74(Suppl.):** 66–9.

32 Meresaar U, Nilsson MI, Holmstrand J, *et al*. Single dose pharmacokinetics and bioavailability of methadone in man studied with a stable isotope method. *Eur J Clin Pharmacol* 1981; **20(6):** 473–8.

33 Bouer R, Barthe L, Philibert C, *et al*. The roles of P-glycoprotein and intracellular metabolism in the intestinal absorption of methadone: *in vitro* studies using the rat everted intestinal sac. *Fund Clin Pharmacol* 1999; **13(4):** 494–500.

34 Wolff K, Sanderson M, Hay AW, *et al*. Methadone concentrations in plasma and their relationship to drug dosage. *Clin Chem* 1991; **37(2):** 205–9.

35 de Castro J, Aguirre C, Rodriguez-Sasiain JM, *et al*. The effect of changes in gastric pH induced by omeprazole on the absorption and respiratory depression of methadone. *Biopharm Drug Dis* 1996; **17(7):** 551–63.

36 Carlos MA, Du Souich P, Carlos R, *et al*. Effect of omeprazole on oral and intravenous RS-methadone pharmacokinetics and pharmacodynamics in the rat. *J Pharm Sci* 2002; **91(7):** 1627–38.

37 Oda Y, Kharasch ED. Metabolism of methadone and levo-alpha-acetylmethadol (LAAM) by human intestinal cytochrome P450 3A4 (CYP3A4): potential contribution of intestinal metabolism to presystemic clearance and bioactivation. *J Pharmacol Exp Ther* 2001; **298(3):** 1021–32.

38 Felder C, Uehlinger C, Baumann P, *et al*. Oral and intravenous methadone use: some clinical and pharmaockinetic aspects. *Drug Alc Depend* 1999; **55(1–2):** 137–43.

39 Kristensen K, Blemmer T, Angelo HR, *et al*. Stereoselective pharmacokinetics of methadone in chronic pain patients. *Ther Drug Monit* 1996; **18(3):** 221–7.

40 Ripamonti C, Zecca E, Brunelli C, *et al*. Rectal methadone in cancer patients with pain. *Annl Oncol* 1995; **6:** 841–3.

41 Bruera E, Watanabe S, Fainsinger RL, *et al*. Custom-made capsules and suppositories of methadone for patients on high-dose opioids for cancer pain. *Pain* 1995; **62:** 141–6.

42 Davis MP, Walsh D, LeGrand SB, *et al*. Symptom control in cancer patients: the clinical pharmacology and therapeutic role of suppositories and rectal suspensions. *Supportive Care in Cancer* 2002; **10(2):** 117–38.

43 Dale O, Hoffer C, Sheffels P, *et al*. Disposition of nasal, intravenous, and oral methadone in healthy volunteers. *Clin Pharmacol Ther* 2002; **72(5):** 536–45.

44 Weinberg DS, Inturrisi CE, Reidenberg B, *et al*. Sublingual absorption of selected opioid analgesics. *Clin Pharmacol Ther* 1988; **44(3):** 335–42.

45 Nilsson MI, Gronbladh L, Widerlov E, *et al*. Pharmacokinetics of methadone in methadone maintenance treatment: characterization of therapeutic failures. *Eur J Clin Pharmacol* 1983; **25(4):** 497–501.

46 Garrido MJ, Aguirre C, Troconiz IF, *et al*. Alpha 1-acid glycoprotein (AAG) and serum protein binding of methadone in heroin addicts with abstinence syndrome. *Int J Clin Pharmacol Ther* 2000; **38(1):** 35–40.

47 Inturrisi CE, Verebely K. Disposition of methadone in man after a single oral dose. *Clin Pharmacol Ther* 1972; **13(6):** 923–30.

48 Inturrisi CE, Verebely K. The levels of methadone in the plasma in methadone maintenance. *Clin Pharmacol Ther* 1972; **13(5):** 633–7.

49 Inturrisi CE, Portenoy RK, Max MB, *et al*. Pharmacokinetic-pharmacodynamic relationships of methadone infusions in patients with cancer pain. *Clin Pharmacol Ther* 1990; **47(5):** 565–77.

50 Abramson FP. Methadone plasma protein binding: alterations in cancer and displacement from alpha 1-acid glycoprotein. *Clin Pharmacol Ther* 1982; **32(5):** 652–8.

51 Gomez E, Martinez-Jorda R, Suarez E, *et al*. Altered methadone analgesia due to changes in plasma protein binding: role of the route of administration. *Gen Pharm* 1995; **26(6):** 1273–6.

52 Eap CB, Berschy G, Baumann P, *et al*. High interindividual variability of methadone enantiomer blood levels to dose ratios. *Arch Gen Psychol* 1998; **55(1):** 89–90.

53 Iribarne C, Dreano Y, Bardou LG, *et al*. Interaction of methadone with substrates of human hepatic cytochrome P450 3A4. *Toxicology* 1997; **117:** 13–23.

54 Foster DJ, Somogyi AA, Bochner F. Methadone N-demethylation in human liver microsomes: lack of stereoselectivity and involvement of CYP3A4. *Br J Clin Pharmacol* 1999; **47(4):** 403–12.

55 Boulton DW, Arnaud P, DeVane L. A single dose of methadone inhibits cytochrome P-4503A activity in healthy volunteers as assessed by the cortisol ratio. *Br J Clin Pharmacol* 2001; **51:** 350–4.

56 Moody DE, Alburges ME, Parker MJ, *et al*. The involvement of cytochrome P450 3A4 in the N-demethylation of L-alpha-acetylmethadol (LAAM), norLAAM, and methadone. *Drug Met Dispos* 1997; **25(12):** 1347–53.

57 Wolff K, Rostami-Hodjegan A, Hay AW. Population-based pharmacokinetic approach for methadone monitoring of opiate addicts: potential clinical utility. *Addiction* 2000; **95(12):** 1771–83.

58 Verebely K, Volavka J, Mule S, *et al*. Methadone in man: pharmacokinetic and excretion studies in acute and chronic treatment. *Clin Pharmacol Ther* 1975; **18(2):** 180–90.

59 Sawe J. High-dose morphine and methadone in cancer patients. *Clin Pharmacol* 1986; **11:** 87–106.

60 Eap CB, Bourquin M, Martin JL, *et al*. Plasma concentrations of the enantiomers of methadone and therapeutic response in methadone maintenance treatment. *Drug Alc Depend* 2000; **61:** 47–54.

61 Prost F, Thormann W. Capillary electrophoresis to assess drug metabolism induced in vitro using single CYP450 enzymes (Supersomes): application to the chiral metabolism of mephenytoin and methadone. *Interscience* 2003; **24(15):** 2577–87.

62 Shiran MR, Chowdry J, Rostami-Hodjegan A, *et al*. A discordance between cytochrome P450 2D6 genotype and phenotype in patients undergoing methadone maintenance treatment. *Br J Clin Pharmacol* 2003; **56(2):** 220–4.

63 Wu D, Otton SV, Sproule BA. Inhibition of human cytochrome P450 2D6 (CYP2D6) by methadone. *Br J Clin Pharmacol* 1993; **35(1):** 30–4.

64 Eap CB, Broly F, Mino A, *et al*. Cytochrome P450 2D6 genotype and methadone steady-state concentrations. *J Clin Psychol* 2001; **21(2):** 229–34.

65 Plummer JL, Gourlay GK, Cherry DA, *et al*. Estimation of methadone clearance: application in the management of cancer pain. *Pain* 1988; **33(3):** 313–22.

66 Wolff K, Rostami-Hodjegan A, Shires S, *et al*. The pharmacokinetics of methadone in healthy subjects and opiate users. *Br J Clin Pharmacol* 1997; **44(4):** 325–34.

67 Kreek MJ, Kalisman M, Irwin M, *et al*. Biliary secretion of methadone and methadone metabolites in man. *Res Comm Chem Path Pharmacol* 1980; **29(1):** 67–78.

68 Bellward GD, Warren PM, Howald W, *et al*. Methadone maintenance: effect of urinary pH on renal clearance in chronic high and low doses. *Clin Pharmacol Ther* 1977; **22(1):** 92–9.

69 Rubenstein RB, Kreek MJ, Mbawa N, *et al*. Human spinal fluid methadone levels. *Drug Alc Depend* 1978; **3(2):** 103–6.

70 Max MB, Inturrisi CE, Kaiko RF, *et al*. Epidural and intrathecal opiates: cerebrospinal fluid and plasma profiles in patients with chronic cancer pain. *Clin Pharmacol Ther* 1985; **38(6):** 631–41.

71 Payne R, Gradert TL, Inturrisi CE. Cerebrospinal fluid distribution of opioids after intraventicular and lumbar subarachnoid administration in sheep. *Life Sci* 1996; **59(16):** 1307–21.

72 Weinberg DS, Inturrisi CE, Reidenberg B, *et al*. Sublingual absorption of selected opioid analgesics. *Clin Pharmacol Ther* 1988; **44(3):** 335–42.

73 Bruera E, Fainsinger R, Moore M, *et al.* Local toxicity with subcutaneous methadone. Experience of two centers. *Pain* 1991; **45(2):** 141–3.

74 Uehlinger C, Hauser C. Allergic reactions from injectable methadone. *Am J Psychol* 1999; **156(6):** 973.

75 Matthew P, Storey P. Subcutaneous methadone in terminally ill patients: manageable local toxicity. *J Pain Symptom Manage* 1999; **18(1):** 49–52.

76 Vormfelde SV, Poser W. Death attributed to methadone. *Pharmacopsychiatry* 2001; **34:** 217–22.

77 Bart PA, Rizzardi PG, Gallant S, *et al.* Methadone blood concentrations are decreased by the administration of abacavir plus amprenavir. *Ther Drug Monit* 2001; **23(5):** 553–5.

78 Gerber JG, Rosenkranz S, Segal Y, *et al.* Effect of ritnavir/saquinavir on stereoselective pharmacokinetics of methadone: results of AIDS Clinical Trials Group (ACTG) 401. *J AIDS* 2001; **27(2):** 153–60.

79 Iribarne C, Picart D, Dreano Y, *et al. In vitro* interactions between fluoxetine or fluvoxamine and methadone or buprenorphine. *Fund Clin Pharm* 1998; **12:** 194–9.

80 Borowsky SA, Lieber CS. Interaction of methadone and ethanol metabolism. *J Pharmacol Exp Ther* 1978; **207(1):** 123–9.

81 Breivik H, Rennemo F. Clinical evaluation of combined treatment with methadone and psychotropic drugs in cancer patients. *Acta Anaesth Scand* 1982; **74:** 135–40.

82 Ventafridda V, Ripamonti C, Bianchi M, *et al.* A randomized study on oral administration of morphine and methadone in the treatment of cancer pain. *J Pain Symptom Manage* 1986; **1(4):** 203–7.

83 Daeninck PJ, Bruera E. Reduction in constipation and laxative requirements following opioid rotation to methadone: a report of four cases. *J Pain Symptom Manage* 1999; **18:** 303–9.

84 Mancini I, Hanson J, Bruera E. Opioid type and other clinical predictors of laxative dose in advanced cancer patients: a retrospective study. *J Pain Symptom Manage* 1998; **15(4):** S16.

85 Krantz MJ, Lewkowiez L, Hays H, *et al.* Torsade de Pointes associated with very-high-dose methadone. *Annl Int Med* 2002; **137:** 501–4.

86 Davis MP, Walsh D. Methadone for relief of cancer pain: a review of pharmacokinetics, pharmacodynamics, drug interactions and protocols of administration. *Supportive Care in Cancer* 2001; **9:** 73–83.

87 Sarhill N, Davis MP, Walsh D, *et al.* Methadone-induced myoclonus in advanced cancer. *Am J Hosp Palliat Care* 2001; **18(1):** 51–3.

88 Bonnet U, Banger M, Wolstein J, *et al.* Choreoathetoid movements associated with rapid adjustment to methadone. *Pharmacopsychiatry* 1998; **31(4):** 143–5.

89 Dittert S, Naber D, Soyka M. Methadone substitution therapy and driving: results of an experimental study. *Nervenarzt* 1999; **70(5):** 457–62.

90 Doverty M, White JM, Somogyi AA, *et al.* Hyperalgesic responses in methadone maintenance patients. *Pain* 2001; **90:** 91–6.

91 Compton P, Charuvastra VC, Ling W. Pain intolerance in opioid-maintained former opiate addicts: effect of long-acting maintenance agent. *Drug Alc Depend* 2001; **63(2):** 139–46.

92 Moryl N, Santiago-Palma J, Kornick C, *et al.* Pitfalls of opioid rotation: substituting another opioid for methadone in patients with cancer pain. *Pain* 2002; **96:** 325–8.

93 Manfredi PL, Gonzales GR, Cheville AL, *et al.* Methadone analgesia in cancer pain patients on chronic methadone maintenance therapy. *J Pain Symptom Manage* 2001; **21(2):** 169–74.

94 Wolff K. Characterization of methadone overdose: clinical considerations and the scientific evidence. *Ther Drug Monit* 2002; **24(4):** 457–70.

95 Kreek MJ. Drug interactions with methadone in humans. In: Braude MC, Ginzburg HM (Eds) *Strategies for Research on the Interactions of Drug of Abuse.* NIDA Research Monograph Series 68. **1986:** 193–225.

96 Novick DM, Kreek MJ, Arns PA, *et al.* Effect of severe alcoholic liver disease on the disposition of methadone in maintenance patients. *Alc Clin Exp Res* 1985; **9(4):** 349–54.

97 Novick DM, Kreek MJ, Fanizza AM, *et al.* Methadone disposition in patients with chronic liver disease. *Clin Pharmacol Ther* 1981; **30(3):** 353–62.

98 Kirby GM, Batist G, Alpert L, *et al.* Overexpression of cytochrome P-450 isoforms involved in aflatoxin B1 bioactivation in human liver with cirrhosis and hepatitis. *Toxicol Pathol* 1996; **24(4):** 458–67.

99 Kreek MJ, Schecter AJ, Gutjahr CL, *et al.* Methadone use in patients with chronic renal disease. *Drug Alc Depend* 1980; **5(3):** 197–205.

100 Furlan V, Hafi A, Dessalles MC, *et al.* Methadone is poorly removed by haemodialysis. *Neph Dial Trans* 1999, **14(1):** 254–5.

101 Jarvis MA, Wu-Pong S, Kniseley JS, *et al.* Alterations in methadone metabolism during late pregnancy. *J Addict Dis* 1999; **18(4):** 51–61.

102 Begg EJ, Malpas TJ, Hackett LP, *et al.* Distribution of R- and S-methadone into human milk during multiple, medium to high oral dosing. *Br J Clin Pharmacol* 2001; **52(6):** 681–5.

103 Wojnar-Horton RE, Kristensen JH, Yapp P, *et al.* Methadone distribution and excretion into breast milk of clients in a methadone maintenance programme. *Br J Clin Pharmocol* 1997; **44(6):** 543–7.

104 Morley JS. Opioid rotation: does it have a role? *Palliat Med* 1998; **12(6):** 464–5.

105 Lawlor PG, Turner KS, Hanson J, *et al.* Dose ratio between morphine and methadone in patients with cancer pain: a retrospective study. *Cancer* 1998; **82(6):** 1167–73.

106 Ettinger DS, Vitale PJ, Trump DL. Important clinical pharmacologic considerations in the use of methadone in cancer patients. *Cancer Treat Rep* 1979; **63(3):** 457–9.

107 Ripamonti C, De Conno F, Groff L, *et al.* Equianalgesic dose/ratio between methadone and other opioid agonists in cancer pain: comparison of two clinical experiences. *Annl Oncol* 1998; **9(1):** 79–83.

108 Vigano A, Fan D, Bruera E. Individualized use of methadone and opioid rotation in the comprehensive management of cancer pain associated with poor prognostic indicators. *Pain* 1996; **67(1):** 115–19.

109 Hunt G, Bruera E. Respiratory depression in a patient receiving oral methadone for cancer pain. *J Pain Symptom Manage* 1995; **10(5):** 401–4.

110 Manfredi PL, Borsook D, Chandler SW, *et al.* Intravenous methadone for cancer pain unrelieved by morphine and hyrdromorphone: clinical observations. *Pain* 1997; **70:** 99–101.

111 Thomas Z, Bruera E. Use of methadone in a highly tolerant patient receiving parenteral hydromorphone. *J Pain Symptom Manage* 1995; **10(4):** 315–17.

112 Fitzgibbon DR, Ready LB. Intravenous high-dose methadone administered by patient controlled analgesia and continuous infusion for the treatment of cancer pain refractory to high-dose morphine. *Pain* 1997; **73:** 259–61.

113 Davis MP. Methadone as a rescue for failed high-dose opiate therapy for catastrophic pain. *Supportive Care in Cancer* 2000; **8:** 138–40.

114 Crews JC, Sweeney NJ, Denson DD. Clinical efficacy of methadone in patients refractory to other mu-opioid receptor agonist analgesics for management of terminal cancer pain. Case presentations and discussion of incomplete cross-tolerance among opioid agonist analgesics. *Cancer* 1993; **72(7):** 2266–72.

115 Paalzow L, Nilsson L, Stenberg P. Pharmacokinetic basis for optimal methadone treatment of pain in cancer patients. *Acta Anaesth Scand* 1982; **Suppl 74:** 55–8.

116 Ayonrinde OT, Bridge DT. The rediscovery of methadone for cancer pain management. *Med J Aust* 2000, **173:** 536–40.

117 Makin MK, O'Donnell V, Skinner JM, *et al*. Methadone in the management of cancer related neuropathic pain: report of five cases. *Pain Clin* 1998; **10(4):** 275–9.

118 Sjogren P, Jensen NH, Jensen TS. Disappearance of morphine-induced hyperalgesia after discontinuing or substituting morphine with other opioid agonists. *Pain* 1994; **59:** 313–16.

119 Mercadante S, Sapio M, Serretta R. Treatment of pain in chronic bowel subobstruction with self-administration of methadone. *Supportive Care in Cancer* 1997; **5:** 327–9.

120 Makin MK, Ellershaw JE. Substitution of another opioid for morphine: methadone can be used to manage neuropathic pain related to cancer. *Br Med J* 1998; **317(7150):** 81.

121 Shir Y, Shenkman Z, Shavelson V, *et al*. Oral methadone for the treatment of severe pain in hospitalized children: a report of five cases. *Clin J Pain* 1998; **14(4):** 350–3.

122 Watanage S, Belzile M, Kuehn N, *et al*. Capsules and suppositories of methadone for patients on high-dose opioids for cancer pain: clinical and economic considerations. *Cancer Treat Rev* 1996; **22(Suppl A):** 131–6.

123 De Conno F, Groff L, Brunelli C, *et al*. Clinical experience with oral methadone administration in the treatment of pain in 196 advanced cancer patients. *J Clin Oncol* 1996; **14(10):** 2836–42.

124 Hagen NA, Wasylenko E. Methadone: outpatient titration and monitoring strategies in cancer patients. *J Pain Symptom Manage* 1999; **18(5):** 369–75.

125 Sawe J, Hansen J, Ginman C, *et al*. Patient-controlled dose regimen of methadone for chronic cancer pain. *Br Med J* 1981; **282:** 771.

126 Hansen J, Ginman C, Hartvig P, *et al*. Clinical evaluation of oral methadone in treatment of cancer pain. *Acta Anaesth Scand* 1982; **Suppl 74:** 124–7.

127 Gourlay GK, Cherry DA, Cousins MJ. A comparative study of the efficacy and phamacokinetics of oral methadone and morphine in the treatment of severe pain in patients with cancer. *Pain* 1986; **25:** 297–312.

128 Grochow L, Sheidler V, Grossman S, *et al*. Does intravenous methadone provide longer lasting analgesia than intravenous morphine? A randomized, double-blind study. *Pain* 1989; **38:** 151–7.

129 Morley JS, Makin MK. The use of methadone in cancer pain poorly responsive to other opioids. *Pain Rev* 1998; **5:** 51–8.

130 Mercadante S, Sapio M, Serretta R, *et al*. Patient-controlled analgesia with oral methadone in cancer pain: preliminary report. *Annl Oncol* 1996; **7:** 613–17.

131 Ripamonti C, Groff L, Brunelli C, *et al*. Switching from morphine to oral methadone in treating cancer pain: what is the equianalgesic dose ratio? *J Clin Oncol* 1998; **16(10):** 3216–21.

132 Gagnon B, Bruera E. Differences in the ratios of morphine to methadone in patients with neuropathic pain versus non-neuropathic pain. *J Pain Symptom Manage* 1999; **18(2):** 120–5.

133 Mercadante S, Casuccio A, Agnello A, *et al*. Methadone response in advanced cancer patients with pain followed at home. *J Pain Symptom Manage* 1999; **18(3):** 188–92.

134 Mercadante S, Casuccio A, Calderone L. Rapid switching from morphine to methadone in cancer patients with poor response to morphine. *J Clin Oncol* 1999; **17:** 3307–12.

135 Scholes CF, Gonty N, Trotman UK. Methadone titration in opioid-resistant cancer pain. *Eur J Cancer Care* 1999; **8(1):** 26–9.

136 Makin MK. Subcutaneous methadone in terminally ill patients. *J Pain Symptom Manage* 2000; **19(4):** 237–8.

137 Mercadante S, Casuccio A, Fulfaro F, *et al*. Switching from morphine to methadone to improve analgesia and tolerability in cancer patients: a prospective study. *J Clin Oncol* 2001; **19(11):** 2898–904.

138 Santiago-Palma J, Khojainova N, Kornick C, *et al*. Intravenous methadone in the management of chronic cancer pain: safe and effective starting doses when substituting methadone for fentanyl. *Cancer* 2001; **92(7):** 1919–25.

Chapter 13

Levorphanol

Mellar P. Davis

Introduction

Levorphanol [(-)-3-hydroxy-N-methyl morphinan] is a morphine analogue that has broad opioid receptor binding capability and is an N-methyl-D-aspartate (NMDA) receptor antagonist, as well as a monoamine reuptake inhibitor. It has been marketed since the 1950s and used anecdotally in advanced cancer patients. Unfortunately, it has become difficult to obtain. A recent positive trial of the use of levorphanol in neuropathic pain has rekindled interest in this opioid.

Pharmacodynamics

Levorphanol is a mu opioid receptor (MOR), delta opioid receptor (DOR) and kappa opioid receptor (KOR_{1+3}) agonist[1]. In animal studies, analgesia is predominantly related to MOR[2]. There is also some analgesia derived from the $kappa_3$ receptor[3]. In mice bred for high and low levorphanol sensitivity, a 1.5–2-fold difference in MOR_1 density was found in the dorsal raphe nucleus, indicating that at least a portion of levorphanol's analgesia is due to brain stem receptor activity[4,5]. Its broad receptor binding appears to explain the unidirectional opioid exhibited tolerance to morphine by levorphanol in animal studies[6,7]. Respiratory depression, which occurs with levorphanol use, is caused by MOR_1 receptor binding[8,9].

In vitro, levorphanol does not cause down-regulation of human KOR, receptor phosphorylation or adenylyl cyclase superactivation, all of which are associated with analgesia tolerance[10]. Levorphanol KOR binding does not initiate receptor modulation or cause rebound adenylyl cyclase activity, although there is data to the contrary[11,12].

Levorphanol is a methyl-levorotatory enantiomer of dextrorphan, a potent NMDA receptor inhibitor. Levorphanol binds to NMDA receptors with less efficiency than its parent drug, dextrophan[13,14]. Levorphanol blocks phencyclidine binding less than ketamine does, but better than dextromethorphan does[15]. Dextrorphan analgesia is not reversed by naloxone, whereas levorphanol analgesia is significantly reversed by naloxone such that the importance of levorphanol NMDA receptor blockade to analgesia is not known[16].

Levorphanol inhibits monoamine reuptake similar to the inhibitory action of methadone and tricyclic antidepressants[17]. The importance of this effect to pain response is not known.

Opioid analgesia and tolerance changes with opioid dose and its stimulus intensity changes in relation to the intrinsic efficacy of the opioid. Intrinsic efficacy directly correlates with functional receptor reserves and reflects the ability of a drug to activate receptors independent of receptor affinity. The intrinsic efficacy of levorphanol is equivalent to that of morphine, which is half that of fentanyl and methadone[18,19]. Mice made tolerant to levorphanol have cerebral concentrates of levorphanol that were higher than those required for pharmacological effects. This indicates that diminishing analgesia is a cellular or subcellular adaptation to levorphanol, and is not caused by altered kinetics or drug levels[20]. This finding conflicts with the previously mentioned *in vitro* pharmacodynamic data, which indicated that levorphanol actually reduced receptor modulation as compared with other opioids.

Levorphanol can sensitize dopamine receptors and increase dopamine agonists responses[21]. Levorphanol, like morphine, will also reduce the impulse frequencies derived from sympathetics and, as a result, reduces blood pressure. This is reversed by naloxone[22]. Levorphanol on the other hand potentates beta adrenergic agonists' actions on cardiac muscle *in vitro* and this is not reversed by opioid receptor blockade unlike its direct action on sympathetic neurons[23]. Overall, levorphanol appears to protect from arrhythmia, as seen by experimental coronary occlusion. This action is independent of opioid receptor interactions. The cardiac protective effects of levorphanol may be related to its action on cardiac muscle repolarization[24].

Levorphanol inhibits the process of calcium binding to synaptic membranes in a dose-dependent fashion[25]. Levorphanol blocks the input to C-fibers in the dorsal horn and decreases the 'wind up' of wide dynamic range neurons. This is fully reversed by naloxone[26,27].

The selective breeding of mice produces large differences in the response to different levels of levorphanol indicating that genetically determined factors are important to levorphanol's analgesia[5].

Finally, levorphanol, like most opioids, increases biliary pressures. The order of effect on isolated biliary ducts *in vitro* is meperidine > levorphanol > morphine and by *in situ* studies levorphanol > morphine > merperidine. Antimuscarinics do not influence opioid-induced biliary spasms[28]. Levorphanol like morphine can cause biliary colic. However, meperidine, often used for biliary procedures will also cause bile duct spasm.

Pharmacokinetics

Levorphanol has triexponential kinetics with a terminal half-life of 11 h[29]. There is a large first pass hepatic clearance of levorphanol of approximately 50%. Peak drug concentrations occur within 30 min of parenteral injection occur and within 1 h after oral dosing. Conjugated levorphanol (morphanol glucuronide) appears rapidly in the blood, independent of the route of adminstration. The glucuronidated metabolites in blood plasma are 5–10 times greater than the parent drug at steady state[29]. This is distinctly different from a related isomer, dextromethorphan, which metabolized through the cytochrome, CYP2D6, and is not conjugated. There is little levorphanol N-demethylation indicating levorphanol metabolism does not occur through type 1 cytochromes. Levorphanol conjugates are found in the stool and, thus, have the potential for enterohepatic circulation and prolonged half-life[30]. This may, in part, account for the triexponential kinetics with chronic dosing (which can have a terminal half-life as much as 16–30 h)[29]. It is not known if the conjugated levorphanol has analgesic activity.

Levorphanol is poorly absorbed sublingually and there is no data as to its rectal bioavailability[31].

Plasma protein binding is 40 + 2.6%[29], which is similar to morphine and oxycodone. The large volume of distribution (10–13 l/kg) and low clearance rate (0.78–1.1 l/kg/h) accounts, in part, for its long half-life[29,32]. Cerebrospinal fluid (CSF) levels are 64–74% of plasma levels. These approximate unbound plasma drug concentrations, which indicates that there is very little drug barrier to central nervous system penetration[29,33]. In mice, only 2% of total central nervous system (CNS) levorphanol stereospecifically binds to membranes and, presumably, binds to opioid receptors[34].

In the few cancer patients studied, pain responses to levorphanol required a minimum plasma concentration of 10 ng/ml for relief. There appears to be 'shallow' and 'steep' patient responders to dose when comparing analgesia to plasma concentrations of levorphanol[29].

Routes of administration and doses

Levorphanol can be taken either by mouth or by parenteral injection, either subcutaneous or intravenous. Levorphanol can produce analgesia by injection at local sites of pain, caused by inflammation without significant systemic absorption[35]. No data exists regarding levorphanol spinal administration, although the rapid appearance of levorphanol in CSF with parenteral/oral routes suggests that there will be little advantage to epidural or intrathecal administration.

Initial doses are 1–2 mg parenterally every 6–8 h or an oral dose of 2 mg every 6–8 h in the opioid naïve. Total daily doses should not exceed 3–8 mg parenteral or 6–12 mg oral[32].

Equivalence

The conversion factor of oral to parenteral levorphanol is 2 : 1. The equivalent dose ratio of parenteral morphine to parenteral levorphanol is 5 : 1[29]. Three milligrams of oral levorphanol is said to be equivalent to approximately 45–90 mg of oral morphine[27]. It is recommended that oral levorphanol should be started at 1/12–1/15th of the total daily oral morphine dose[32]. At the present time, there are no equivalent levorphanol comparisons to other opioids (including fentanyl, methadone or oxycodone).

Drug interactions and toxicity

There is little data as to drug interactions involving levorphanol. The fact that it is conjugated drug suggests that there is a potential for drug interaction at glucuronidation (UGT) enzyme sites. It is unknown whether the parent drug or the conjugated metabolite of levorphanol binds to type 1 cytochrome enzymes. Potential, although unproven drug interactions include non-steroidal anti-inflammatory, valproic acid and lorazepam, which may compete for levorphanol binding sites on UGT. Rifampin, which stimulates glucuronidation, could potentially increase levorphanol clearance. Pentobarbitol sedation is greatly lengthened by levorphanol for which there is no tolerance with chronic dosing[36]. Hence, the use of sedative medication with levorphanol should be avoided[32]. Pharmaceutical incompatabilities include aminophylline, amobarbital, heparin, methicillin, pentobarbital, phenobarbital, phenytoin, secobarbital, sodium bicarbonate and thiopental[32].

Side effects recorded in a randomized trial of levorphanol for neuropathic pain include pruritus, dry mouth, sweating, sedation, euphoria, mental cloudiness, personality changes, weakness, confusion and dizziness. This list does not significantly differ from other opioids[27].

Dosing and special populations

There is no data as to levorphanol dosing in patients with organ failure or in the elderly patient. Glucuronidation of levorphanol is relatively preserved in patients with hepatic failure such that drug half-life would also be relatively well preserved until late stages of hepatic failure, which is similar to morphine actions. Bioavailability of this drug is anticipated to be increased with portal hypertension and reduced hepatic blood flow, since levorphanol has significant first pass clearance. Levorphanol's half-life is three times that of morphine, which makes it less attractive in liver failure than morphine. The influence of renal failure upon drug clearance is completely unknown. Levorphanol should be used cautiously in renal failure until further data is available.

Levorphanol, like morphine, may have its drug half-life prolonged in the elderly due to age-related reduction in hepatic blood flow and renal function. However, there is no data available to confirm this theory.

Evidence base for cancer pain

Levorphanol has been used to treat chronic non-malignant pain and cancer pain, as well as postoperative pain[37–39]. There are no perspective cohort single drug studies or retrospective series using levorphanol for cancer pain. A recent randomized prospective trial of levorphanol for peripheral or central non-cancer neuropathic pain syndromes demonstrates a dose-dependent decrease in pain. Peripheral neuropathic pain was more likely to respond than central pain syndromes. Both touch-induced allodynia and spontaneous neuropathic pain improved with levorphanol use. The mean daily doses in this study were 2.7 mg in the low dose group and 8.9 mg in the high dose group, which produced a mean blood level of 1.4 and 4.8 ng/ml, respectively. Analgesia was experienced in this group of patients at doses lower than previously reported levels in cancer patients[27,29]. In this study, prior opioid exposure, age and duration of pain were not factors influencing levorphanol response.

Summary

There are many potential advantages to the use of levorphanol in cancer pain that require further study. Positive aspects include its long half-life, fewer daily doses and multiple opioid receptor spectrum. In addition, levorphanol prevents monoamine reuptake, blocks calcium influx, as well as blocks NMDA receptors. It has a similar profile to methadone. However, its intrinsic efficacy and metabolism differs from methadone and is unique. It is conjugated and would have fewer anticipated drug–drug interactions than methadone (unless the parent drug or metabolite binds and blocks cytochrome enzymes). Levorphanol rapidly penetrates the central nervous system and has evidence-based benefits in the treatment of neuropathic pain. Levorphanol is available in oral and parenteral preparations, which adds versatility to its benefits. Levorphanol appears to be a forgotten opioid for some unknown reason, for which the full benefits in cancer pain have not yet been realized[40].

Dose and route

Levorphanol is available as 2-mg tablets of levorphanol tartrate, and as 2 mg/ml ampules (10 and 1 ml) for intravenous or subcutaneous injection.

References

1 Fiorica E, Spector S. Opioid binding site in EL-4 thymoma cell line. *Life Sci* 1988; **42**(2): 199–206.

2 Gatch MB, Liguori A, Negus SS, *et al.* Naloxonazine antagonism of levorphanol-induced antinociception and respiratory depression in rhesus monkeys. *Eur J Pharmacol* 1996; **298**(1): 31–6.

3 Tive L, Ginsberg K, Pick CG, *et al.* Kappa 3 receptors and levorphanol-induced analgesia. *Neuropharmacology* 1992; **31**(9): 851–6.

4 Prado WA, Roberts MH. Antinociception from a stereospecific action of morphine microinjected into the brainstem: a local or distant site of action? *Br J Pharmacol* 1984; **84**(4): 877–82.

5 Belknap JK, Laursen SE, Sampson KE, *et al.* Where are the mu receptors that mediate opioid analgesia? An autoradiographic study in the HAR and LAR selection lines. *J Addict Dis* 1991; **10**(1–2): 29–44.

6 Moulin DE, Ling GS, Pasternak GW. Unidirectional analgesic cross-tolerance between morphine and levorphanol in the rat. *Pain* 1988; **33**(2): 233–9.

7 Foley KM. Opioids and chronic neuropathic pain. *N Engl J Med* 2003; **348**(13): 1279–81.

8 Liguori A, Morse WH, Bergman J. Respiratory effects of opioid full and partial agonists in rhesus monkeys. *J Pharmacol Exp Therapeut* 1996; **277**(1): 462–72.

9 Howell LL, Bergman J, Morse WH. Effects of levorphanol and several kappa-selective opioids on respiration and behavior in rhesus monkeys. *J Pharmacol Exp Therapeut* 1988; **245**(1): 364–72.

10 Blake AD, Bot G, Li S, *et al.* Differential agonist regulation of the human kappa-opioid receptor. *J Neurochem* 1997; **68(5)**: 1846–52.

11 Li JG, Zhang F, Jin XL, *et al.* Differential regulation of the human kappa opioid receptor by agonists: etorphine and levorphanol reduced dynorphin A- and U50, 488H-induced internalization and phosphorylation. *J Pharmacol Exp Therapeut* 2003; **305(2)**: 531–40.

12 Carter BD, Medzihradsky F. Receptor mechanisms of opioid tolerance in SH-SY5Y human neural cells. *Molec Pharmacol* 1993; **43(3)**: 465–73.

13 Choi DW, Peters S, Visesul V. Dextrorphan and levorphanol selectively block N-methyl-D-aspartate receptor-mediated neurotoxicity and cortical neurons. *J Pharmacol Exp Therapeut* 1987; **242(2)**: 713–20.

14 Church J, Lodge D, Berry SC. Differential effects of dextrorphan and levorphanol on the excitation of rat spinal neurons by amino acids. *Eur J Pharmacol* 1985; **111(2)**: 185–90.

15 Murray TF, Leid ME. Interaction of dextrorotatory opioids with phencyclidine recognition sites in rat brain membranes. *Life Sciences* 1984; **34(20)**: 1899–911.

16 Stevens CW, Pezalla PA. Naloxone blocks the analgesic action of levorphanol but not of dextrorphan in the leopard frog. *Brain Research* 1984; **301(1)**: 171–4.

17 Rojas-Corrales MO, Berrocoso E, Gilbert-Rahola J, *et al.* Antidepressant-like effects of tramadol and other central analgesics with activity on monoamines reuptake, in helpless rats. *Life Sci* 2002; **72(2)**: 143–52.

18 Morrison JD, Loan WB, Dundee JW. Controlled comparison of the efficacy of fourteen preparations in the relief of postoperative pain. *Br Med J* 1971; **3(769)**: 287–90.

19 Adams JU, Paronis CA, Holtzman SG. Assessment of relative intrinsic activity of mu-opioid analgesics *in vivo* by using beta-funaltrexamine. *J Phamacol Exp Therapeut* 1990; **255(3)**: 1027–32.

20 Richter JA, Goldstein A. Tolerance to opioid narcotics, II. Cellular tolerance to levorphanol in mouse brain. *Proc Nat Acad Sci USA* 1970; **66(3)**: 944–51.

21 Martin JR, Takemori AE. Modification of the development of acute opiate tolerance by increased dopamine receptor sensitivity. *J Pharmacol Exp Therapeut* 1987; **241(1)**: 48–55.

22 Jurna I, Rummel W. Depression by morphine and levorphanol of activity in sympathetic nerve fibres in anaesthetized rats. *Eur J Pharmacol* 1984; **101(1–2)**: 75–82.

23 Kindman LA, Kates RE, Ginsburg R. Opioids potentiate contractile response of rabbit myocardium to the beta adrenergic agonist isoproterenol. *J Cardiovas Pharmacol* 1991; **17(1)**: 61–7.

24 Sarne Y, Flitstein A, Oppenheimer E. Anti-arrhythmic activities of opioid agonists and antagonists and their stereoisomers. *Br J Pharmacol* 1991; **102(3)**: 696–8.

25 Ross DH, Cardenas HL. Levorphanol inhibition of Ca^{++} binding to synaptic membranes *in vitro*. *Life Sci* 1977; **28(8)**: 1455–62.

26 Dickenson AH, Sullivan AF, Stanfa LC, *et al.* Dextromethorphan and levorphanol on dorsal horn nociceptive neurones in the rat. *Neuropharmacology* 1991; **30(12A)**: 1303–8.

27 Rowbotham MC, Twilling L, Davies PS, *et al.* Oral opioid therapy for chronic peripheral and central neuropathic pain. *N Engl J Med* 2003; **348(13)**: 1223–32.

28 Crema A, Benzi G, Frigo GM, *et al.* The responses of the terminal bile duct to morphine and morphine-like drugs. *J Pharmacol Exp Therapeut* 1965; **149(3)**: 373–8.

29 Dixon R, Crews T, Inturrisi C, *et al.* Levorphanol: pharmacokinetics and steady-state plasma concentrations in patients with pain. *Res Comm Chem Pathol Pharmacol* 1983; **41(1)**: 3–17.

30 Leinweber FJ, Szuna AJ, Loh AC, *et al.* Pharmacodynamic studies with (-)-3-phenoxy-N-methyl-morphinan in rats. *Biochem Pharmacol* 1982; **31(4)**: 553–9.

31 **Weinberg DS, Inturrisi CE, Reidenberg B,** *et al.* Sublingual absorption of selected opioid analgesics. *Clin Pharmacol Therapeut* 1988; **44(3):** 335–42.

32 **Pharmacy Network Group.** *Levo dromoran dosage and indications/levorphanol.* http://www.pharmacynetworkgroup.com/i/levo-dromoran-indicatior.

33 **Leinweber FJ, Szuna AJ, Williams TH,** *et al.* The metabolism of (-)-3-phenoxy-N-methylmorphinan in dog. *Drugs Metab Dispos* 1981; **9(3):** 284–91.

34 **Goldstein A, Lowney LI, Pal BK.** Stereospecific and nonspecific interactions of the morphine congener levorphanol in subcellular fractions of mouse brain. *Proc Nat Acad Sci USA* 1971; **68(8):** 1742–7.

35 **Joris JL, Dubner R, Hargreaves KM.** Opioid analgesia at peripheral sites: a target for opioids released during stress and inflammation. *Anesth Analg* 1987; **66(12):** 1277–81.

36 **Pechnick RN, Terman GW.** The role of opiate receptors in the potentiation of pentobarbital sleeping time by the acute and chronic administration of opiates. *Neuropharmacology* 1987; **26(11):** 1589–93.

37 **Portenoy RK, Moulin DE, Rogers A,** *et al.* IV infusion of opioids for cancer pain: clinical review and guidelines for use. *Cancer Treat Rep* 1986; **70(5):** 575–81.

38 **Portenoy RK, Foley KM.** Chronic use of opioid analgesics in non-malignant pain: report of 38 cases. *Pain* 1986; **25(2):** 171–86.

39 **Banister EH.** Six potent analgesic drugs. *Anaesthesia* 1974; **29:** 158–62.

40 **Coniam SW.** Withdrawal of levorphanol. *Anaesthesia* 1991; **46(1):** 71–2.

Chapter 14

Diamorphine

Janet R. Hardy

Diamorphine (di-acetyl morphine, heroin) is a semisynthetic derivative of morphine. It is not an active drug in its own right, but a pro-drug or opioid delivery system. The active metabolites, 6-monoacetylmorphine (6-AM) and morphine are responsible for the analgesic effects of the drug.

Diamorphine was first produced commercially in the late 1890s as a treatment for a variety of respiratory conditions, including dyspnea, pharyngitis, laryngitis, bronchitis, asthma and tuberculosis. It was marketed by the Bayer Company under the trade name 'heroin'. It was also recommended as a remedy for morphine dependence. In 1924 it was banned from medicinal use in the USA when its potential for abuse and addiction was recognized[1]. Diamorphine is used widely and remains the parenteral opioid of choice for the treatment of chronic cancer pain in the UK, but is not used elsewhere because of these concerns.

Physicochemical properties

Diamorphine (di-acetyl morphine, heroin) is a semisynthetic derivative of morphine, having acetyl groups, rather than hydroxyl groups at the 3 and 6 positions of the morphine molecule (Fig. 14.1). The acetylation of the 3 and 6 positions of the morphine molecule affect both the physical and chemical properties of the molecule. Any differences in activity between morphine and diamorphine are related to these differences in molecular structure. In contrast to morphine and 6-AM, diamorphine is highly soluble in water and chloroform (hence, its usefulness in parenteral delivery and in chronic subcutaneous administration). At the temperature at which 1.6 ml is required to dissolve 1 g of diamorphine, the volumes required to dissolve hydromorphone, morphine acetate and morphine sulfate are 3, 2.5 and 21 ml, respectively[1]. Although more lipid soluble than morphine, it is 440 times less lipid soluble than fentanyl and should not be classed as a lipid-soluble opioid.

Diamorphine is rapidly de-acetylated in the body to the active metabolites 6-monoacetylmorphine (6-AM) and morphine. Like many other members of the morphine alkaloid series, the diamorphine molecule has a T-shaped three-dimensional configuration that is thought to be important for the analgesic effect. It has no intrinsic analgesic activity; however, as an unsubstituted phenolic hydroxyl group at the

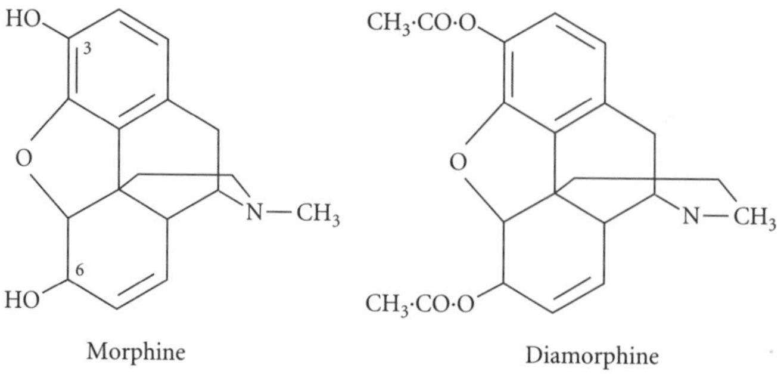

Fig. 14.1 Molecular structure.

3-position of the morphine molecule is considered essential for opioid receptor activation. Current evidence suggests that both morphine and 6-AM are responsible for the pharmacological action of diamorphine[2]. 6-AM does bind to mu receptors and analgesic activity has been shown to correlate with the concentration of 6-AM and to decline following transformation[3]. The late effects of diamorphine are likely to be due to morphine, however, as very low levels of 6-AM are detected before termination of the analgesic effect.

Pharmacokinetics/pharmacodynamics

Oral delivery

After oral administration, diamorphine passes readily across mucous membranes, e.g. the buccal mucosa and upper gastrointestinal tract, and is well absorbed. In one study of repeated oral administration of diamorphine elixir, 77% of the drug was excreted in the urine as total morphine. A similar amount was excreted in the urine after intravenous administration, suggesting that diamorphine is well absorbed from the gastrointestinal tract in man[4]. It then undergoes extensive first pass metabolism, and is rapidly converted to 6-AM and morphine. Following oral administration, only morphine can be measured in substantial amounts in the plasma of patients with no detectable levels of diamorphine or 6-AM[3]. Moreover, the amount of circulating morphine provided by an oral dose of diamorphine is only about 80% of that available from an equal dose of morphine[3]. Oral diamorphine is therefore considered to be an inefficient means of delivering morphine[3–5].

Parenteral delivery

When given parenterally, diamorphine has greater analgesic potency, a more rapid onset and a shorter duration of action compared to morphine[6]. It is rapidly absorbed from injection sites and, upon reaching the blood stream, is converted to 6-AM with a half-life of 9 min, then to morphine with a half-life of about 60 min[7]. The plasma concentration of unchanged diamorphine reduces very rapidly ($t\frac{1}{2} < 5$ min). Thirty minutes after intramuscular injection, plasma concentrations of parent drug are no longer measurable. Because of its lipid solubility and degree of ionization at plasma pH, diamorphine passes rapidly across the blood–brain barrier. It therefore provides a highly efficient delivery system for uptake into the brain following parenteral administration.

There are no formal studies measuring plasma levels of diamorphine or its metabolites following subcutaneous infusion, but a wealth of clinical evidence pointing to its effectiveness.

Intrathecal and epidural delivery

There are no enzymes in the cerebrospinal fluid (CSF) capable of converting diamorphine to its active metabolites[7]. De-acetylation occurs following diffusion of the parent molecule into the spinal cord. At the same time, diamorphine is absorbed into the bloodstream from both CSF and neural tissue leading to systemic effects. These are generally minimal, however, as the amount of drug delivered intrathecally is usually very small. Following intrathecal injection, morphine diffuses out to the systemic circulation very slowly in view of its low lipid solubility. Late respiratory depressant effect following intrathecal diamorphine probably reflects the slow release of morphine following rapid uptake as diamorphine. When given epidurally, diamorphine diffuses into the CSF and then the substance of the spinal cord.

Other routes of delivery

Since it is readily absorbed from the oral or nasal mucosa, administration in the form of a snuff or sublingual tablet should avoid first pass liver metabolism and be very efficient[7]. One study has shown much lower levels of urinary morphine following two modes of inhalation than after intravenous diamorphine. The authors surmise that inhalation is not an effective route for administering diamorphine[8].

Metabolism

Diamorphine is a prodrug and is rapidly deacetylated to 6-AM, then more slowly to morphine in liver, kidney, brain and blood. It undergoes complete first pass metabolism after oral administration. Esterases are responsible for the de-acetylation of diamorphine, but the exact enzyme or enzyme systems responsible for metabolism has not been clearly established. It is thought to be an active process, rather than spontaneous hydrolysis, however[4].

Excretion

Diamorphine is excreted mainly as conjugated morphine in the urine.

Relative potency

There has been much controversy regarding the relative potency of morphine, but most would agree that parenteral diamorphine is about two to three times more potent than parenteral morphine[7,9,10].

Drug interactions and toxicity

Some studies have suggested that diamorphine produces more euphoria and fewer side effects than morphine. Other have described mental clouding, euphoria and talkativeness, but reduced friendliness to others[7], and that these subjective effects may develop more quickly and have greater intensity than those of morphine[11]. Others have refuted these findings[10]. A single intramuscular dose study comparing diamorphine with morphine showed that doses with equal analgesic effect provided comparable improvements in mood, particularly in feelings of peacefulness. Peak mood improvement occurred earlier after diamorphine than after morphine (1.2 versus 1.8 h), but was less sustained. There was no difference in other side effects[10]. Similarly, there is no evidence to support the hypothesis that diamorphine causes less nausea and vomiting than morphine, as shown in a study by Dundee and colleagues[12].

Like other opioids, diamorphine has a marked effect on gastrointestinal smooth muscle, delaying gastric transit and inhibiting gastric emptying. It may therefore influence the absorption of other drugs. As with morphine, diamorphine can cause respiratory depression by reducing the responsiveness of respiratory centers to carbon dioxide. Toxic doses can reduce responsiveness to hypoxia leading to life-threatening hypoventilation. Diamorphine acts as a cough suppressant via a direct effect on the cough center in the medulla independent of its respiratory depressant effect[7].

Dosing in special populations

The caution taken when administering diamorphine to the elderly, and patients with renal and liver impairment is as applies to morphine (see Chapter 8).

Evidence base

The effect of diamorphine on the pain of myocardial infarction has been compared with morphine, methadone and pentazocine. At the doses tested, diamorphine produced greater pain relief at 10 min, but all drugs were equally effective at 30 min[13].

In 1974, Twycross presented the experience of St Christophers Hospice in London in using both oral and intravenous diamorphine in patients with advanced disease[14]. In 1977, the same author demonstrated that morphine was a satisfactory substitute for orally-administered diamorphine and showed the practical advantage of parenteral diamorphine over morphine because of increased solubility[5].

In cancer patients with postoperative pain, diamorphine was found to be about twice as potent as morphine, and produced its peak analgesic and mood-improving effects sooner. Both effects lasted longer with morphine however[10].

In the double-blind cross-over study of intramuscular diamorphine and morphine by Beaver and colleagues[9], diamorphine was found to be 2.4–2.6 times as potent as morphine with a slightly more rapid onset and shorter duration of action.

Diamorphine was compared with hydromorphone in a randomized double-blind study in cancer patients by Wallenstein and colleagues in 1990. Both drugs were found to be potent, relatively short-acting analgesics with similar efficacy and side effect profiles[15].

There have been very few studies of diamorphine as an analgesic in recent years, presumably because of its limited use outside the UK.

Doses and routes of administration

Diamorphine has been produced in liquid and tablet form, but is rarely used as it offers no advantage over oral morphine as described above. It is available as a 10-mg diamorphine hydrochloride tablet and as an elixir containing diacetyl diamorphine in chloroform. For injection, it is produced as a powder for reconstitution as 5-, 10-, 30-, 100- and 500-mg vials.

The ratio of oral morphine to parenteral diamorphine is said to be 1 : 3. As with many opioid conversions, however, the potency ratios are controversial, and vary according to the patient and circumstances in which the opioid is used[16]. Most clinicians use a ratio of 1 : 3 when converting oral morphine to subcutaneous diamorphine and a 1 : 1 ratio when converting oral morphine to oral diamorphine.

Controversies

Diamorphine was first synthesized in 1874 and marketed as a cough suppressant. When it first became apparent that dependence was a feature of prolonged morphine use, diamorphine was promoted as a safer alternative. This premise was soon proved to be untrue and when its addictive potential with consequent social implications were realized, it was banned from medicinal use. Federal Law prevents its manufacture in North America, but there is no evidence that it is more dangerous or more open to misappropriate use than other drugs of addiction or other opioids described in this text. Equipotent doses of morphine and diamorphine have identical potential for both tolerance and physical addiction[7]. The analgesic properties of diamorphine are long-established and remain the sole indication for its use. In the UK it is widely used as the parenteral opioid of choice and is recognized as such in the guidelines of the European Association of Palliative Care (EAPC)[17]. Restrictions on its use are no different from those of any similar agent and, consequently, it is used routinely in clinical practice. The greater solubility of diamorphine as compared with morphine sulfate has long been considered a practical advantage when large parenteral doses are required. It is, however, not much more soluble than hydromorphone so offers little advantage in those countries where the latter drug is available. Much of the controversy has focused on the belief that diamorphine is a better analgesic than morphine[6,18,19]. It is now generally accepted that there is no difference between the analgesic efficacy of the two drugs. Similarly, there is no strong evidence to support a better side effect profile. In summary, diamorphine does not appear to have unique advantages or disadvantages compared with other opioids when used for the relief of pain, although the evidence to back this premise is wanting[6].

References

1 Twycross R. Pain relief in advanced cancer. In: Twycross R (Ed.) *Strong Opioids*. Edinburgh: Churchill Livingstone 1994.

2 Intrussi C, Schultz M, Shin S, *et al.* Evidence from opiate binding studies that heroin acts through its metabolites. *Life Sci* 1983; **33**: 773–6.

3 Intrussi C, Max M, Foley K, *et al.* The pharmacokinetics of heroin in patients with chronic pain. *N Engl J Med* 1984; **310**: 1213–17.

4 Stevens L, Wootton C. The pharmacokinetic properties of diamorphine. In: Scott DB (Ed.) *Diamorphine, Its Chemistry, Pharmacology and Clinical Use*. Cambridge: Woodhead-Faulkner Ltd in association with Evans Medical Ltd, 1988, pp. 15–43.

5 Twycross R. Choice of strong analgesic in terminal cancer: diamorphine or morphine? *Pain* 1977; **3**: 93–104.

6 Levine M, Sackett D. Heroin vs morphine for cancer pain? *Arch Intern Med* 1986; **146**: 353–6.

7 Hull C. The pharmacodynamics of diamorphine. In: Scott DB (Ed.) *Diamorphine, Its Chemistry, Pharmacology and Clinical Use*. Cambridge: Woodhead-Faulkner Ltd in association with Evans Medical Ltd, 1988, pp. 44–54.

8 Mo B, Way E. An assessment of inhalation as a mode of administration of heroin by addicts. *J Pharm Exp Therapeut* 1966; **154**: 142–7.

9 Beaver W, Schein P, Hext M. Comparison of the analgesic effects of intramuscular heroin and morphine. *Am Soc Clin Pharm Therapeut* 1981; **29(2)**: 232.

10 Kaiko R, Wallenstein S, Rogers A. Analgesic and mood effects of heroin and morphine in cancer patients with postoperative pain. *N Engl J Med* 1981; **304**: 1501–5.

11 Smith G, Beecher H. Subjective effects of heroin and morphine in normal subjects. *J Pharmacol Exp Ther* 1962; **136**: 47–52.

12 Dundee J, Clarke R, Loan W. Comparative toxicity of diamorphine, morphine and methadone. *Lancet* 1967; **2**: 221–3.

13 Scott M, Orr R. Effects of diamorphine, methadone, morphine and phenazocine in patients with suspected myocardial infarction. *Lancet* 1969; **1**: 1065–7.

14 Twycross R. Clinical experience with diamorphine in advanced malignant disease. *Int J Clin Pharm* 1974; **9**: 184–98; *Pain* 1990; **41**: 5–13.

15 Wallenstein S, Houde R, Portenoy R, *et al.* Clinical analgesic assay of repeated and single doses of heroin and hydromorphone. *Pain* 1990; **41**: 5–13.

16 Amesbury B. Converting from oral morphine to subcutaneous diamorphine. *Palliat Med* 2000; **14**: 165–7.

17 **Hanks G, de Conno F, Cherny N, *et al*.** Expert working group of the European Association for Palliative Care. Morphine and alternative opioids in cancer pain: the EAPC recommendations. *Br J Cancer* 2001; **84(5):** 587–93.

18 **Foley K.** Controversies in cancer pain. *Cancer* 1989; **63:** 2257–65.

19 **McCarthy R, Montagne M.** The argument for therapeutic use of heroin in pain management. *Am J Hosp Pharm* 1993; **50:** 992–6.

Chapter 15

Oxymorphone

Paul Glare

Pharmacology

Oxymorphone (dihydrohydroxymorphinone) is a potent semisynthetic derivative of morphine that is available commercially in the USA and Canada, but not the UK or Australia. It is available as a solution for injection and as a rectal suppository (US trade name, Numorphan). Oxymorphone is synthesized from morphine by replacing the hydroxyl group at C6 with a methyl group and, like many other derivatives, there is a double bond between C7 and C8, and a hydroxyl group added to C14[1]. Oxymorphone is also the -O demethylated metabolite of oxycodone, but is present in only small concentrations after oxycodone doses. It is believed to play a role in analgesia in rats administered oxycodone but not in humans[2].

Pharmacodynamics

Oxymorphone produces many of the same effects as its parent compound morphine. Parenteral administration produces analgesia within 5–10 min and rectal administration within 15–30 min. The duration of analgesia is 3–4 h. Oxymorphone has about eight to 10 times the potency of morphine, i.e. 1–1.5 mg oxymorphone is equivalent to 10 mg of morphine[3,4].

Pharmacokinetics

Absorption

Oxymorphone is well absorbed from both the subcutaneous (s.c.) and intramuscular (i.m.) routes. Oral absorption does occur, but the bioavailability (BA) is poor, approximately 1/6th that of i.m. oxymorphone[3]. Rectal absorption does also occur, but the BA is only 1/10th of i.m.[4]

Elimination

Oxymorphone undergoes hepatic metabolism and is then excreted as the glucuronide by the kidney. There is insufficient data to establish its safety during breast-feeding and caution is advised by the American Academy of Pediatrics[5].

Half-life

Two to three hours, as for morphine and its other short-acting derivatives.

Metabolism

Oxymorphone is extensively metabolized by humans (and many other species, e.g. rat, dog and guinea pig, and to a lesser extent by rabbit)[6]. Being a close synthetic derivative of morphine, oxymorphone is metabolized primarily by uridine diphosphate glucuronosyl transferase (UGT) enzymes in the liver. The most abundant metabolite in urine is conjugated oxymorphone (accounting for between 13 and 82% of an administered dose), followed by small amounts of 6-beta- and 6-alpha-oxymorphol (<5%), produced by the 6-keto reduction of oxymorphone. Stereoselectivity of 6-keto reduction was observed for all species with the 6-beta-carbinol metabolite being most abundant. Small amounts of free oxymorphone (<10%) are also excreted. Overall recoveries of oxymorphone and metabolites from urine ranges from 15 to 96%, of which more than 80% is excreted in the first 24 h. Considerable individual variability occurred in the excretion of free and conjugated oxymorphone by six human subjects following oraldosing[6].

It is difficult to make conclusions about pharmacokinetic drug–drug interactions with oxymorphone. *In vivo* drug–drug interaction studies with oxymorphone have not been carried out.As it is a semisynthetic derivative of morphine and has a 6-glucuronide metabolite, other agents that inhibit or induce UGT enzymes could alter levels of oxymorphone and its metabolites, but the clinical relevance of this is not known at this time.

Routes of administration

There is no oral preparation of oxymorphone currently commercially available. The drug is usually given parenterally. Rectal suppositories will produce a lower and more delayed peak analgesia, and longer duration than parenteral routes and the rectal dose has about 1/10th the potency of parenteral oxymorphone. Laboratory data indicate oxymorphone hydrochloride appears to have the solubility, potency and absorption properties required for efficient nasal and transdermal delivery as alternatives to injections, but there is no data for its efficacy[7,8]. Oxymorphone is administered spinally in veterinary anesthesia, but not in man.

Drug interactions and toxicity

Interactions

Oxymorphone has the same sort of drug–drug interactions as morphine with other central nervous system (CNS) depressants like barbiturates, alcohol and other opioids (sedation, respiratory). The cardiorespiratory effects of concomitant administration of oxymorphone, phenobarbitol and tetrahydrocannabinol have been reported to be severe[9,10]. Oxidative metabolism of oxymorphone may be induced by cyctochrome

P450 enzyme inducers like rifabutin, requiring an increase in the oxymorphone dose. Agents such as quinidine and fluoxetine have been shown in human microsomal preparations to produce inhibition of conversion of oxycodone to oxymorphone[11], implicating a role for the CYP2D6 isoenzyme. However, other isoenzymes have been implicated[12].

Toxicity

Oxymorphone has been traditionally said to cause more nausea than morphine[13], but this has not been confirmed in more recent clinical trials. During routine anesthetic inductions, moderately large doses of oxymorphone (0.2 mg/kg) administered by infusion do not appear to stimulate release of clinically significant plasma levels of histamine[14]. Oxymorphone may have less effect on the cough reflex than other strong opioids. It is rated US Food and Drug Administration's Pregnancy Category B or D if used for prolonged periods or in high doses at term[15].

Dosing in special populations

There are no known studies of the safety/efficacy of oxymorphone in pediatrics. It is presumed that oxymorphone glucuronide accumulates in renal failure, but it is unclear if this is clinically important.

Evidence-based use for cancer pain

There have been very few studies of the use of oxymorphone in cancer pain. The only clinical trial was conducted by Beaver and colleagues more than 30 years ago[3]. Those authors evaluated the relative analgesic potency of oral and intramuscular oxymorphone in a double-blind cross-over comparison of graded single doses in patients with chronic pain due to cancer. When both duration and intensity of analgesia are considered (total effect), oral oxymorphone was 1/6th as potent as the intramuscular form. In terms of peak effect, however, oral oxymorphone was only 1/14th as potent. These values are almost identical to those obtained in a previous study comparing oral with intramuscular morphine. The analgesic effect of oral oxymorphone rose to a peak later and had a longer duration than the effect of intramuscular oxymorphone. Intramuscular oxymorphone and morphine were also compared in a similar patient group. Intramuscular oxymorphone proved to be 8.7 times as potent as morphine in terms of total analgesic effect and 13 times as potent in terms of peak effect. In roughly equianalgesic doses, the occurrence of side effects was qualitatively and quantitatively similar for oral and intramuscular oxymorphone, and for intramuscular oxymorphone and morphine.

These investigators also investigated the relative analgesic potency of single doses of oxymorphone by rectal suppository and intramuscular injection in 136 patients with postoperative pain[4]. In these subjects, rectal oxymorphone was 1/10th as potent as the intramuscular form; in peak effect, it was only 1/16–1/20th as potent. However, because intramuscular oxymorphone is 9–10 times as potent as intramuscular morphine, 5–10 mg oxymorphone by suppository provides analgesia comparable to that provided by the usually used doses of parenteral narcotics. Rectal oxymorphone produced no more and perhaps somewhat fewer side effects than doses of intramuscular oxymorphone producing equivalent total analgesic effect. None of the patients objected to the rectal route of analgesic administration. This study suggested that the rectal route is an acceptable and practical way of administering potent analgesics, and is probably being under-utilized by physicians in the control of moderate to severe pain.

Subsequently, oxymorphone was used in one of 46 continuous i.v. infusion (CI) of opioids in 36 patients with cancer pain reviewed by Portenoy et al. The specific results of the oxymorphone case were not given, but overall the CIs were safe and effective in most cases[16]. Other groups have reported the safety and efficacy of oxymorphone in other clinical groups. Sinatra et al. reported the analgesic efficacy and adverse effects of morphine and oxymorphone in 64 patients following cesarean delivery, 32 of whom received oxymorphone[17]. Half the subjects in the study received traditional patient-controlled analgesia (PCA) and were compared with the other half receiving the same agents via PCA plus basal opioid infusion (PCA + BI). Patients utilizing PCA + BI noted significant reductions in resting pain scores with oxymorphone and decreased pain during movement with both opioids when compared with individuals using PCA alone ($p < 0.05$). There were no significant differences between treatment groups in 24-h dose requirements or patient satisfaction with therapy ($p = $ NS).

Similarly, White et al. reported 120 patients undergoing major orthopedic (e.g. total hip replacement), urological (e.g. radical prostatectomy) or gynecological (e.g. total abdominal hysterectomy) procedures who were randomly assigned to receive either morphine or oxymorphone postoperatively using a patient-controlled analgesic (PCA) delivery system[18]. The opioid analgesic was administered either intravenously (i.v. PCA) or subcutaneously (s.c. PCA) during the 72-h study period. Oxymorphone, 0.65 ± 0.42 mg/h (0–24 h), 0.53 ± 0.35 mg/h (24–48 h), and 0.42 ± 0.31 mg/h (48–72 h), was as effective as morphine, 2.2 ± 1.6 mg/h (0–24 h), 1.6 ± 1.2 mg/h (24–48 h), and 1.2 ± 1.1 mg/h (48–72 h), in providing postoperative pain relief (mean values ± SD). Although the average opioid dosage requirements were 10–28% higher with s.c. PCA, it is an acceptable alternative to conventional i.v. PCA for pain control after major surgical procedures. Postoperative analgesia scores and patient satisfaction were similar in all four PCA treatment groups. Thus, s.c. PCA with either oxymorphone or morphine represents a clinically acceptable alternative to i.v. PCA in the treatment of postoperative pain.

Dose and routes

Intramuscular or subcutaneous: 1–1.5 mg every 4–6 h.
Intravenous: 0.5 mg every 4–6 h.
PR: 5 mg every 4–6 h.

References

1 Jaffe J, Martin WR. Opioid analgesics. In: Hardman J, Limbird L (Eds) *Goodman & Gilman's the Pharmacological Basis of Therapeutics*, 9th edn. New York: McGraw-Hill, 1996; pp. 361–96.

2 Poyhia R, Vannio A, Kalso E. A review of oxycodone's pharmacokinetics and pharmacodynamics. *J Pain Sympt Manag* 1993; **8**: 63–7.

3 Beaver WT, Wallenstein SL, Houde RW, *et al.* Comparisons of the analgesic effects of oral and intramuscular oxymorphone and of intramuscular oxymorphone and morphine in patients with cancer. *J Clin Pharmacol* 1977; **17**: 186–98.

4 Beaver WT, Feise GA. A comparison of the analgesic effect of oxymorphone by rectal suppository and intramuscular injection in patients with postoperative pain. *J Clin Pharmacol* 1977; **17**: 276–91.

5 Anon. American Academy of Pediatrics Committee on Drugs: the transfer of drugs and other chemicals into human milk. *Pediatrics* 2001; **108**: 776–89.

6 Cone EJ, Darwin WD, Buchwald WF, *et al.* Oxymorphone metabolism and urinary excretion in human, rat, guinea pig, rabbit, and dog. *Drug Metab Dispos* 1983; **11**: 446–50.

7 Aungst BJ, Blake JA, Rogers NJ, *et al.* Transdermal oxymorphone formulation development and methods for evaluating flux and lag times for two skin permeation-enhancing vehicles. *J Pharmaceut Sci* 1990; **79**: 1072–6.

8 Hussain MA, Aungst BJ. Intranasal absorption of oxymorphone. *J Pharmaceut Sci* 1997; **86**: 975–6.

9 Johnstone RE, Lief PL, Kulp RA, *et al.* Combination of delta9-tetrahydrocannabinol with oxymorphone or pentobarbital: effects on ventilatory control and cardiovascular dynamics. *Anesthesiol* 1975; **42**: 674–84.

10 Armstrong SC, Cozza KL. Pharmacokinetic drug interactions of morphine, codeine, and their derivatives: theory and clinical reality, part I. *Psychosomatics* 2003; **44**: 167–71.

11 Otton S, Wu D, Joffe RT, *et al.* Inhibition of fluoxetine of cytochrome P450 2D6 activity. *Clin Pharmacol Ther* 1993; **53**: 401–9.

12 Cleary J, Mikus G, Somogyi A, *et al.* The influence of pharmacogenetics on opioid analgesia: studies with codeine and oxycodone in the Sprague–Dawley/Dark agouti rat model. *J Pharmacol Exp Ther* 1994; **271**: 1528–34.

13 Keats AS, Telford J. Studies of analgesic drugs: V. The comparative subjective effects of oxymorphone and morphine. *Clin Pharmacol Ther* 1960; **1(6)**: 703–7.

14 Warner MA, Hosking MP, Gray JR, *et al.* Narcotic-induced histamine release: a comparison of morphine, oxymorphone, and fentanyl infusions. *J Cardiothor Vasc Anesth* 1991; **5**: 481–4.

15 Briggs GG, Freeman RK, Yaffe SJ. *Drugs in Pregnancy and Lactation: a reference guide to fetal and neonatal risk*, 6th edn. Philadelphia: Lippincott Williams & Wilkins, 2002.

16 Portenoy RK, Moulin DE, Rogers A, *et al.* I.v. infusion of opioids for cancer pain: clinical review and guidelines for use. *Cancer Treat Rep* 1986; **70**: 575–81.

17 Sinatra R, Chung KS, Silverman DG, *et al.* An evaluation of morphine and oxymorphone administered via patient-controlled analgesia (PCA) or PCA plus basal infusion in postcesarean-delivery patients. *Anesthesiol* 1989; **71**: 502–7.

18 White PF. Subcutaneous-PCA: an alternative to IV-PCA for postoperative pain management. *Clin J Pain* 1990; **6**: 297–300.

Chapter 16

Choice of opioids and the WHO ladder

Paul Glare

Approximately one-third of patients with advanced cancer receiving anticancer treatment and 70–90% of patients with far-advanced cancer experience moderate to severe pain[1]. For such patients, guidelines recommend a trial of opioids[2–6]. Which opioid they should receive and how it is best delivered remains controversial.

Prior to the 1970s, neurosurgical and neurolytic techniques were the mainstay of cancer pain management. In 1976, Balfour Mount *et al.* showed that Brompton's cocktail was superior to these traditional methods of pain relief[7], and by the late 1970s pharmacological management became the mainstay, with a resulting decline in neurosurgical procedures[8]. By 1980, oral morphine was recommended by Robert Twycross as the 'narcotic analgesic of choice' in far advanced cancer, although it was also recognized by others that alternatives were available that varied in their potency and duration of action[9,10].

In 1989, Foley challenged the primacy of morphine amongst the opioids[11]. In its favor, morphine provides reliable analgesia, is inexpensive and has the most flexibility of dosage and routes of administration[12]. However, morphine is far from an 'ideal analgesic'. Its oral bioavailability is highly variable, resulting in a broad spectrum of response and wide dosing requirements. It has pharmacologically active metabolites, notably morphine-6-glucuronide (M6G) that can accumulate particularly in the presence of renal dysfunction[12]. Some types of pain (e.g. neuropathic pain, muscle spasm) do not always respond well to morphine and there is a stigma attached to taking morphine.

In the past 5 years, oxycodone, hydromorphone and fentanyl have become more widely available, and there has been a resurgence in the use of methadone as an analgesic, raising new clinical questions and options[13,14]. In addition to severity of pain, coexisting disease, response to previous therapy, the drug's pharmacokinetics and available formulations influence the choice of an opioid agent. Short half-life drugs, such as morphine, hydromorphone, fentanyl, oxycodone and oxymorphone, are generally favored initially because they are easier to titrate than long half-life agents. Long-acting controlled-release opioid preparations can lessen the inconvenience of around-the-clock administration of drugs with a short duration of action. In recent years, several new formulations have been developed, including:

+ controlled-release morphine suppositories and suspensions;
+ controlled-release tablets of oxycodone, hydromorphone and codeine;
+ transdermal fentanyl, a patch that allows 3-day dosing and avoids the first-pass effect of the liver.

Most patients who receive controlled-release opioids should be provided with a rescue dose of an immediate-release opioid to treat pain that may break through the controlled-release schedule.

Considerable interest has been generated recently in the use of methadone for the treatment of cancer pain[15]. Previously, the use of methadone for this patient population had waned with the development of long-acting opioid preparations of morphine, oxycodone and fentanyl. Methadone is a unique opioid that possesses many attractive features[16]. Not only is methadone a mu-opioid receptor agonist, but it also possesses delta and kappa-opioid receptor activity[17,18]. It is also an inhibitor of serotonin reuptake and the d-isomer is an N-methyl D-aspartate (NMDA) receptor antagonist. These properties make methadone particularly suited to the treatment of neuropathic pain. Methadone can also be administered via many routes of administration, including orally, rectally, subcutaneously and intravenously. Because methadone has a long half-life, it can be conveniently dosed with an interval of every 8–12 h. Methadone is also inexpensive, particularly relative to the other long-acting opioid preparations, and this feature is of particular interest to US hospices and other settings that are required to provide palliative care and medications with limited resources. However, there are a number of disadvantages to methadone[16]. Methadone remains stigmatized as a medication used to treat heroin addiction. Because of multiple pharmacokinetic and pharmacodynamic issues, prescribing methadone both safely and effectively can be challenging. Some of these issues are:

+ its biphasic elimination, which can result in accumulation and potential side effects/toxicity;
+ its multiple potential drug–drug interactions, due to the activities of the cytochrome P450 (CYP) enzymes CYP 3A4, CYP 2D6 and CYP 1A2[19];
+ its dynamic potency based on previous opioid exposure;
+ its high protein binding to alpha-1-acid glycoprotein, an acute phase reactant that can impact the free fraction of methadone in the bloodstream.

The culmination of these and other issues surrounding methadone may be the primary barrier to the prescribing of methadone. With greater clinical experience or as the result of experimental findings, oxycodone, hydromorphone, fentanyl or methadone may replace morphine as the preferred strong opioid in the future.

In critically ill patients with cancer, there are other issues to consider. Cardiovascular stability observed with fentanyl and sufentanil indicates their use in hemodynamically compromised patients[20]. Short-acting remifentanil offers several advantages in patients requiring prolonged infusions. The organ-independent metabolism of this newer molecule may be valuable in patients with multiple organ failure[20].

In the 1980s there was vigorous debate about the legalization of heroin for cancer pain. Heroin was promoted as a superior analgesic and there were animal data that it retards tumor growth. Oral heroin is not superior to oral morphine[21]. Subcutaneous heroin is commonly administered in British hospices. Opponents argue that, while heroin may be a safe and effective opioid analgesic, it has few advantages over other available drugs and the social implications of legalization outweigh any clinical benefits. Recently, there has been some revival of this controversy[22].

Strong versus weak opioids: the WHO ladder

In 1982, a WHO consultation in Milan, Italy, brought together a group of experts in the management of cancer pain. At the time, there was much concern about the inadequacies of cancer pain management—due largely to physician-related barriers in developed countries and restricted access of cancer patients to strong opioids in many developing countries. In many parts of the world, not a single dose of oral morphine was available. The reasons for this were complex and included social, cultural and political ones[23]. It was estimated that millions of people worldwide were suffering needlessly and this could be easily fixed if only strong opioids were made available. For many of these patients, there was (and still is) no prospect for cure, and the only realistic, humane approach to their illness was to offer pain relief and palliative care. The WHO Ladder was ultimately a global public health exercise.

They expressed the consensus that through a limited number of drugs, pain relief was a realistic target for the majority of cancer patients. Subsequently, another meeting was held in Milan in 1984, which resulted in the publication of *Cancer Pain Relief*[2]. This contained the 'method for pain relief', a structured approach to drug selection, which has become known as the 'WHO Analgesic Ladder'. This consists of three basic steps:

- patients with mild cancer-related pain should be treated with a non-opioid analgesic, which should be combined with adjuvant drugs if a specific indication for this exists;
- patients who are relatively non-tolerant and present with moderate pain, or fail to achieve adequate relief after a trial of non-opioid, should be treated with an opioid conventionally used for mild to moderate pain (formerly known as weak opioids);
- patients who present with severe pain, or who fail to achieve adequate relief following appropriate administration of drugs on the second step of the analgesic ladder should receive an opioid conventionally used for moderate to severe pain (formerly known as a strong opioid).

According to these guidelines, a trial of opioid therapy should be given to all patients with pain of moderate or greater severity. Some 20 years on, authorities continue to widely endorse the guiding principle behind the ladder, that analgesic selection should be primarily determined by the severity of the pain[4,5,6,24].

Despite widespread promulgation of the ladder, surveys indicate that many patients appear to still have inadequate analgesia. There are several possible explanations for this discrepancy. On one hand, there might be barriers to the implementation of the ladder. On the other hand, the ladder might not be as applicable, effective or acceptable as was originally expected. Undoubtedly, the WHO Ladder—in combination with the hard work of many individuals—has been very effective as a public health measure, as legislative change in many of these countries to increase the availability of pain-killings drugs has now been achieved. The evidence for its efficacy as a clinical practice guideline is less clear. Its usefulness as a method of pain relief in individual patients throughout the course of the cancer illness has also been challenged.

Evidence for the ladder

Evidence for the recommendations in the ladder

Step 1: non-opioids for mild cancer pain

Current cancer pain guidelines recommend that patients with mild pain should receive a non-steroidal anti-inflammatory drug (NSAID) or acetaminophen/paracetamol[3,5]. The choice of drug is based on a risk/benefit analysis for individual patients. Much of the evidence for the safety and efficacy of NSAIDs comes from the non-cancer pain literature[25]. A systematic review of the safety and efficacy of NSAIDs in cancer pain carried out more than decade ago included 25 studies of both single and repeated dosing of various agents[26]. Single dose studies found NSAIDs to be roughly equivalent to 5–10 mg i.m. morphine. There was some evidence of a dose–response effect with a ceiling effect to analgesia. A lack of comparable studies precluded testing the hypothesis that NSAIDs are particularly effective for malignant bone pain.

Step 2: weak opioids for moderate cancer pain

As discussed in the chapter on dextropropoxyphene (Chapter 7), there has been controversy about whether weak opioids alone or in combination with non-opioids are more effective than non-opioids alone. While the efficacy achieved by single doses of weak opioids such as codeine is poor, multiple doses may perform better. Paracetamol in combination with an opioid for mild to moderate pain appears to be marginally more effective than paracetamol alone[27].

At therapeutic doses there is no evidence of superiority for one opioid for mild to moderate pain over another[28]. Tramadol is an opioid with additional effects on the monaminergic system[29]. At therapeutic doses, its analgesic effect is similar to that of an opioid for mild to moderate pain in combination with a non-opioid[30]. The extent to which the dose can be titrated is limited, as at doses just above the normal tramadol can cause convulsions and produces serious psychiatric reactions at therapeutic doses in some patients[29]. For these reasons, it appears to offer little over existing opioids for mild to moderate pain in patients with advanced cancer.

More recently, low dose formulations of opioids traditionally used for severe pain have been used for the management of mild–moderate pain. This, together with the introduction of new agents such as tramadol, has widened the repertoire of agents suitable for the management of moderate pain. Indeed, many authorities now advocate the use of the same opioid for all pains of moderate or greater intensity[4,6,31,32].

Step 3: strong opioids for severe cancer pain

A recent systematic review has concluded that oral morphine is effective for cancer pain, although the body of randomized trial literature was small[33]. The opioid of choice for oral use is morphine[4]. The reasons are:

- the majority of patients tolerate morphine well;
- it is usually effective, dose titration to a suitable level of analgesia usually being achievable;
- for long term use, the oral route is preferable to parenteral or rectal;
- a wide variety of oral formulations are available, allowing flexibility of dosing intervals;
- there is less long-term safety data on alternative opioids.

A trial of an alternative opioid should be considered for moderate to severe pain where dose titration is limited by the side effects of morphine. The main candidates are oxycodone, hydromorphone, fentanyl and methadone.

There are a number of strong opioids that are widely available, but not usually recommended for the treatment of moderate to severe pain in patients with cancer. The drugs and the reasons they are not thought to be suitable are[5]:

- *meperidine/pethidine*: on the WHO Essential Drug list, but short acting and with repeated dosing there is accumulation of neurotoxic metabolite, normeperidine;
- *dextromoramide*: methadone analogue that is twice as potent as morphine and can be given sublingually, too short-acting for regular use, but may be of some use in controlling incident pain;
- *buprenorphine*: mixed agonist/antagonist with ceiling dose that prevents continuing dose titration;
- *nalbuphine and pentazocine*: mixed agonist/antagonists with ceiling dose that prevents continuing dose titration; also may cause psychotomimetic side effects in some patients;
- *dipipanone*: only available in combination with cyclizine and leads to cyclizine toxicity with dose titration.

Evidence for the efficacy of the WHO ladder

A recent systematic review has criticized the evidence for the efficacy of the ladder[34]. Eight primary studies were included[35–42]. All were case series with no control groups, precluding a meta-analysis being performed. While all claimed efficacy of >70%, there were a number of methodological problems with all the studies, including:

- no information on conditions in which the pain was assessed;
- two were retrospective;
- two had short or variable follow-up periods;
- three had high withdrawal rates.

The review concluded that the evidence provided is insufficient to be able to estimate the efficacy of the ladder. Carefully designed controlled studies are needed before the ladder can be rightly used to evaluate clinical outcomes or determine policy.

Applicability of the ladder

A problem with the WHO ladder is that it is too simplistic to be a useful tool for managing cancer pain in individual patients, particularly in developed countries.

Even ignoring the lack of evidence for its recommendations and the controversy for the need for a second rung, there are three conceptual problems with the WHO Ladder in its current format:

1. It ignores the importance of identifying the noxious stimulus

Not all pain experienced by people with cancer is due to the disease. It can be due to a side effect of treatment, debilitation or totally unrelated to the cancer or its treatment. Many of these other pains have specific treatments that need to be considered. Patients with cancer who are in pain need a comprehensive, multidimensional assessment. This means taking a careful history followed by a focused physical examination, supplemented by appropriate investigations. Psychosocial assessment should be included.

2. It focuses too much on pharmacological management of cancer pain, especially with opioids

The reason for a multi-dimensional assessment is to plan multi-modal treatment. The Ladder ignores the importance of psychosocial assessment and support, physiotherapy and occupational therapy, anti-neoplastic therapies, and invasive procedures like spinal opioids, nerve blocks and neurosurgical techniques.

3. It implies a one-way escalation of opioids

The Ladder implies a one-way, inexorable increase in opioid potency, with patients ending up on morphine until they die. While this may be the case in far advanced cancer, many patients with newly diagnosed cancer present with severe pain that requires a strong opioid from the outset, which can be stopped once effective anticancer treatment has been initiated.

A better approach to cancer pain management?

Two alternative approaches to the WHO ladder have been developed. The most well known is the 'pyramid-plus-ribbon' approach, advocated in recent US Dept of Health Agency for Health Care Policy and Research (AHCPR) Guidelines for Cancer Pain Management guidelines is preferable (see Fig. 16.1)[3]. The pyramid depicts a hierarchy of pain management strategies from least invasive (at base) to most invasive (at apex). Therapies depicted on the ribbon may benefit patients receiving 'pyramid' therapies at any level of invasiveness. Pain-killing drugs remain the corner stone—the base of the pyramid—but the multidisciplinary approach to assessment and treatment that is needed to optimize pain relief is much more explicit with this approach than with the Ladder. This is particularly helpful when analgesics are ineffective and other options need to be considered. Research is needed to determine the effectiveness of these other modalities, alone or in combination, in various populations. The distribution of these guidelines has led to the increased awareness of cancer pain as a problem and increasing uptake of rational management strategies, especially among target providers such as oncologists in the US[43].

The other is the so-called four-step 'Sydney Stickman' approach, based on a cartoon figure, which combines a multidimensional patient assessment with individualized

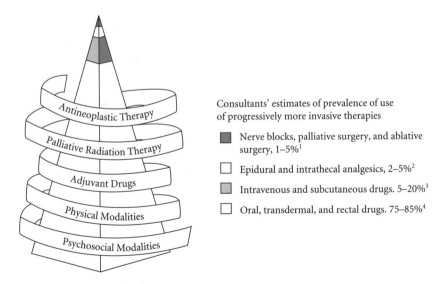

Consultants' estimates of prevalence of use of progressively more invasive therapies

■ Nerve blocks, palliative surgery, and ablative surgery, 1–5%[1]

☐ Epidural and intrathecal analgesics, 2–5%[2]

▨ Intravenous and subcutaneous drugs. 5–20%[3]

☐ Oral, transdermal, and rectal drugs. 75–85%[4]

Fig. 16.1 Pyramid plus ribbon[3].

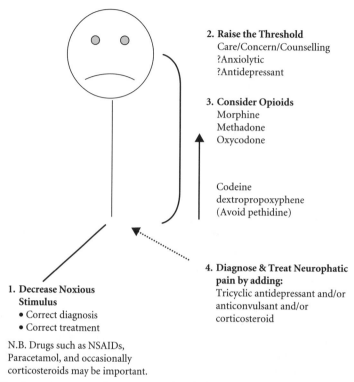

2. Raise the Threshold
Care/Concern/Counselling
?Anxiolytic
?Antidepressant

3. Consider Opioids
Morphine
Methadone
Oxycodone

Codeine
dextropropoxyphene
(Avoid pethidine)

4. Diagnose & Treat Neurophatic pain by adding:
Tricyclic antidepressant and/or
anticonvulsant and/or
corticosteroid

1. Decrease Noxious Stimulus
• Correct diagnosis
• Correct treatment

N.B. Drugs such as NSAIDs,
Paracetamol, and occasionally
corticosteroids may be important.

Fig. 16.2 The four-step approach to cancer pain relief.

application of various treatment modalities (Fig. 16.2)[44]. The four steps are best undertaken in chronological order, even if all are approached in a short period of time. This approach emphasizes communication with patient, the patient 'telling the self'. Both the 'pyramid and ribbon' and the 'Stickman' approaches adopt similar four-step methods:

◆ *Assess and reduce the noxious stimulus.* The physician should take a careful pain history followed by a focused physical examination and then order appropriate investigations. As the author states, the pain diagnosis may be made in 5 min or may evolve over several days. Treatment includes peripherally-acting agents like paracetamol or a NSAID, and possibly anti-tumour therapy.

◆ *Raise the patient's pain threshold.* There are various models of the relationship between pain, pain behavior and suffering. All patients will benefit from simple psychological support (e.g. explanation, reassurance). Encouraging the patient to tell the story of themselves in relation to the cancer and their pain has the potential for self-healing and reducing some distress. Some patients have significant anxiety, depression and other emotions, and may benefit from specific therapy (antidepressants, psychological therapy).

- *Exploit the opioid receptor system.* Opioids should be prescribed appropriately, along the lines advocated by the analgesic ladder and in the various cancer pain guidelines. This includes anticipating and preventing side effects like constipation[44].

- *Recognize and treat neuropathic pain.* Despite the controversy regarding the efficacy of opioids and neuropathic pain states[12], this step recognizes the role of co-analgesic drugs as opioid-sparing agents in the management of neuropathic pain.Due consideration needs to be given to polypharmacy, side effects and drug interactions when prescribing these co-analgesics. In some cases, invasive techniques like spinal opioids or neurosurgical techniques need to be considered.

Can guidelines improve cancer pain management?

In 1999, Du Pen *et al.* reported a study evaluating whether the AHCPR guidelines improved cancer pain management when implemented in a community setting[45]. The prospective, longitudinal, randomized controlled study involved 81 cancer patients from the outpatient clinic settings of 26 western Washington-area medical oncologists. A multilevel treatment algorithm based on the guideline was compared with standard-practice (control) pain and symptom management therapies used by community oncologists. Patients randomized to the pain algorithm group achieved a statistically significant reduction in usual pain intensity, measured as slope scores, when compared with standard community practice. Concurrent chemotherapy and patient adherence to treatment were significant mediators of worst pain. There were no significant differences in other symptoms or quality of life between the two treatment groups. The results of this study support the use of algorithmic decision making in the management of cancer pain. These findings suggest that comprehensive pain assessment and evidence-based analgesic decision-making processes do enhance usual pain outcomes.

Subsequently, a tailored cost-effectiveness analysis has been used to compare three approaches to cancer pain, guideline-based care (GBC), oncology-based care (OBC) and usual care (UC)[46]. The model found that after 1 month of treatment, the percentage of cancer pain patients with effective pain management and the cost of each strategy were estimated as follows:

- GBC, 80% and $579;
- OBC, 55% and $466;
- UC, 30% and $315.

Compared with OBC, GBC had an incremental cost-effectiveness ratio of $452 per additional patient relieved of cancer pain. Compared with UC, OBC had an incremental cost-effectiveness ratio of $601 per additional patient relieved of cancer pain. It was concluded that guideline-based cancer pain management leads to improved pain control with modest increases in resource use.

Cost of opioid therapy

While clinical issues like pain severity, comorbidities, response to previous therapy, the drug's pharmacokinetics and available formulations should be the factors that influence the choice of an opioid agent, there are many patient-related and system-wide factors that influence choice, and one of these may be cost.

Opioid costs and availability varied widely in both developing and developed countries. In the United States, average wholesale price (AWP) are used and a 30-day supply of morphine long-acting tablets dosed at 100 mg/12 h has an AWP of approximately $294.00; a 30-day supply of methadone at a comparable dose of 10 mg/12 h (using a 10 : 1 ratio) has an AWP of approximately $9.00[16]. In the UK and Australia, drug costs are subsidized by the government and the cost of these drugs sold to hospitals is discounted. The costs of various formulations dosed at 200 mg oral morphine equivalents per day in an Australian hospital are shown in Table 16.1. Considering the differences in the exchange rate, the Australian prices are approximately one-third those of the AWP in the USA. It is also seen that, in the Australian hospital, oral methadone is approximately half the price of normal release morphine (but not the injection), modified release morphine is double the price of normal release and the injections are double again. The different formulations of morphine, oxycodone, hydromorphone and fentanyl are all similarly priced.

The actual importance of drug costs is controversial. A cost effectiveness study was carried out in the UK some 10 years ago to estimate the cost of managing

Table 16.1 Comparative cost to hospitals in Central Sydney, Australia, of 200 mg oral morphine/day, in Australian dollars, 2004 prices ($A1.00 approximately equal to $US 0.70)

Drug	Formulation	30-day cost*
Morphine hydrochloride	NR liquid, 5 mg/ml	$56
Morphine sulfate	MR tablet	$130.50
Morphine sulfate	Injection, 10 mg/ml	$231
Oxycodone	NR tablet	$81.50
Oxycodone	MR tablet	$2.82
Hydromorphone	NR liquid	$141
Hydromorphone	Injection, 2 mg/ml	$211
Fentanyl	Transdermal patch	$151
Fentanyl	Lozenge	$16.00 each
Methadone	NR tablet[†]	$25
Methadone	Injection	$288

* 200 mg oral morphine (or equivalents)/day.

† Methadone liquid supplied free to hospital.

NR, normal release; MR, modified release.

terminally-ill cancer patients after they switched from a weak to a strong opioid[47]. The expected cost ranged from £2391 sterling to £3701 at 1995/1996 prices, depending primarily on the patient's duration of survival. It was estimated that the drugs themselves accounted for only 2–8% of expected costs, and that factors other than economic issues, such as tolerability profile, patient preference and convenience of use, should form the basis of clinical decision-making between opioids with similar analgesic efficacy.

Opioid costs in developing countries have been reported to be higher than those in developed nations and would appear to be an important consideration. In one study, the median cost of opioids (calculated in US dollars) differed substantially between developed and developing countries ($53 and $112, respectively) and suggest that in developing countries opioid access for the majority of patients is likely to be limited by cost, and development of palliative care programs will require heavy or total subsidization of opioid costs[48]. The relative cost of opioids to income is also higher in developing countries. The median costs of all opioid preparations as a percentage of GNP *per capita* per month were 36% for developing and 3% for developed nations; the difference was statistically significant ($p < 0.001$). In developing countries, 23 of 45 (51%) of opioid dosage forms cost more than 30% of the monthly GNP *per capita*, versus only three of 76 (4%) in developed countries.

References

1 **Foley KM.** Acute and chronic pain syndromes. In: Doyle D, Hanks GW, Cherny N, *et al.* (Eds). *Oxford Textbook of Palliative Medicine*, 3rd edn. Oxford: Oxford University Press, 2004, pp. 298–9.

2 **World Health Organization.** *Cancer Pain Relief.* Geneva: WHO, 1986.

3 **Jacox A, Carr DB, Payne R** (Eds). *Management of Cancer Pain*, Clinical Practice Guideline No.9. Washington: US Dept Health and Human Services AHPCR Publication No. 94–0592, 1994.

4 **Hanks GW, Conno F, Cherny N,** *et al.* Morphine and alternative opioids in cancer pain: the EAPC recommendations. *Br J Cancer* 2001; **84:** 587–93.

5 **Scottish Intercollegiate Guideline Network (SIGN).** *Control of Pain in Patients with Cancer,* a National Clinical Guideline. SIGN, June 2000. Available at: www.sign.ac.uk.

6 **Benedetti C, Brock C, Cleeland C,** *et al.* NCCN Practice guidelines for cancer pain. *Oncology* 2000; **14:** 135–50.

7 **Mount BM, Melzack R, Mackinnon KJ.** The management of intractable pain in patients with advanced malignant disease. *Trans Am Ass Genito-Urin Surg* 1977; **69:** 84–91.

8 **Black P.** Management of cancer pain: an overview. *Neurosurgery* 1979; **5:** 507–18.

9 **Twycross RG.** Medical treatment of chronic cancer pain. *Bull Cancer* 1980; **67:** 209–16.

10 **Shimm DS, Logue GL, Maltbie AA,** *et al.* Medical management of chronic cancer pain. *J Am Med Ass* 1979; **241:** 2408–12.

11 **Foley KM.** Controversies in cancer pain. Medical perspectives. *Cancer* 1989; **63:** 2257–62.

12 **McQuay H.** Opioids in pain management. *Lancet* 1999; **353:** 2229–32.

13 **Cherny N.** New strategies in opioid therapy for cancer pain. *J Oncol Manag* 2000; **9:** 8–15.

14 **Glare P, Aggarwal G, Clark K.** Ongoing controversies in the pharmacological management of cancer pain. *Intern Med J* 2004; **34:** 45–9.

15 Fishman SM, Wilsey B, Mahajan G, *et al.* Methadone reincarnated: novel clinical applications with related concerns. *Pain Med* 2002; **3**: 339–48.

16 Weschules DJ, McMath JA, Gallagher R, *et al.* Methadone and the hospice patient: prescribing trends in the home-care setting. *Pain Med* 2003; **4**: 269–76.

17 Davis MP, Walsh D. Methadone for relief of cancer pain: a review of pharmacokinetics, pharmacodynamics, drug interactions and protocols of administration. *Support Care Cancer* 2001; **9**: 73–83.

18 Garrido MJ, Trocóniz IF. Methadone: a review of its pharmacokinetic/pharmacodynamic properties. *J Pharmacol Toxicol Meth* 1999; **42**: 61–6.

19 Bernard SA, Bruera E. Drug interactions in palliative care. *J Clin Oncol* 2000; **18**: 1780–99.

20 Mastronardi P, Cafiero T. Rational use of opioids. *Minerva Anesthesiolog* 2001; **67**: 332–7.

21 Twycross RG. Choice of strong analgesic in terminal cancer: diamorphine or morphine? *Pain* 1977; **3**: 93–104.

22 Baumrucker SJ. Clinical research on heroin in cancer pain control. *Am J Hospice Palliat Care* 2000; **17**: 8–9.

23 World Health Organization. *Cancer Pain Relief and Palliative Care*, Technical Report Series 804. Geneva: WHO, 1990.

24 Hanks G, Cherny NI, Fallon M. Opioid analgesic therapy. In: Doyle D, Hanks G, Cherny N, *et al.* (Eds) *Oxford Textbook of Palliative Medicine*, 3rd edn. Oxford: Oxford University Press, 2004, pp. 318–321.

25 McQuay H, Moore A. *An Evidence Based Resource for Pain Relief.* Oxford: Oxford University Press, 1999.

26 Eisenberg E, Berkey CS, Carr DB, *et al.* Efficacy and safety of NSAIDs for cancer pain: a meta-analysis. *J Clin Oncol* 1994; **12**: 2756–65.

27 Moore A, Collins S, Carrol D, *et al.* Paracetamol with and without codeine in acute pain: a quantitative systematic review. *Pain* 1997; **70**: 193–201.

28 De Conno F, Ripamonti C, Sbanotto A, *et al.* A clinical study of the use of codeine, oxycodone, dextropropoxyphene, buprenorphine and pentazocine in cancer pain. *J Pain Sympt Manag* 1991; **6**: 423–7.

29 Anon. Tramadol—a new analgesic. *Drug Ther Bull* 1994; **32**: 85–7.

30 Moore A, McQuay HJ. Single patient data meta-analysis of 3453 post-operative patients: oral tramadol versus placebo, codeine and combination analgesics. *Pain* 1997; **69**: 287–94.

31 Cleary JF. Cancer pain management. *Cancer Control* 2000; **7**: 120–31.

32 Walsh D. Pharmacological management of cancer pain. *Sem Oncol* 2000; **27**: 45–63.

33 Whiffen PJ, Edwards JE, Barden J, *et al.* Oral morphine for cancer pain (Cochrane review), *Cochrane Library*, 2003; 4.

34 Jadad AR, Browman GP. The WHO analgesic ladder for cancer pain management. *J Am Med Ass* 1995; **274**: 1870–3.

35 Ventafridda V, Tamburini M, Caraceni A, *et al.* A validation study of the WHO method for cancer pain relief. *Cancer* 1987; **59**: 850–6.

36 Walker VA, Hoskin PJ, Hanks GW, *et al.* Evaluation of WHO analgesic guidelines for cancer pain in a hospital-based palliative care unit. *J Pain Symptom Manage* 1988; **3**: 145–9.

37 Goisis A, Gorini M, Ratti R, *et al.* Application of a WHO protocol on medical therapy for oncologic pain in an internal medicine hospital. *Tumori* 1989; **75**: 470–2.

38 Ventafridda V, Caraceni A, Gamba A. Field-testing of the WHO guidelines for cancer pain relief. In: Foley KM, Bonica JJ, Ventafridda V, *et al.* (Eds) *Advances in Pain Research and Therapy*, Vol. 16. Baltimore: Raven Press, 1990, pp. 451–64.

39 **Takeda F.** Japan's WHO cancer pain relief program. In: Foley KM, Bonica JJ, Ventafridda V, *et al.* (Eds) *Advances in Pain Research and Therapy*, Vol. 16. Baltimore: Raven Press, 1990, pp. 475–83.

40 **Wenk R, Diaz C, Echeverria M, *et al.*** Argentina's WHO cancer pain relief: a patient care model. *J Pain Sympt Manag* 1991; **6:** 40–3.

41 **Siguan SS, Damole A, Megarito A.** Results of cancer pain treatment at Southern islands Medical center, Cebu, Philippines. *Philipp J Surg Spec* 1992; **47:** 173–6.

42 **Zech DF, Grond S, Lynch J, *et al.*** Validation of WHO guidelines for cancer pain relief: a 10-yr prospective study. *Pain* 1995; **63:** 65–76.

43 **Rischer JB, Cildress SB.** Cancer pain management: pilot implementation of the AHPCR guideline in Utah. *Jt Comm J Qual Improv* 1996; **22:** 683–700.

44 **Lickiss JN.** Approaching cancer pain relief. *Eur J Pain* 2001; **5(suppl):** 5–14.

45 **Du Pen SL, Du Pen AR, Polissar N, *et al.*** Implementing guidelines for cancer pain management: results of a randomized controlled clinical trial. *J Clin Oncol* 1999; **17:** 361–70.

46 **Abernethy AP, Samsa GP, Matchar DB.** A clinical decision and economic analysis model of cancer pain management. *Am J Managed Care* 2003; **9:** 651–64.

47 **Guest JF, Hart WM, Cookson RF.** Cost analysis of palliative care for terminally ill cancer patients in the UK after switching from weak to strong opioids. *Palliat Care Advis Comm Pharmacoeconom* 1998; **14:** 285–97.

48 **De Lima L, Sweeney C, Palmer JL, *et al.*** Potent analgesics are more expensive for patients in developing countries: a comparative study. *J Pain Palliat Care Pharmacother* 2004; **18:** 59–70.

Chapter 17

Opioid rotation

Janet R. Hardy

Introduction

Morphine is the opioid of choice for moderate to severe cancer pain[1] and can be used successfully to control pain in the majority of cancer patients. Although criticized for a lack of formal validation[2], there is a wealth of clinical experience in the use of morphine in the context of the WHO analgesic ladder and claims of efficacy above 80%[3].

Some patients, however, experience intolerable adverse effects before adequate analgesia is achieved or, more rarely, have no analgesic benefit at all. It has been estimated that 10–30% of all patients have a poor response and/or unacceptable toxicity when started on morphine[4]. This is often due to factors such as co-morbid medical disorders predisposing to toxicity, the pathophysiology of the pain and specific pharmacological effects of individual drugs. To reduce toxicity and improve pain control, one might consider the more aggressive treatment of side effects (e.g. parenteral antiemetics or psychostimulants for somnolence), the use of co-analgesics (e.g. anticonvulsants for neuropathic pain), intravenous hydration, anesthetic procedures (e.g. nerve blocks) and the use of non-pharmacological interventions (e.g. acupuncture and relaxation therapy). An alternative approach is to change or switch to an alternative opioid in an attempt to allow titration to adequate pain control, whilst limiting side effects. Although the most common reason for opioid rotation is opioid-related toxicity often associated with suboptimal pain control, other practical issues often apply, e.g. cost, drug volume (the relatively poor solubility of some drugs renders it difficult to give large doses by subcutaneous infusion), drug availability, convenience, familiarity and experience along with physician and patient preference. This practice is becoming increasingly common, and is generally known as 'opioid rotation'.

Terminology

The practice of changing from one opioid to another has been called opioid 'switching', 'rotation', or 'substitution'. These terms are generally used interchangeably, although some 'rotate' opioids in sequential therapeutic trials to identify the opioid that provides the best pain control, whereas others 'switch' or 'substitute' to alleviate side effects. This may not only involve a change of drug, but also a change in route of drug delivery, e.g. a rotation from oral morphine to rectal morphine or subcutaneous fentanyl.

Clinical experience

The reported use of opioid rotation varies widely, ranging in frequency from less than 10%[5,6] to 80% of patients[7]. One suspects the practice has become more frequent over recent years, and has been facilitated by the release of a number of new opioids and opioid formulations. This is likely to be influenced by drug availability in different centers, experience of individual practitioners and cost issues. The use of opioid rotation has been reported widely in the literature.

In some cases, the primary aim of the rotation has been to improve pain control[8–12]. In others, the primary indication has been to improve toxicity[6,13–23], or both pain control and toxicity[4,24–30]. Cherney and colleagues[4] have highlighted some of the other indications, e.g. patient convenience, convenience of route, wish for a reduction in invasiveness and cost.

Possible mechanisms

It has not been established how opioid rotation might work and there is little hard evidence that it does work. There is much anecdotal evidence, however, to support the practice and several theories to explain why it might work.

Toxicity

The primary metabolite of morphine, morphine-6-glucuronide (M6G), is an active compound, considerably more potent than the parent compound morphine. It accumulates in renal failure and is a common cause of opioid-related toxicity in patients who develop renal impairment[31]. The metabolites of other opioids, e.g. dextropropoxyphene and tramadol also accumulate in renal failure, and will contribute to toxicity in the absence of dose reduction. Other opioids, e.g. fentanyl and alfentanil, are metabolized in the liver to inactive products and are therefore safer to use in renal failure than morphine. Thus, in a patient with renal impairment, rotating from morphine to an opioid with pharmacodynamics not dependent on renal function should allow for the clearance of toxic metabolites, and at the same time, the maintenance or improvement in pain control. Renal impairment is very common in palliative care, often related to co-morbidity, disease progression, dehydration and/or the co-administration of other nephrotoxic drugs, e.g. NSAIDs. It is often unrecognized and it is often inappropriate to test for it. The benefit of an opioid rotation in this situation may simply reflect the use of drugs better tolerated in renal failure. This factor must always be taken into consideration in the design of any formal study assessing opioid rotation.

Glucuronidation is not affected by cirrhosis[32], therefore morphine metabolism should not be impaired in patients with liver metastases. The elimination half-life of other opioids, e.g. oxycodone, pentazocine and propoxyphene is significantly prolonged in end-stage liver disease. Although dose reduction or extended dose intervals would probably suffice to avoid toxicity in patients with end-stage liver disease, a rotation to morphine has theoretical logic.

Pain pathophysiology

The mechanism of pain may influence the pattern of response to different opioids. Neuropathic pain does not have the same pathophysiology as nociceptive pain. It appears relatively opioid insensitive, and is likely to be influenced by drugs that inhibit neuronal hyperexcitability and associated intracellular events such as the NMDA receptor antagonists[33]. In addition to being opioid receptor agonists, ketobemidone, methadone, dextropropoxyphene and pethidine are all weak non-competitive NMDA antagonists in animal models[34]. If these drugs have clinically significant NMDA antagonistic activity in man, they may be more likely to be effective in the control of pain with a prominent neuropathic component.

Genetic factors

It is becoming increasingly clear that there is considerable genetic variability between individuals, and their ability to metabolize and respond to drugs. Codeine is ineffective as an analgesic in about 10% of the Caucasian population due to genetic polymorphisms in the enzyme necessary to o-methylate codeine to morphine, the active metabolite. Other polymorphisms can lead to enhanced metabolism and thus increased sensitivity to codeine's effects[35]. Genetic variability in the expression or density of opioid receptors, receptor affinity or in secondary messenger activation, could explain the inter-individual variation seen in the response to morphine. Similarly, variability in the expression of enzymes responsible for the metabolism of different opioids could contribute to the differences seen in dose requirements and toxicity. In the future, pharmacogenetic mapping may allow us to predict in advance which opioid is best suited to a particular individual[36].

Drug interactions

The metabolism of many opioids is dependent on the cytochrome P450 system. Moreover, many drugs commonly used in palliative care are inducers, inhibitors or substrates for cytochrome P450 isoforms 3A4 and 2D6 (see Table 17.1). Therefore, co-medication with known P450 inhibitors or inducers will effect opioid metabolism, and thus dose requirements and toxicity. Any beneficial or deleterious outcome following rotation may reflect changing drug interactions[37].

Incomplete cross-tolerance

This is the mechanism of action most commonly quoted to explain the perceived benefits of opioid rotation[8,38,39]. Analgesic tolerance is defined as a reduction in potency of opioids after repeated administration, i.e. the need for higher doses over time to get the same analgesic effect, a shift of the dose response curve to the right. Tolerance to side effects is also seen with time, for example, the nausea and somnolence seen in about one-third of patients when started on morphine usually resolves after 2–3 days and does not always recur when the patient is changed to another opioid.

Table 17.1 Interaction between analgesics, inducers and inhibitors of the cytochrome P450 system

Cytochrome	Substrate	Inhibitor	Inducer
3A4	Alfentanil	Fluconazole	Carbamazepine
	Fentanyl	Ketoconazole	Phenytoin
		Itraconazole	Rifampicin
		Metronidazole	Erythromycin
		Norfloxacin	Omeprazole
		Fluoxetine	Cyclophosphamide
		Fluvoxamine	Dexamethasone
		Sertraline	Phenobarbitol
		Clarithromycin	St John's Wort
		Erythromycin	
		Cannabinoids	
2D6	Oxycodone	Paroxetine	Phenytoin
	Methadone	Cimetidine	Carbamazepine
	Morphine	Desipramine	Phenobarbitol
	Tramadol	Fluoxetine	
	Codeine	Haloperiodol	
		Sertraline	
		Celecoxib	

Incomplete cross-tolerance has been postulated as the mechanism, whereby a patient remains tolerant to the side effects, but not to the analgesic effect of an opioid when rotating from one opioid to another. It is dependent on the rate and magnitude of tolerance to side effects being different from the rate and magnitude of tolerance to pain. A patient would only benefit from a change of opioid if the cross-tolerance to the analgesic effect was less than the cross-tolerance to the adverse effects.

Although there are both animal and human studies showing less effect from the same dose of opioid after repeated dosing[33], there remains controversy as to how often tolerance occurs when using systemic opioids for the treatment of cancer pain and how it can be differentiated from increasing analgesic need in the face of progressive disease[40]. Similarly, it is not clear why tolerance develops to some side effects (e.g. nausea and somnolence), but not to others, e.g. constipation.

Postulated mechanisms for incomplete cross-tolerance include involve preferential binding to different receptor subtypes and/or the use of different secondary messenger systems by different opioids perhaps related to differences in their chemical structure and receptor binding properties[38].

Incomplete cross-tolerance is difficult to explain at the cellular level in that most of the clinically used opioids are relatively selective for mu receptors, reflecting their similarity to morphine. Moreover, activation of the mu receptor results in both the analgesic effects and many of the adverse effects (respiratory depression, reduced gut motility and sedation). Side effects related to opioid receptor activation will not be improved by changing to an equianalgesic dose of a different opioid that acts on the same receptors[33]. Some side effects can be attributed to activation of delta or kappa receptors (see Chapter 2), and it has been suggested from animal studies that some opioids have minor effects on receptors other than mu. Furthermore, drugs that are relatively selective at standard doses will interact with additional receptor types when given at sufficiently high dose[41]. Whether this is clinically relevant or not in man is unknown.

Differential activation of receptor subtypes has been put forward as a possible explanation for cross-tolerance[42]. Two subtypes of the mu receptor have been postulated: mu1, thought to mediate supraspinal analgesia, and mu2, which mediates analgesia at the spinal level. There is some evidence that the mu1 receptor has no role in respiratory depression[43] and that the mu2 receptor mediates the central effect of morphine on the GI tract[44]. In animal models, differences in time to developing tolerance to effects mediated by different mu subtypes have been demonstrated[45], but there is no evidence to date to suggest that different opioids acts preferentially with any one subtype in man.

Recent work has suggested the existence of receptor heterodimers—a high affinity mu/delta complex[46]. It has been proposed that some of the pharmacological diversity observed between different opioids might result from a modified specificity for opioid ligands due to heterodimerization of receptors.

Dose equivalence

There remains great uncertainty as to the exact dose equivalence of different opioids as illustrated in many case reports[13,25,27]. There is considerable variation between equianalgesic doses of opioids quoted in the literature[47] and wide ranges of published dose equivalence of some drugs, e.g. the morphine equivalence for transdermal fentanyl preparations. Similarly, standard dose conversions when changing from one opioid to another do not always apply when changing back as has been demonstrated with methadone[48], and with the lipophilic drugs such as fentanyl and sufentanil. It may be that, in many instances, opioid rotation is perceived as successful (at least with respect to a lessening of side effects) because the switch has resulted in an opioid dose reduction. Many health professionals will routinely recommend a dose reduction when rotating because of concerns regarding opioid toxicity[49]. This factor has to be considered in any formal study of the efficacy of opioid rotation.

Evidence

No large randomized controlled study has proven definitively the benefit of opioid rotation. There are several uncontrolled prospective studies, however, together with many retrospective studies and case reports giving a wealth of anecdotal evidence to suggest a benefit in selected patients, and highlighting the inter-individual variability in analgesic effect and propensity to side effects.

Rotation in general

The pain service within the Memorial Sloan-Kettering Cancer center in New York acquired data prospectively from 100 consecutive in-patients. Eighty of the 100 patients underwent 182 changes in drug, route or both before discharge or death. Twenty patients required 2 or more changes (range 2–6). These therapeutic changes were associated with improvement in physician-recorded pain intensity and a lower prevalence of cognitive impairment, hallucinations, nausea and vomiting, and myoclonus among patients who were discharged from hospital[7].

In an uncontrolled, prospective study, Lee and colleagues[28] documented the reasons for opioid rotation and the subsequent outcome. They describe 80 opioid changes in 70 cancer patients. The main reason for change was drowsiness, nausea and vomiting, uncontrolled pain, confusion and hallucinations. In 64% of cases, the rotation resulted in resolution of the main opioid-induced side effect. There was also improvement in 56% of those patients whose opioid was changed in order to improve pain control. A number of patients underwent dose reduction at the time of rotation.

In a similar study, Ashby et al.[20] completed a prospective audit of consecutive palliative care patients undergoing opioid substitution because of intolerable side effects. Prior to rotation, standard supportive measures were instituted as indicated, e.g. rehydration, neuroleptic drugs, sedatation, antiemetics. A trial of dose reduction was also attempted, but discontinued if the pain worsened. Pain and confusion were formally assessed pre- and postrotation. The substitution produced partial or complete relief from confusion in 18/25 cases, nausea in 13/19 and drowsiness in 8/15 patients.

In a retrospective study, Bruera[25] assessed the reason for change, the analgesic dose and pain intensity in patients rotating from morphine to hydromorphone, and hydromorphone to methadone, and calculated dose ratios following each conversion.

De Stoutz and colleagues[17] undertook a retrospective note review of 80 patients who underwent opioid rotation because of toxicity or persistent pain. The leading symptom was said to improve in 73% of patients and pain control to be improved at doses significantly lower than predicted to be equianalgesic.

Galer[42] presents detailed descriptions of variable responses to different opioid drugs within the context of sequential therapeutic trials in individual patients.

Rotation to specific drugs

Several uncontrolled studies point to beneficial effects following specific opioid switches. Methadone is used as the alternative opioid of first choice in many centers as discussed by Mancini and colleagues[50]. It is a logical choice in that it lacks active metabolites, is not dependent on renal function for clearance, has good oral availability and low cost[51], although others are more wary because of its long half-life and the uncertainty surrounding the best means of dose titration (see Chapter 12).

Pain control and adverse effects were assessed in a prospective study of 52 cancer patients with uncontrolled pain or intolerable side effects from morphine who were switched to methadone[51]. Pain intensity was assessed by a patient's self-reported 10-point visual analogue scale and opioid-related side effects by a 4-point verbal scale. Switching to methadone was considered effective if the pain decreased to 4 or less, and the intensity of other symptoms was reduced to a 'clinically acceptable' level. Switching was considered effective in 80% of the patients in an average of 3.65 days. Significant improvements were found in pain intensity, nausea and vomiting, constipation and drowsiness. In a subsequent study, the same group measured opioid plasma concentrations when switching from morphine to methadone[30].

Other case reports describe successful rotations from morphine/hydromorphone to methadone[9,10,21,24–27,52], fentanyl to methadone[22,29], multiple prior opioids to methadone[8,42] and were reviewed by Morley in 1998[54].

Unsuccessful rotations are less likely to be reported. Santiago-Palma and colleagues[29] have illustrated some of the potential pitfalls of opioid rotation in their description of problems encountered in 12 out of 13 patients when converting from methadone to some other opioid. A similar experience has been described by Lawler[52], who suggests the need for a highly individualized cautious approach when rotating from morphine to methadone.

Oxycodone has a more favorable pharmacokinetic profile than morphine with greater oral bioavailability, less variability in plasma concentration and metabolites that are not thought to contribute significantly to the pharmacological effects of the drug[55]. It would therefore seem to be a logical drug to use in the context of an opioid rotation (see Chapter 15). In a prospective uncontrolled study, Maddocks reported a significant improvement in side effects in patients changed from morphine to an oxycodone infusion[18]. Gagnon and colleagues have reported their experience in using intermittent subcutaneous injections of oxycodone in patients with prior opioid toxicity[56]. Delirium settled in about one-third of these patients. Surprisingly, few other case reports have been published[57].

Fentanyl is a popular choice of alternative opioid; it is better tolerated than morphine in renal failure and offers an alternative route of administration. In a study of 19 patients 'distressed as a result of morphine toxicity'[23], who were rotated to transdermal fentanyl (TTS), patients' global assessment of well-being was significantly improved over the 14-day study period. Pain control was maintained, and there were improvements in cognitive function and dizziness. Ellershaw and colleagues also report successful switches to TTS fentanyl[58]. Johnson reports a case of a patient demonstrating tolerance to high dose morphine who required a much smaller dose of fentanyl following rotation. This was attributed to an absence of cross-tolerance[59]. In a retrospective analysis of

11 patients rotated from subcutaneous, epidural or oral morphine to subcutaneous fentanyl or sufentanil, Paix and colleagues describe an improvement in morphine adverse events in all patients and 'adequate pain relief' in all but one[16].

In three cases, severe CNS side effects resolved without detrimental effect on pain control following a rotation from hydromorphone to a reduced dose of morphine[13]. Fainsingers group in Edmonton also reported their experience of morphine to hydromorphone and hydromorphone to morphine rotations to improve toxicity[6].

Change of route

Some believe that a change of route rather than a change of opioid *per se* is the most logical means of instigating an opioid rotation[33]. The issue is whether changing the route allows for a dose increase and effective analgesia without an increase in side effects. This may hold true for those drugs with active metabolites that undergo extensive first-pass metabolism when given orally. Kalso *et al.*[11] have published a small, double-blind cross-over studies in which patients were randomized to receive epidural and subcutaneous morphine. There was no difference in effectiveness or acceptability between arms and both treatments provided better pain relief with less adverse effects compared to the prestudy oral morphine treatment. Enting and colleagues[12] evaluated the efficacy of parenteral opioids (morphine, fentanyl and sufentanil) in 100 patients who had failed conventional opioids (codeine, tramadol, morphine, methadone and fentanyl TTS). The authors report an improved balance between analgesia and side effects in 71% of the patients. Furthermore, there was no difference between the patients who changed opioid and route and those who changed route alone.

The uncontrolled studies describing the benefit of rotating to transdermal fentanyl[23,58,59] and from morphine to subcutaneous oxycodone[18,56] have been described above.

Conclusion

Although randomized controlled trials have shown some minor differences in side effect profile between different opioids, there is no strong evidence to suggest that any one drug is superior to another[4]. In general, all opioids have similar adverse effects and equal analgesic efficacy when given in equianalgesic dosage. In an evidence-based report, an expert working group of the European Association of Palliative Care (EAPC)[4] found no reason to suggest that morphine should no longer be regarded as the opioid of first choice in cancer pain management. Despite this, there is a plethora of clinical experience suggesting that opioid rotation is of benefit and the EAPC have acknowledged this by including alternative opioids in their guidelines for the management of cancer pain[60]. It would appear that some patients tolerate some opioids better than others. This can be attributed to a multitude of reasons including age, co-morbidity, inter-individual variation in pharmacodynamics and pharmacogenetics as discussed above. There is unlikely to be a single explanation for the improved pain control and reduction in side effects so often seen following an opioid switch. Moreover, there is no controlled study to show that a rotation is better than an opioid dose reduction or rigorous treatment of side effects, and unsuccessful switches are less likely to be reported. In those centers fortunate enough to be able to use a range of different opioids and opioid formulations, however, it would seem worthwhile to undertake therapeutic substitutions of different drugs in an attempt to find the opioid "best suited" to the patient. This should not replace the symptomatic treatment of side effects, the optimal use of co-analgesics, or the use of anesthetic or non-pharmacological means of pain control, but is an added means of attempting to improve the quality of life of cancer patients.

References

1 Hanks GW, de Conno F, Ripamonti C, *et al.* Morphine in cancer pain: modes of administration. *Br Med J* 1996; **312:** 823–6.

2 Jadad A, Browman G. The WHO ladder for cancer pain management. *J Am Med Ass* 1995; **274(23):** 1870–3.

3 Zech D, Grond S, Lynch J, *et al.* Validation of WHO guidelines for cancer pain relief: a 10-year prospective study. *Pain* 1995; **63:** 65–76.

4 Cherny N, Ripamonti C, Pereira J, *et al.* Strategies to manage the adverse effects of oral morphine: an evidence-based report. *J Clin Oncol* 2001; **19(9):** 2542–54.

5 Hawley P, Forbes K, Hanks GW. Opioids, confusion and opioid rotation. *Palliat Med* 1998; **12:** 63–4.

6 Fainsinger R. Opioids, confusion and opioid rotation. *Palliat Med* 1998; **12:** 463–4.

7 Cherny NJ, Chang V, Frager G, *et al.* Opioid pharmacotherapy in the management of cancer pain. *Cancer* 1995; **76:** 1283–93.

8 Crews JC, Sweeney NJ, Denson DD. Clinical efficacy of methadone in patients refractory to other mu-opioid receptor agonist analgesics for management of terminal cancer pain. *Cancer* 1993; **72:** 2266–72.

9 Morley J, Watt J, Wells J, *et al.* Methadone in pain uncontrolled by morphine. *Lancet* 1993; **342:** 1243.

10 Leng G, Finnegan M. Successful use of methadone in nociceptive cancer pain unresponsive to morphine. *Palliat Med* 1994; **8:** 153–5.

11 Kalso E, Heiskanen T, Rantio M, *et al.* Epidural and subcutaneous morphine in the management of cancer pain: a double-blind cross-over study. *Pain* 1996; **67:** 443–9.

12 Enting R, Oldenmenger W, van der Rijt C, *et al.* A prospective study evaluating the response of patients with unrelieved cancer pain to parenteral opioids. *Cancer* 2002; **94:** 3049–56.

13 MacDonald N, Der L, Allan S, *et al.* Opioid hyperexcitability: the application of alternate opioid therapy. *Pain* 1993; **53:** 353–5.

14 Sjogren P, Jensen N, Jensen T. Disappearance of morphine-induced hyperalgesia after discontinuing or substituting morphine with other opioid agonists. *Pain* 1994; **59(2):** 313–16.

15 Bruera E, Franco JJ, Maltoni M, *et al.* Changing pattern of agitated impaired mental status in patients with advanced cancer: association with cognitive monitoring, hydration, and opioid rotation. *J Pain Sympt Manag* 1995; **10:** 287–91.

16 Paix A, Coleman A, Lees J, *et al.* Subcutaneous fentanyl and sufentanil infusion substitution for morphine intolerance in cancer pain management. *Pain* 1995; **63(2):** 263–9.

17 De Stoutz ND, Bruera E, Suarez-Almazor M. Opioid rotation for toxicity reduction in terminal cancer patients. *J Pain Sympt Manag* 1995; **10:** 378–84.

18 Maddocks I, Somogyi A, Abbott F, *et al.* Attenuation of morphine-induced delirium in palliative care by substitution with infusion of oxycodone. *J Pain Sympt Manag* 1996; **12:** 182–9.

19 Mercadante S. Opioid rotation for cancer pain. Rational and clinical aspects. *Cancer* 1999; **86:** 1856–66.

20 Ashby MA, Martin, Jackson KA. Opioid substitution to reduce adverse effects in cancer pain management. *Med J Am* 1999; **170:** 68–71.

21 Daeninck P, Bruera E. Reduction in constipation and laxative requirements following opioid rotation to methadone: a report of four cases. *J Pain Sympt Manag* 1999; **18(4):** 303–9.

22 Del Rosario M, Feria M. Reversible delirium during opioid switching from transdermal fentanyl to methadone. *J Pain Sympt Manag* 2001; **21:** 177–8.

23 McNamara P. Opioid switching from morphine to transdermal fentanyl for toxicity reduction in palliative care. *Palliat Med* 2002; **16(5):** 425–34.

24 Vigano A, Fan D, Bruera E. Individualised use of methadone and opioid rotation in the comprehensive management of cancer pain associated with poor prognostic factors. *Pain* 1996; **67(1):** 115–19.

25 Bruera E, Pereira J, Watanabe S, *et al.* Opioid rotation in patients with cancer pain. A retrospective comparison of dose ratios between methadone, hydromorphone and morphine. *Cancer* 1996; **78:** 852–7.

26 Fitzgibbon D, Ready L. Intravenous high-dose methadone administered by patient controlled analgesia and continuous infusion for the treatment of cancer pain refractory to high-dose morphine. *Pain* 1997; **73(2):** 259–61.

27 Manfredi PL, Borsook D, Chandler SW, *et al.* Intravenous methadone for cancer pain unrelieved by morphine and hydromorphone: clinical observations. *Pain* 1997; **70:** 99–101.

28 Lee B, Cole C, Gwilliam B, *et al.* A survey of the use of alternative strong opioids. *Palliat Med* 2000; **14(3):** 238–9.

29 Santiago-Palmer J, Khojainova N, Fischberg D, *et al.* Intravenous methadone in the management of chronic cancer pain: safe and effective starting doses when substituting methadone for fentanyl. *Cancer* 2001; **92(7):** 1919–25.

30 Mercadante S, Bianchi M, Villari P, *et al.* Opioid plasma concentration during switching from morphine to methadone: preliminary data. *Support Care Cancer* 2003; **11(5):** 326–31.

31 Osborne R, Joel S, Slevin M. Morphine intoxication in renal failure: the role of morphine-6-glucuronide. *Br Med J* 1986; **292:** 1548–9.

32 Patwardhan R, Johnson R, Hoyumpa A, *et al.* Normal metabolism of morphine in cirrhosis. *Gastroenterology* 1981; **81:** 1006–11.

33 McQuay H. Opioids in pain management. *Lancet* 1999; **353:** 2229–32.

34 Ebert B, Thorkilsden C, Andersen S, *et al.* Opioid analgesics as noncompetitive N-Methyl-D-aspartate (NMDA) antagonists. *Biochem Pharm* 1998; **56:** 553–9.

35 **Eichelbaum M, Evert B.** Influence of pharmacogenetics on drug disposition and response. *Clin Exp Pharmacol Physiol* 1996; **23**: 983–5.

36 **Roses A.** Pharmacogenetics and future drug development and delivery. *Lancet* 2000; **355**: 1358–61.

37 **Bernard S, Bruera E.** Drug interactions in palliative care. *J Clin Oncol* 2000; **18**: 1780–99.

38 **Fallon M.** Opioid rotation: does it have a role? *Palliat Med* 1997; **11**: 177–8.

39 **Mercadante S, Casuccio A, Calderone L.** Rapid switching from morphine to methadone in cancer patients with poor response to morphine. *J Clin Oncol* 1999; **17**: 3307–12.

40 **Zeppetella G, Bates C.** Scientific evidence and expert clinical opinion for the utility of opioid switching. In: Hillier R, Finlay I, Milea A (Eds) *The Effective Management of Cancer Pain*, 2nd edn, UK Key Advances in Clinical Practice Series. San Francisco: Aesculapius Medical Press, 2002.

41 **Gutstein H, Akil H.** Opioid analgesics. In: Hardman JG, Limbird LE (Eds) *Goodman and Gilman's the Pharmacological Basis of Therapeutics*, 10th edn. New York: McGraw Hill Publishers, 2001, pp. 569–619.

42 **Galer BS, Coyle N, Pasternak GW, et al.** Individual variability in the response to different opioids: report of five cases. *Pain* 1992; **49**: 87–91.

43 **Ling G, Speigel K, Lockhart S, et al.** Separation of opioid analgesia from respiratory depression: evidence for different opioid mechanisms. *J Pharmacol Exp Ther* 1985; **230**: 341–8.

44 **Heyman J, Williams C, Burks T, et al.** Dissociation of opioid antinociception and central gastrointestinal propulsion in the mouse. *J Pharmacol Exp Ther* 1988; **245**: 238–43.

45 **Ling G, Paul D, Simantov R, et al.** Differential development of acute tolerance to analgesia, respiratory depression, gastrointestinal transit and hormone release in a morphine infusion model. *Life Sci* 1989; **45(18)**: 1627–36.

46 **Gomes I, Jordan B, Gupta A, et al.** Heterodimerization of mu and delta opioid receptors: a role in opiate synergy. *J Neurosci* 2000; **20**: RC110(1–5).

47 **Anderson R, Saiers JH, Abram S, et al.** Accuracy in equianalgesic dosing: conversion dilemmas. *J Pain Sympt Manag* 2001; **21(5)**: 397–406.

48 **Moryl N, Santiago-Palmer J, Kornick C, et al.** Pitfalls of opioid rotation: substituting another opioid for methadone in patients with cancer pain. *Pain* 2002; **96(3)**: 325–8.

49 **Indelicato R, Portenoy R.** Opioid rotation in the management of refractory cancer pain. *J Clin Oncol* 2002; **20(1)**: 348–52.

50 **Mancini I, Lossignol D, Body J.** Opioid switch to oral methadone in cancer pain. *Curr Opin Oncol* 2000; **12(4)**: 308–13.

51 **Mercadante S, Casuccio A, Fulfaro F, et al.** Switching from morphine to methadone to improve analgesia and tolerability in cancer patients: a prospective study. *J Clin Oncol* 2001; **19(11)**: 2898–904.

52 **Lawlor P, Turner K, Hanson J, et al.** Dose ratio between morphine and methadone in patients with cancer pain: a retrospective study. *Cancer* 1998; **82(6)**: 1167–73.

53 **Morley J.** Opioid rotation: does it have a role? *Palliat Med* 1998; **12**: 464–5.

54 **Morley J, Makin M.** The use of methadone in cancer pain poorly responsive to other opioids. *Pain Rev* 1998; **5**: 51–8.

55 **Shah S, Hardy J.** Oxycodone: a review of the literature. *Eur J Pall Care* 2001; **8(3)**: 93–6.

56 **Gagnon B, Bielech M, Watanabe S, et al.** The use of intermittent subcutaneous injections of oxycodone for opioid rotation in patients with cancer pain. *Support Care Cancer* 1999; **7(4)**: 265–70.

57 **Mercadante S.** Oxycodone in a patient reporting toxicities with multiple trials of opioids. *Palliat Med* 1998; **12(6)**: 466–7.

58 **Ellershaw J, Smith J, O'Donnell V, *et al*.** Opioid substitution with transdermal fentanyl (abstract). *Palliat Med* 1998; **12:** 489.

59 **Johnson S.** The absence of 'cross-tolerance' when switching from oral morphine to transdermal fentanyl. *Palliat Med* 1997; **11(6):** 494–5.

60 **Hanks GW, de Conno F, Cherny N, *et al*.** Morphine and alternative opioids in cancer pain: the EAPC recommendations. *Br J Cancer* 2001; **84(5):** 587–93.

Chapter 18

Opioids equianalgesia: dynamics and kinetics

Mellar P. Davis

Introduction

In the past two decades knowledge about opioid pharmacology has dramatically increased, which has altered our understanding of opioid–receptor interactions. The development of genetic studies with antisense mapping and cloning have improved our understanding of opioid pharmacokinetics, receptor gene expression, gene polymorphisms and individual differences in opioid responses. Such differences are influenced by opioid metabolism and receptor genetics[1–4]. A better understanding of opioid pharmacology from published clinical experience apart from laboratory studies has improved prescribing guidelines. Opioid titration, rescue and around the clock dosing principles are founded on clinical experience, rather than the present day understanding of opioid receptor physiology. Such experience has established the relative lack of complete cross-tolerance between various potent opioids.

Most patients with cancer pain are effectively managed with low to moderate doses of opioids. Some require high doses or require a change in dosing strategy due to side effects and or lack of response. Several strategies have improved resistant cancer pain:

- opioid 'sparing' by the addition of adjuvant analgesics;
- opioid 'conversion' to an alternative route;
- opioid 'rotation' to a different opioid using equianalgesic dosing guidelines;
- treatment of dose limiting side effects particularly for those who are actively dying[5–9].

The success of opioid rotation is based upon the incomplete cross-tolerance between opioid analgesics implying a distinctly different pharmacodynamic and receptor interaction between opioids[2–4]. The practice of opioid rotation, however, depends upon the accuracy of equianalgesic tables and the accuracy of equianalgesic dosing is subject to individual genetic variability, which influence both opioid metabolism and response (Tables 18.1 and 18.2)[5,6,9]

Table 18.1 Factors which influence equianalgesia

Intrinsic	Extrinsic
Age	Interacting medication
Gender	Reasons for rotation
Pharmacogenetics	
UGT regulator gene	
CYP3A4 regulator gene	
MDR1 polymorphism	
MOR receptor polymorphism	Type of pain
Co-morbidities	
End organ function	
Enterohepatic circulation	
Opioid	
Intrinsic efficacy	
Tolerance	
Physiochemical characteristics	
Dose and routes of administration	
Order of opioid rotation	
Opioid half-life	
Method	
Pain Intensity	
Number of patients studied	
Acute or steady state dosing	
Population hetergeneity	

UGT–uridine glucuronyl tranferase

CYP–cyochrome

Pharmacogenetics

Genetic polymorphisms within a population (by definition occurring in greater than 1% of the normal population) can influence the individual patient's metabolism and response to various opioids (Table 18.3). Such genetic polymorphisms account for individual variations in opioid pharmacokinetics and dynamic[10]. The recent advancement in our understanding opioid receptor pharmacogenetics have provided a rational basis to incomplete cross-tolerance and sequential trials of opioids when morphine fails[11–16]. Drug development, predictions about drug interactions and individual responses will hopefully be better served by future pharmacogenetic studies using microarray techniques and opioid receptor profiling, which would preclude empiric drug trials[17–25].

Table 18.2 Unique features of opioid equivalents

Wide variability among studies
- morphine:oxycodone 2.5:1 to 1:1
- morphine:fentanyl 68.1:85.1

Linear changes with dose
- morphine:methadone 4:1 (<90 mg)
- morphine:methadone 8:1 (90–300 mg)

Gender differences with oxycodone

Time dependent changes in potency ratios

Bidirectional differences in equivalent ratios
- morphine→hydromorphone 5:1
- hydromorphone→morphine 3.5:1
- morphine→oxycodone 2:3
- oxycodone→morphine 3:4

Table 18.3 Pharmacogenetics and opioid kinetics

UGT2B7 promoter gene (morphine, hydromorphone)

CYP3A4 promoter gene (methadone, fentanyl)

CYP2D6 structural gene (codeine, tramadol)

CYP1A2 promoter (methadone)

UGT—uridine glucuronyl tranferase

CYP— cytochome

Pharmacokinetics

The pharmacogenetics of the hepatic cytochrome and conjugase systems influence drug metabolism and clearance, which in turn determines the duration of drug response and drug-drug interactions (Table 18.4)[26]. For instance, codeine, hydrocodone, oxycodone and tramadol are all metabolized through the cytochrome isoenzyme CYP2D6. However, the parent drugs, hydrocodone and oxycodone are active analgesics, whereas codeine and tramadol require O-demethylation before becoming mu opioid receptor (MOR) agonists.[26–28] CYP2D6 isoenzyme polymorphisms can be associated with poor drug metabolism particularly when both alleles are mutated.[29] Poor metabolizers produce little morphine from codeine and little O-demethyl-tramadol from tramadol resulting in poor pain relief among poor metabolizers[26,29]. Rotating from codeine or tramadol to a potent opioid like morphine in a poor metabolizer by using published equivalence can result in an over-estimation of the amount of potent opioid dose necessary for pain relief resulting in opioid toxicity. Certain ethnic groups have a high prevalence of slow metabolizing CYP2D6 isoenzymes. Asians have CYP2D6#10 and Africans have CYP2D6#17, which both slowly metabolize CYP2D6 dependent drugs.

Table 18.4 Medications and opioid interactions

Drug	Enzyme	Opioid
Rifampin	UGT$^+$, CYP3A4$^+$, CYP1A2$^+$	Morphine, methadone, fentanyl, hydromorphone
Selective serotonin reuptake Inhibitors	CYP2D6$^-$, CYP3A4$^-$	Codeine, Tramadol, Methadone, Fentanyl, oxycodone
Tricyclic antidepressants	CYP2D6$^-$, UGT$^+$	Methadone, morphine
Carbamazepine, phenytoin	CYP3A4$^+$	Methadone, fentanyl
Phenobarbital	CYP3A4$^+$, UGT$^+$	Morphine, methadone, fentanyl
Quinine/quinidine	CYP2D6$^-$	Codeine, tramadol, oxycodone
Imidazole	CYP3A4$^-$	Methadone, fentanyl
Phenothiazines	UGT$^-$, CYP2D6$^-$	Morphine, codeine, tramadol, oxycodone

−, Inhibitory; +, inducer.

Tramadol is reported to be a less effective in African and African American populations with the CYP2D6#17 allele[30,31].

The pregnane-X receptor initiates CYP3A4 transcription[32]. Thirty-eight single nucleotide polymorphisms are described with this promoter site. These polymorphisms determine both CYP3A4 basal level activity and inducibility[32,33]. Certain medications have the ability to induce CYP3A4 and influence opioid clearance dependent upon CYP3A4 transcription metabolism[34]. Both the basal rate and the inducibility of CYP3A4 determine fentanyl and methadone elimination, and duration of drug action[35,36]. CYP3A4 activity determines the equivalence of methadone and fentanyl as compared with other opioids.

Glucuronosyl transferase (UGT)

Glucuronosyl transferase is responsible for conjugating morphine and hydromorphone[37]. UGT2B7, which is the conjugase responsible for much of morphines metabolism is expressed in both the liver and the intestinal mucosa[37–40]. UGT expression in the gastrointestinal mucosa is subject to promoter site polymorphic variations, which are responsible for the 7-fold difference between the individual with morphine glucuronidation[40]. Tissue specific UGT expression and individual polymorphic regulatory genes within the small bowel influence prehepatic morphine metabolism and explains, in part, the large differences in morphine bioavailability among individuals[39–41]. UGT2B7 structural polymorphisms have been described, but at the present time, their clinical importance is unknown[40,42].

P-glycoprotein, *MDR-1* gene and opioid distribution

P-glycoprotein the product of the *MDR-1* gene, is found in blood brain capillaries, bile ducts, renal tubules and intestinal columnar epithelium. P-glycoprotein effluxes xeno-biotic toxins from cells as a protective mechanism. P-glycoprotein is also responsible for multi-drug resistance to chemotherapy and is an important determinant to the bioavailability and elimination of commonly used medications. MDR-1 poly-morphisms have been identified in humans and are clinically significant[43]. Morphine-6 glucuronide, a major active morphine metabolite, is subject to P-glycoprotein efflux from the central nervous system (CNS)[44]. The enhanced activity of P-glycoprotein or inhibitors, such as verapamil or vincristine, will influence the CNS levels of certain opioids[45,46]. Morphine, methadone and fentanyl analgesia improved in MDR-1 knock-out mice compared with normal controls[47]. MDR-1 knockout mice have a net CNS influx of morphine 2.3 times that of normal mice[47,48]. Blocking P-glycoprotein increases parenteral morphine analgesia in experimental animals, but diminishes spinal morphine analgesia, perhaps indicating that peripheral redistribution and peripheral opioid receptor binding is an important factor with spinal analgesia[49–51]. Up-regulation of MDR-1 by rifampin stimulates gastrointestinal and brain morphine efflux, reducing both serum and CNS morphine and morphine 6-glucuronide levels, thereby inducing opioid withdrawal[46,50,52]. The use of P-glycoprotein inhibitors or inducers could theoret-ically either enhance or diminish analgesia associated with P-glycoprotein-dependent opioids relative to non-P-glycoprotein-dependent opioids. Single nucleotide MDR-1 genetic polymorphisms are common in humans. Allelic frequencies of these polymor-phisms differ between populations, some of which have been associated with altered P-glycoprotein function[53–56]. While individual and population-related allelic MDR expressions differ, and could possibly influence the distribution of opioids in humans, the clinical significance of P-glycoprotein genetics is relatively unknown[57–63].

Opioid receptor genetics, G-proteins and homologous tolerance

There are differences in MOR expression and activation among individuals[2–4,64]. Overall reduction in MOR will reduce morphine responses. The end result of reduced receptor expression is a shift to the right in dose–response curves as seen in animal studies[65]. Morphine responses in some mice can persist despite a 90% inactivation of MOR by irreversible antagonists, while in others responses are attenuated with inactiva-tion of only a minority of receptors[65].

Qualitative changes in MOR activity influence opioid-binding affinity and receptor activation. For instance, CXB mice are insensitive to morphine, but respond normally to methadone as a result of changes in their opioid exons responsible for morphine binding and receptor activation[66]. MOR receptor subtypes, which are derived from four different exons, determine opioid interactions[3,4,67–70]. Receptor heterodimers between MOR, kappa opioid receptor (KOR) and delta opioid receptor (DOR) have been described, which will also influence opioid responses and opioid intrinsic efficacy[71,72]. Non-cross-tolerance between opioids reflects subtle differences in opioid receptor binding, which causes changes in receptor conformation, G-protein activation, and influence receptor desensitization, internalization and down-regulation[72–76].

Single nucleotide polymorphisms have been discovered within the human MOR. For instance, 20% of individuals have a single nucleotide polymorphism at position 118 (A118G)[77]. The A118G polymorphism reduces receptor-binding affinity for morphine-6-glucuronide[78]. Homozygotes for A118G tolerate high doses of morphine despite significant levels of morphine-6-glucuronide, which have been reported to cause opioid toxicity in some patients[79]. Reduced receptor binding in this instance was proposed to account for differences in opioid toxicities between individuals on morphine.

Receptor desensitization internalization and down regulation are also dependent upon receptor conformations induced by the opioid which is independent of the ability of the opioid G-proteins to activate[80]. Internalization of opioid receptors through endocytosis requires beta-2 arrestin and phosphorylation of the receptor C-terminus. Receptor desensitization occurs through phosphorylation of the intracellular loop-3 by G protein[81]. Both internalization and desensitization are governed by the activity of various kinases. Opioids with high intrinsic efficacy, promote receptor internalization (which are 'resensitized'), whereas partial agonists, such as morphine, cause desensitization without internalization[81]. Receptor internalization leads to receptor dephosphorylation and recovery of membrane bound receptor function or down-regulation with receptor destruction[81]. As a result, there can be a relative increase in analgesic potency with dose and pain intensity for high intrinsic efficacy opioids, which are capable of inducing internalization, as compared with low intrinsic efficacy opioids which cause receptor desensitization without receptor internalization[81,84,86,87]. Methadone and fentanyl have greater intrinsic efficacy than morphine, which accounts for the change in equianalgesia with morphine dose when rotating from morphine to methadone[88–91]. Equianalgesic guidelines at usual doses may therefore not be accurate when rotating from a low intrinsic efficacy opioid to high intrinsic efficacy opioid at high doses[92].

Loss of receptor function can occur as a result of changes in the G protein heterotrimeric complexes from inhibitory to excitatory. This adaptive response reduces opioid analgesia and increases opioid tolerance despite stable opioid doses and receptor density. Altered G-protein-receptor interactions influence analgesic responses with chronic dosing[67,82–85]. Opioid receptor genetics, receptor G-protein interactions and counter-adaptative responses will influence opioid equivalences. Opioid pharmacodynamics account for most of the individual differences in opioid responses. Predicting G-protein interactions with opioid receptors are highly variable, since there are potentially over 800 different G-protein heterotrimeric combinations possible[84].

Heterologous analgesic tolerance

Analgesic tolerance can be due to changes in drug metabolism, P-glycoprotein or an adaptive heterologous receptor response that is pronociceptive[93–102]. Opioids will induce phosphorylation of NMDA receptors, which results in receptor activation. Certain opioids, such as methadone and levorphanol, block the heterologous pronociceptive receptor responses involving NMDA receptor activation resulting in reduced analgesic tolerance. Adjuvant analgesics such as ketamine reduce pronociceptive NMDA responses and enhance opioid analgesia. NMDA receptor antagonists have synergistic interactions with MOR and DOR, but not with KOR[101]. Certain adjuvants may be 'more opioid sparing' with particular opioids and with in particular pain syndromes. This difference will influence equal effective dosing based upon the adjuvant. Some adjuvants will reduce or accelerate opioid kinetics, which worsens or improves opioid analgesia. An example of this, amitriptyline, which improves morphine analgesia and delays morphine clearance[103]. As a result, adjuvant analgesics will have a greater analgesic potential with certain opioids and certain types of pain, which will alter opioid equivalents.

Physical chemical properties and routes of administration

The physical chemical properties of opioids are not predictive of opioid receptor affinity or intrinsic efficacy, but do influence the drug's bioavailability and clearance[104]. Differences in oral bioavailability lead to differences in equivalents when there are changes in routes of administration. For instance, morphine has an oral bioavailability of 30–34% and oxycodone has a 60% oral bioavailability[104]. Oral equianalgesic doses are 1.5–1 (morphine to oxycodone), but when changed to parenteral, the ratio is 0.7:1[103].

Opioids with bi-exponential pharmacokinetics and large volumes of distribution will require a longer time to reach stable state, which leads to an apparent increase in potency with time relative to opioids with smaller volumes of distribution and a shorter half-life. Equivalents between short- and long-acting opioids will be different with acute dosing than at stable state[105]. Potency ratios of methadone compared with those of morphine by single dose studies are 1:1, but with multiple dose studies, equivalents can range from 1:4 and 1:20[106]. Methadone has both a larger volume of distribution and a longer half-life than morphine[104,107].

Spinal opioids are used for their presumed regional benefits to limit certain side effects. Opioid receptors on the dorsal horn and within the dorsal root ganglion are exposed to increased opioid concentrations with spinal opioids in the hopes of improving analgesia and limiting side effects. Systemic opioid exposure is theoretically limited and lower doses are required. Ideally, opioids limited to the spinal canal would avoid side effects. However, all spinal opioids do redistribute systemically. This is by absorption through spinal arteries, veins and into fat. Lipophilic opioids preferably bind to myelin and epidural fat. Redistribution will also be subject to P-glycoprotein efflux as previously mentioned. Intrathecal opioids have higher concentrations around dorsal root ganglion than around spinal cord gray matter based upon anatomical studies and may be the primary site of action[107,108]. Epidural and intrathecal opioids must reach the dorsal horn by transversing multiple barriers—epidural fat, collagen, arachnoid cells, membranes, intracellular orginales, cerebral spinal fluid, neuron cell bodies, extracellular fluid and the glycoprotein matrix[103,107,108]. Highly fat-soluble opioids will have limited diffusion into the hydrophilic dorsal horn and are preferentially sequestered onto epidural fat, and absorbed into spinal veins, artery and spinal cord myelin[103,108]. Redistribution of liphophilic opioids occurs rapidly, while hydrophilic opioids such as morphine gradually ascend in the CSF and are relatively confined to the CSF[103,109]. As a result, intrathecal analgesic potency will be inversely related to lipid solubility where the onset to action will directly depend on lipid solubility and rate distribution.[109] As lipid solubility decreases spinal opioid potency increases and accounts for 70% of the differences in analgesic potency when converting various opioids to spinal analgesia[109]. Therefore, because of rapid distribution, highly lipophilic opioids like fentanyl and methadone will have little advantage when given by spinal administration. Blood levels of both opioids will be the same as if given by parenteral administeration[110–112]. Morphine produces pain relief at doses that are 20-fold lower than anticipated compared with fentanyl based upon systemic equivalents[104].

Drug interactions

Drug interactions alter opioid kinetics or dynamics, and will influence equivalents. Drug interactions may be favorable as with adjuvant analgesics (Figs 18.1 and 18.2).[1] Analgesic tolerance to adjuvants does not usually develop as opposed to opioids. Adjuvants may either shift 'right' opioid dose toxicity curves or shift 'left' opioid dose responses. For instance, methylphenidate reduces opioid sedation whereas NSAIDs improve opioid analgesia. While adjuvants improve opioid responses, opioid kinetics may be altered by inhibiting or accelerating opioid metabolism. For instance, methadone clearance is accelerated by carbamazepine[104,113] Medications with opioid drug interactions may change drug absorption, metabolism, or alter elimination to a different extent for each opioid and indirectly change opioid equivalence. Examples of particular pharmacokinetic interactions are:

- absorption (kaolin with morphine);
- distribution (rifampin and morphine)[114,115].

The cytochrome P-450 enzyme system, which is responsible for most serious kinetic drug interactions either enhances or diminishes opioid analgesia or toxicity through enzyme inhibition or induction[116]. Most opioid drug interactions involve cytochrome CYP3A4, CYP2D6, CYP1A2, CYP2C9 and CYP2C19. A few involve the conjugases UGT2B7 and UGT1A2[114–118]. Opioid interactions occur from induction of CYP3A, CYP1A and UGT2B7 activity or inhibition of CYP3A4, CYP2D6 or

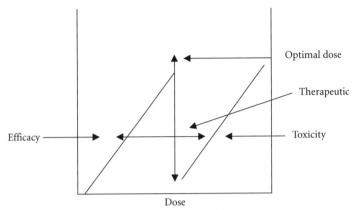

Fig. 18.1 Drug response (efficacy) has a linear relationship between the log dose at 20% and 80% response (EC20 and EC80). The onset to toxicity can be grafted in the same relationship. The area between efficacy and toxicity is the therapeutic 'window'. The therapeutic index can be determined by the equation EC50 toxicity/EC50 efficacy, where EC50 is the dose at 50% efficacy or toxicity. The higher the number the greater the therapeutic index.

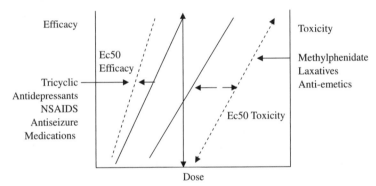

Fig. 18.2 Adjuvant analgesic either shift-left opioid close response or shift-right opioid toxicity resulting in improved opioid therapeutic index (EC50 toxicity)/(EC50 efficacy).

UGT2B7 enzyme activity. Such interactions depend upon the affinity of the competing drug for the isoenzyme and drug concentration relative to the opioid for the same enzyme. Inhibition can be competitive or non-competitive requiring enzyme regeneration for resolution and recovery of normal drug metabolism. Some opioids are metabolized by several cytochrome isoenzymes, as is methadone, which increases the risk for drug–drug interactions[113]. Drug interactions will phenocopy the genetic prototype of rapid or poor metabolizers. Paradoxically, genetically poor 'metabolizers' have fewer drug interactions. Interactions are unique to the particular opioid and rotating 'into' or 'out' of a drug interaction will change equivalences relative to non-interacting opioids.

Organ failure

Organ failure variably influences the clearance of opioids. The degree to which elimination is influenced depends upon the particular opioid used. Morphine clearance is relatively insensitive to liver dysfunction, but quite sensitive to renal function since morphine-6-glucuronide accumulates quickly in renal failure[104]. Methadone is relatively insensitive to renal and hepatic failure. The delayed clearance of morphine and morphine-6-glucuronide in both renal failure will alter morphine to methadone ratios, since patients will fail to clear morphine and even more morphine-6-glucuronide.

Liver failure

Opioid clearance is dependent upon hepatic blood flow, hepatic enzyme reserve, first pass clearance, the activity of extrahepatic cytochromes and conjugases, and plasma protein binding (albumin and alpha-1 acid glycoprotein), as well as type of opioid[114,119]. The isoenzyme CYP3A4 and UGT are found extensively in extrahepatic tissues, but CYP2D6 is found in small amounts within the intestinal wall and brain[37,120]. Hepatic shunting due to portal hypertension increases the oral bioavailability of highly liver extracted opioids such as morphine such that oral bioavailability increases with portal hypertension[119]. Total enzyme reserve determines opioid clearance with opioids that have low hepatic extraction such as oxycodone[119]. CYP2D6 metabolizes oxycodone and has less of a reserve with hepatic failure compared with CYP3A4 and UGT2B7. As a result, oxycodone's half-life increases 4-fold with liver failure, while morphine clearances are relatively normal[120-123]. Reduced albumin protein binding increases at the enzyme site, but also increases opioid volume of distribution without increasing serum levels as occurs with fentanyl[119]. The balance between increased cytochrome metabolism due to the availability of unbound drug and the volume of distribution that extends the drug half-life preserves opioid clearance in hepatic failure as occurs with fentanyl.

Kidney failure

Kidney disease increases tubule P-glycoprotein in the kidney, but decreases brain P-glycoprotein[124]. The result is an increase in opioid tubular secretion of morphine and morphine-6-glucuronide, which partially compensates for decreased elimination through diminished glomerular filtration rate (GFR). The central nervous system morphine and morphine-6-glucuronide may increase due to reduced efflux[124,125]. Therefore, a complex relationship evolves with renal failure between morphine dynamics and kinetics, which may not be adequately reflected by serum concentrations and may not correlate with diminishing GFR. Hemofiltration and hemodialysis will normalize the clearance of morphine-6-glucuronide and morphine, whereas peritoneal dialysis does not. As a result, the dose–response curves of morphine are altered in renal failure and the correction of this will be dependent upon the type of renal replacement therapy used[126–129]. Renal failure slightly influences the kinetics of fentanyl and methadone[125]. As a result morphine equivalence will change with renal failure and will be additionally determined by the type of renal replacement therapy.

Clinical relevance

Opioid equivalences are usually derived from population studies, but are applied to individuals with cancer experiencing different degrees of pain intensity who may or may not be opioid naïve, and who are usually on multiple medications that potentially interact with opioids. Opioid rotation involves sequentially administered opioids where population studies usually involve parallel designs with simultaneous opioid dosing. Clinical differences between the study population and the single patient in whom opioid equivalences are applied leads to risks of inaccurately determined equianalgesic doses. Cancer patients frequently have hepatic or renal dysfunction related to disease, or have co-morbidities that influence opioid metabolism. The individual cancer patient may have little in common with the population from whom opioid equivalence was determined.

Individual genetics govern opioid kinetics and dynamics, which accounts for the individual variability in equivalents. Population polymorphisms will influence opioid metabolism and receptor function and unpredictably alters opioid equivalents for the single individual.

Summary

Clinical decisions involve more than simply taking published results and directly applying them at the bedside. Physicians need to consider the similarities of their patients to the study population from whom equivalents were derived. Current equianalgesic tables are clinically useful. Tables provide a rough guideline, but cannot be used in a rote fashion without taking patient characteristics into account. It is important to consider intrinsic and extrinsic factors with dosing schedules and selections for rotating opioids. Recommended dose reductions with rotation of 1/10th for methadone to 2/3rds for other opioids are based upon clinical experience and incomplete analgesic cross-tolerance[1]. The elderly, and those with severe renal and hepatic failure should have doses reduced by at least 50% or more when rotating opioids[130]. Equianalgesic dosing should be based upon steady state dosing tables to be useful for chronic pain. Equivalences change with doses when rotating from low to high intrinsic efficacy opioids. Polypharmacy changes equivalence and dose ratios depending upon the opioid. A good understanding of opioid pharmacology is essential for safe and effective opioid rotation.

References

1 Intrussi C. Clinical pharmacology of opioids for pain. *Clin J Pain* 2002; **18:** S3–13.

2 Synder SH, Pasternak GW. Historical review: opioids receptors. *Trends Pharmacol Sci* 2003; **24(4):** 198–205.

3 Pasternak GW, Standifer KM. Mapping of opioid receptors using antisense oligodeoxynuclieotides: correlating their molecular biology and pharmacology. *Trends Pharmacol Sci* 1995; **16:** 344.

4 Pasternak GW. Incomplete cross tolerance and multiple mu opioid peptide receptors. *Trends Pharmacol Sci* 2001; **22(2):** 67.

5 Anderson R, Saiers J, Abram S, *et al.* Accuracy in Equianalgesic Dosing: Conversion Dilemmas. *J Pain Sympt Manag* 2001; **21:** 397–406.

6 Pereira J, Lawlor P, Vigano A, *et al.* Equianalgesic dose ratios for opioids: a critical review and proposals for long-term dosing. *J Pain Sympt Manag* 2001; **22:** 672–86.

7 Inturrisi CE. Clinical pharmacology of opioids for pain. *Clin J Pain* 2002; **18:** S3–13.

8 Mercandante S, Portenoy RK. Opioid poorly-responsive cancer pain Part 3. Clinical strategies to improve opioid responsiveness. *J Pain Sympt Manag* 2001; **21(4):** 338–54.

9 Mercandante S. Opioid rotation for cancer pain. Rationale and aspects. *Cancer* 1999; **86:** 1856–66.

10 Pasternak GW. Insights into mu opioid pharmacology the role of mu opioid receptor subtypes. *Life Sci* 2001; **68:** 2213–19.

11 Flores CM, Mogil JS. The pharmacogenetics of analgesia: toward a genetically-based approach to pain management. *Pharmacogenomics* 2001; **2(3):** 177–94.

12 Breivik H. Opioids in cancer and chronic non-cancer pain therapy-indications and controversies. *Acta Anaesthesiol Scand* 2001; **45(9):**1059–66.

13 Bloan EA, Tallarida RJ, Pasternak GW. Synergy between m opioid ligands: evidence for functional interactions among m opioid receptor subtypes. *J Pharm Exp Therapeut* 2002; **303(2):** 557–62.

14 Pan XY, Xu J, Mahurter L, *et al.* Generation of the mu opioid receptor (MOR-1) protein by three new splice variants of the Oprm gene. *Proc Natl Acad Sci USA* 2001; **98(24):** 14084–9.

15 Rossi GC, Leventhal L, Pan YX, *et al.* Antisense mapping of MOR-1 in rats: distinguishing between morphine and morphine-6b-glucoronide antinociception. *J Pharm Exp Therapeut* 1997; **281:** 109–14.

16 Rossi GC, Brown GP, Leventhal L, *et al.* Novel receptor mechanisms for heroin and morphine-6b-glucuronide analgesia. *Neurosci Lett* 1996; **216:** 1–4.

17 Chicurel ME, Dalma-Weiszhausz DD. Microarrays in pharmacogenomics—advances and future promise. *Pharmacogenomics* 2002; **3(5):** 589–601.

18 Ferentz AE. Integrating pharmacogenomics into drug development. *Pharmacogenomics* 2002; **3(4):** 453–67.

19 Lindpainter K. The impact of pharmacogenetics and pharmacogenomics on drug discovery. *Nature Rev Drug Discov* 2002; **1(6):** 463–9.

20 Shi J, Chen S. Pharmacogenomics genomics approaches to optimizing drug therapy. *Chung-Hua i Hsueh i Chuan Hseuh Tsa Chih* 2002; **19(2):** 156–8.

21 Ozawa S. Drug–drug interaction in pharmacogenetics and pharmacogenomics. *Rinsho Byori—Japan J Clin Pathol* 2002; **50(2):** 146–50.

22 McLeod H. Genetic Strategies to Individualize Supportive Care. *J Clin Oncol* 2002; **20(12):** 2765–7.

23 Evans WE, Johnson JA. Pharmacogenomics: the inherited basis for interindividual differences in drug response. *Ann Rev Genom Hum Genet* 2001; **2:** 9–39.

24 Lichtermann D, Franke P, Maier W, *et al*. Pharmacogenomics and addiction to opiates. *Eur J Pharmacol* 2000; **410(2–3):** 269–79

25 Phillips K, Veensstra D, Oren E, *et al*. Potential role of pharmacogenomics in reducing adverse drug reactions: a systematic review. *J Am Med Ass* 2001; **286(18):** 2270–9.

26 Daly AK. Pharmacogenetics of the major polymorphic metabolizing enzymes. *Fund Clin Pharmacol* 2003; **17(1):** 27–41.

27 Mikus G, Somogyi AA, Bochner F, *et al*. Polymorphic metabolism of opioid narcotic drugs: possible clinical implications. *Annl Acad Med, Sing* 1991; **20(1):** 9–12.

28 Caraco Y, Sheller J, Wood A. Pharmacogenetic determination of the effects of the codeine and prediction of drug interactions. *J Pharm Exp Therapeut* 1996; **278(3):** 1165–74.

29 Fagerlund TH, Braaten O. No pain relief from codeine . . . ? An introduction to pharmacogenomics. *Acta Anaesthesiol Scand* 2001; **45(2):** 140–9.

30 Ogunleye DS. Investigation of racial variations in the metabolism of tramadol. *Eur J Drug Metab Pharmackinet* 2001; **26(1–2):** 95–8.

31 Bradford LD, Gaedigk A, Leeder JS. High frequency of CYP2D6 poor and 'intermediate' metabolizers in black populations: a review and preliminary data. 1998; **34(3):** 797–84.

32 Zhang J, Kuehl P, Green ED, *et al*. The human pregnane X receptor: genomic structure and identification and functional characterization of natural allelic variants. *Pharmacogenetics* 2001; **11(7):** 555–72.

33 Luo G, Cunningham M, Kim S, *et al*. CYP3A4 Induction by drugs: correlation between a pregnane X receptor reporter gene assay and CYP3A4 expression in human hepatocytes. *Drug Metab Dispos* 2002; **30(7):** 795–804.

34 Raucy J, Warfe L, Yueh MF, *et al*. A cell-based reporter gene assay for determining induction of CYP3A4 in a high-volume system. *J Pharmacol Exp Therapeut* 2002; **303:** 412–23.

35 Feierman DE, Lasker JM. Metabolism of fentanyl, a synthetic opioid analgesic, by human liver microsomes. Role of CYP3A4. *Drug Metab Dispos* 1996; **24(9):** 932–9.

36 Raucy J, Warfe L, Yeuh MF, *et al*. A cell-based reporter gene assay for determining induction of CYP3A4 in a high-volume system. *J Pharm Exp Therapeut* 2002; **303:** 412–23.

37 Tukey RH, Strassburg CP. Human UDP-glucuronosyltransferases: metabolism, expression, and disease. *Ann Rev Pharmacol Toxicol* 2000; **40:** 581–616.

38 Tukey RH, Strassburg CP. Genetic multiplicity of the human UDP-glucuronosyltransferases and regulation in the gastrointestinal tract. *Mol Pharmacol* 2001; **59(3):** 405–14.

39 Strassburg CP, Strassburg A, Nguyen N, *et al*. Regulation and function of family 1 and family 2 UDP-glucuronosyltransferase genes (UGT1A, UGT2B) in human esophagus. *Biochem J* 1999; **338(2):** 489–98.

40 Strassburg CP, Kneip S, Topp J, *et al*. Polymorphic gene regulation and interindividual variation of UDP-glucuronosyltransferase activity in human small intestine. *J Biol Chem* 2000; **275(46):** 36164–71.

41 Strassburg CP, Strassburg A, Kneip S, *et al*. Developmental aspects of human hepatic drug glucuronidation in young children and adults. *Gut* 2002; **50(2):** 259–65.

42 Bhasker R, McKinnon W, Stone A, *et al*. Genetic polymorphism of UDP-gluconosyltransferase 2B7 (UGT2B7) at amino acid 268: ethnic diversity of alleles and potential clinical significance. *Pharmacogenetics* 2000; **10(8):** 679–85.

43 Cascorbi I, Gerloff T, Johne A, *et al*. Frequency of single nucleotide polymorphisms in the P-glycoprotein drug transporter MDR1 gene in white subjects. *Clin Pharmacol Therapeut* 2001; **69(3):** 169–74.

44 Huwyler J, Drewe J, Klusemann C, *et al*. Evidence for P-glycoprotein-modulated penetration of morphine-6-glucuronide into brain capillary endothelium. *Br J Pharmacol* 1996; **118(8):** 1879–85.

45 Huwyler J, Drewe J, Gutman H, et al. Modulation of morphine-6-glucuronide penetration into the brain by P-glycoprotein. *Int J Clin Pharmacol Therapeut* 1998; **36(2)**: 69–70.

46 Gutmann H, Torok M, Fricker G, et al. Modulation of multidrug resistance protein expression in porcine brain capillary endothelial cells *in vitro*. *Drug Metab Dispos* 1999; **27(8)**: 937–41.

47 Lotsch J, Tegeder I, Angst MS, et al. Antinociceptive effects of morphine-6-glucuronide in homozygous MDR1a P-glycoprotein knockout and in wildtype mice in the hotplate test. *Life Sci* 2000; **66(24)**: 2393–403.

48 Thompson SJ, Koszdin K, Bernards CM. Opiate-induced analgesia is increased and prolongs in mice lacking P-glycoprotein. *Anesthesiology* 2000; **92(5)**: 1392–9.

49 Xie R, Hammarlund-Udenaes M, de Boer AG, et al. The role of P-glycoprotein in blood-brain barrier transport of morphine: transcortical microdialysis studies in mdr1a ($-/-$) and mdr1a ($+/+$) mice. *Br J Pharmacol* 1999; **128(3)**: 563–8.

50 Zong J, Pollack GM. Morphine antinociception is enhanced in mdr1a gene-deficient mice. *Pharm Res* 2000; **17(6)**: 749–53.

51 King M, Su W, Chang A, et al. Transport of opioids from the brain to the periphery by P-glycoprotein: peripheral actions of central drugs. *Nat Neurosci* 2001; **4(3)**: 268–74.

52 Drewe J, Ball H, Beglinger C, et al. Effect of P-glycoprotein modulation on the clinical pharmacokinetics and adverse effects of morphine. *Br J Clin Pharmacol* 2000; **50(3)**: 237–46.

53 Schinkel AH, Wagenaar E, van Deemter L, et al. Absence of the mdr1a P-Glycoprotein in mice affects tissue distribution and pharmacokinetics of dexamethasone, digoxin, and cyclosporin A. *J Clin Invest* 1995; **96(4)**: 1698–705.

54 Kim RB, Leake BF, Choo EF, et al. Identification of funtionally variant MDR1 alleles among European Americans and African Americans. *Clin Pharmacol Therapeut* 2001; **70(2)**: 189–99.

55 Kerb R, Hoffmeyer S, Brinkmann U. ABC drug transporters: hereditary polymorphisms and pharmacological impact in MDR1, MRP1 and MRP2. *Pharmacogenomics* 2001; **2(1)**:51–64.

56 Hoffmeyer S, Burk O, von Richter O, et al. Functional polymorphisms of the human multi-drug-resistance gene: multiple sequence variations and correlation of one allele with P-glycoprotein expression and activity *in vivo*. *Proc Nat Acad Sci USA* 2000; **97(7)**: 3473–8.

57 Matheny C, Lamb M, Brouwer K, et al. Pharmacokinetic and Pharmacodynamic Implications of P-glycoprotein Modulation. *Pharmacotherapy* 2001; **21(7)**: 778–96.

58 Fromm MF, Eckhardt K, Li S, et al. Loss of analgesic effect of morphine due to coadministration of rifampin. *Pain* 1997; **72(1–2)**: 261–7.

59 Fromm MF. The influence of MDR1 polymorphisms on P-glycoprotein expression and function in humans. *Adv Drug Deliv Rev* 2002; **45(10)**: 1295–310.

60 Kim RB, Wandel C, Leake B, et al. Interrelationship between substrates and inhibitors of human CYP3A and P-glycoprotein. *Pharmaceut Res* 1999; **16(3)**: 408–14.

61 Fromm MF. P-glycoprotein: a defense mechanism limiting oral bioavailability and CNS accumulation of drugs. *Int J Clin Pharmacol Therapeut* 2000; **38(2)**: 69–74.

62 Fromm MF. The influence of MDR1 polymorphisms on P-glycoprotein expression and function in humans. *Adv Drug Deliv Rev* 2002; **54(10)**: 1295–310.

63 Fromm MF, Kaufmann HM, Burk O, et al. The effect of rifampin treatment on intestinal expression of human MRP transporters. *Am J Pathol* 2000; **157(5)**: 1575–80.

64 Uhl GR, Sora I, Wang Z. The mu opiate receptor as a candidate gene for pain: polymorphisms, variations in expression, nociception, and opiate responses. *Proc Nat Acad Sci USA* 1999; **96(14)**: 7752–5.

65 Sora I, Elmer G, Funada M, et al. Mu opiate receptor gene dose effects on different morphine actions: evidence for differential *in vivo* mu receptor reserve. *Neuropsychopharmacology* 2001; **25**: 41–54.

66 Chang A, Emmel DW, Rossi GC, *et al.* Methadone analgesia in morphine-insensitive CXBK mice. *Eur J Pharmacol* 1998; **351(2):** 189–91.

67 Pasternak G. Incomplete cross tolerance and multiple mu opioid peptide receptors. *Trends Pharmacol Sci* 2001; **22(2):** 67–70.

68 Pan YX, Xu J, Bolan E, *et al.* Identification and characterization of three new alternatively spliced mu-opioid receptor isoforms. *Mol Pharmacol* 1999; **56(2):** 396–403.

69 Pan YX, Xu J, Bolan E, *et al.* Isolation and expression of a novel alternatively spliced mu opioid receptor isoform, MOR-1F. *FEBS Lett* 2000; **466(2–3):** 337–40.

70 Pan YX, Xu J, Mahurter L, *et al.* Generation of the mu opioid receptor (MOR-1) protein by three new splice variants of the Oprm gene. *Proc Nat Acad Sci USA* 2001; **98(24):** 14084–9.

71 Narita M, Khoitb J, Suzuki M, *et al.* Heterologous m-opioid receptor adaptation by repeated stimulation of k-opioid receptor: up-regulation of G-protein activation and antinociception. *J Neurochem* 2003; **85:** 1171–9.

72 Law PY, Wong YH, Loh HH. Molecular mechanisms and regulation of opioid receptors. *Ann Rev Pharmacol Toxicol* 2000; **40:** 389–430.

73 Pasternak, G. Insights into mu opioid pharmacology: the role of mu opioid receptor subtypes. *Life Sci* 2001; **68:** 2213–19.

74 Schuller AG, King MA, Zhang J, *et al.* Retention of heroin and morphine-6 beta-glucuronide analgesia in a new line of mice lacking exon 1 of MOR-1. *Nat Neurosci* 1999; **2(2):** 151–6.

75 Rossi GC, Leventhal L, Pan YX, *et al.* Antisense mapping of MOR-1 in rats: distinguishing between morphine and morphine-6-beta-glucuronide antinociception. *J Pharmacol Exp Therapeut* 1991; **281:** 109–14.

76 Bolan E, Tallrida R, Pasternak G. Synergy between opioid ligands: evidence for functional interactions among opioid receptor subtypes. *J Pharmacol Exp Therapeut* 2002; **303(2):** 557–62.

77 Grosch S, Niederberger E, Lotsch J, *et al.* A rapid screening method for a single nucleotide polymorphism (SNP) in the human MOR gene. *Br J Clin Pharmacol* 2001; **52(6):** 711–14.

78 Lotsch J, Skarke C, Grosch S, *et al.* The polymorphism A118G of the human mu-opioid receptor gene decreases the pupil constrictory effect of morphine-6-glucuronide but not that of morphine. *Pharmacogenetics* 2002; **12:** 3–9.

79 Lotsch J, Zimmermann M, Darimont J, *et al.* Does the A118G Polymorphism at the [mu]-opioid Receptor Gene Protect against Morphine-6-Glucuronide Toxicity? *J Am Soc Anesthesiologists* 2002; **97(4):** 814–19.

80 Befort K, Filliol D, Decaillot FM, *et al.* A single nucleotide polymorphic mutation in the human [micro]-opioid receptor severely impairs receptor signaling. *J Biol Chem* 2001; **276(5):** 3130–7.

81 Von Zastrow M, Svingos A, Haberstock-Debic H, *et al.* Regulated endocytosis of opioid receptors: cellular mechanisms and proposed roles in physiological adaptation to opiate drugs. *Curr Opin Neurobiol* 2003; **13:** 348–53.

82 Borgland SL, Connor M, Osborne P, *et al.* Opioid agonists have different efficacy profiles for G protein activation, rapid desensitization, and endocytosis of mu-opioid receptors. *J Biol Chem* 2003; **278(21):** 18776–84.

83 Traynor JR, Clark MJ, Remmers AE. Relationship between rate and extent of G protein activation: comparison between full and partial opioid agonists. *Pharmacol Exp Therapeut* 2002; **300(1):** 157–61.

84 Law PY, Loh HH. Regulation of opioid receptor activities. *J Pharmacol Exp Therapeut* 1999; **289(3):** 607.

85 Standifer KM, Pasternak GW. G proteins and opioid receptor-mediated signalling. *Cell Signal* 1997; **9(3/4):** 237–48.

86 Taylor DA, Fleming WW. Unifying perspectives of the mechanisms underlying to development of tolerance and physical dependence to opioids. *J Pharmacol Exp Therapeut* 2001; **297(1):** 11–18.

87 Liu JG, Prather PL. Chronic exposure to m-opioid agonists produces constitutive activation of m-opioid receptors in direct proportion to the efficacy of the agonist used for pretreatment. *Mol Pharmacol* 2001; **60(1):** 53–62.

88 Kissin I, Brown P, Bradley Jr E. Magnitude of acute tolerance to opioids is not related to their potency. *Anesthesiology* 1991; **75:** 813–16.

89 Paktor J, Vaught JL. Differential analgesic cross-tolerance to morphine between lipophilic and hydrophilic narcotic agonists. *Life Sci* 1984; **34:** 13–21.

90 Paronis CA, Holtzman SG. Development of tolerance to the analgesic activity of mu agonists after continuous infusion of morphine, meperidine or fentanyl in rats. *J Pharmacol Exp Therapeut* 1992; **262:** 1–9.

91 Ripamonti C, Bianchi M. The use of methadone for cancer pain. *Hematol Oncol Clin N Am* 2002; **16(3):** 543–55.

92 Twycross R, Wilcox A, Charlesworth S, *et al. Palliative Care Formulary*. Oxford: Radcliffe Medical Press. Volume 1. 1998.

93 Fundytus ME. Glutamate receptors and nociception: implications for the drug treatment of pain. *CNS Drugs* 2001; **15:** 29–58.

94 Hsu MM, Wong, CS. The roles of the pain facilitatory systems in opioid tolerance. *Acta Anaesthesiol Sinica* 2000; **38(3):** 155–66.

95 Vanderah TW, Gardell LR, Burgess SE, *et al.* Dynorphin promotes abnormal pain and spinal opioid antinociceptive tolerance. *J Neurosci* 2000; **20(18):** 7074–9.

96 Ueda H, Inoue M, Takeshima H, *et al.* Enhanced spinal nociceptin receptor expression develops morphine tolerance and dependence. *J Neurosci* 2000; **20(20):** 7640–7.

97 Aquilante CL, Letrent SP, Pollack GM, *et al.* Increased brain P-glycoprotein in morphine tolerant rats. *Life Sci* 2000; **66(4):** PL47–51.

98 Ossipov MH, Lai J, Vanderah TW, *et al.* Induction of pain facilitated by sustained opioid exposure: relationship to opioid antinociceptive tolerance. *Life Sci* 2003; **73:** 783–800.

99 Pasternak GW, Kolesnikov YA, Babey AM. Perspectives on the N-methyl-D-aspartate/nitric oxide cascade and opioid tolerance. *Neuropsychopharmacology* 1995; **13:** 309–13.

100 Dickenson AH. Neurophysiology of opioid poorly responsive pain. *Cancer Surv* 1994; **21:** 5–16.

101 Mao J. NMDA and opioid receptors: their interactions in antinociception, tolerance and neuroplasticity. *Brain Res Rev* 1999; **30:** 289–304.

102 Ueda H, Inoue M, Mizuno K. New approaches to study the development of morphine tolerance and dependence. *Life Sci* 2003; **74:** 313–20.

103 Donnelly S, Davis M, Walsh D, Naughton M. Morphine in cancer pain management: a practical guide. *Support Care Cancer* 2002; **10:** 13–35.

104 Bernards CM. Clinical Implications of physicochemical properties of opioids. In: Stein C. (Ed.) *Opioids in Pain Control Basic and Clinical Aspects*. Cambridge: Cambridge University Press, 1999, pp. 166–87.

105 Paalzow LK. Pharmacokinetic aspects of optimal pain treatment. *Acta Anesthiol Scand* 1982; **74:** 37–43.

106 Ripamonti C, Groff L, Brunelli C, *et al.* Switching from morphine to oral methadone in treating cancer pain: what is the equianalgesic dose ratio? *J Clin Oncol* 1998; **16(10):** 3216–21.

107 Hogan Q. Distribution of solution in the epidural space: examination by cryomicrotome section. *Reg Anesthiol Pain Med* 2002; **27(2):** 150–6.

108 Hogan Q. Anatomy of spinal anesthesia: some old and new findings. *Reg Anesthiol Pain Med* 1998; **23(4):** 340–3.

109 McQuay HJ, Sullivan AF, Smallman K, Dickenson AH. Intrathecal opioids, potency and lipophilicity. *Pain* 1989; **36:** 111–15.

110 Chrubasik J, Chrubasik S, Martin E. The ideal epidural opioid–fact or fantasy? *Eur J Anaesthesiol* 1993; **10(2):** 79–100.

111 Ellis DJ, Millar WL, Reisner LS. A randomized double-blind comparison of epidural versus intravenous fentanyl infusion for analgesia after cesarean section. *Anesthesiology* 1990; **72(6):** 981–6.

112 Loper KA, Ready LB, Downey M, *et al.* Epidural and intravenous fentanyl infusions are clinically equivalent after knee surgery. *Anesth Analg* 1990; **70:** 72–5.

113 Davis M, Walsh D. Methadone for relief of cancer pain: a review of pharmacokinetics, pharmacodynamics, drug interactions and protocols of administration. *Support Care Cancer* 2001; **9:** 73–83.

114 Lennard M. Genetically determined adverse drug reactions involving metabolism. *Drug Safety Concepts* 1993; **9:** 60–77.

115 Bernard S. The interaction of medications used in palliative care. *Hematol Oncol Clin N Am* 2002; **16:** 641–55.

116 Johnson M, Newkirk G, White Jr J. Clinically significant drug interactions: What you need to know before writing prescriptions. *Postgrad Med* 1999; **105(2):** 193–222.

117 Davis M, Homsi J. The importance of cyctochrome P450 monooxygenase CYP2D6 in palliative medicine. *Support Care Center* 2001; **9:** 442–51.

118 Bernard S, Bruera E. Drug interactions in palliative care. *J Clin Oncol* 2000; **18(8):** 1780–99.

119 Tegeder I, Lotsch J, Geisslinger G. Pharmacokinetics of opioids in liver disease. *Clin Pharmcokinet* 1999; **37(1):** 17–50.

120 Davis MP, Varga J, Dickerson D, *et al.* Normal-release and controlled-release oxycodone: pharmacokinetics, pharmacodynamics, and controversy. *Support Care Cancer* 2003; **11(2):** 84–92.

121 Tallgren M, Olkkola K, Seppala T, *et al.* Pharmacokinetics and ventilatory effects of oxycodone before and after liver transplantation. *Clin Pharmacol Therapeut* 1997; **61(6):** 655–60.

122 Mazoit J, Sandouk P, Zetlaoui P, *et al.* Pharmacokinetics of unchanged morphine in normal and cirrhotic subjects. *Anesth Analg* 1987; **66:** 293–8.

123 Patwardhan R, Johnson R, Hoyumpa Jr A, *et al.* Normal metabolism of morphine in cirrhosis. *Gastroenterology* 1981; **81:** 1006–11.

124 D'Honneur G, Gilton A, Sandouk P, *et al.* Plasma and cerebrospinal fluid concentrations of morphine and morphine glucuronides after oral morphine. The influence of renal failure. *Anesthesiology* 1994; **81:** 87–93.

125 Davies G, Kingswood C, Street M. Pharmacokinetics of opioids in renal dysfunction. *Clin Pharmacokinet* 1996; **6:** 410–22.

126 Bodd E, Jacobsen D, Lund E, *et al.* Morphine-6-glucuronide might mediate the prolonged opioid effect of morphine in acute renal failure. *Hum Exp Toxicol* 1990; **9(5):** 317–21.

127 Osborne RJ, Joel SP, Slevin ML. Morphine intoxication in renal failure: the role of morphine-6-glucuronide. *Br Med J Clin Res* 1986; **292(6535):** 1548–9.

128 Farrell A, Rich A. Analgesic use in patients with renal failure. *Eur J Palliat Care* 2000; **7(6):** 201–5.

129 Angst M, Buhrer M, Lotsch J. Insidious intoxication after morphine treatment in renal failure: delayed onset of morphine-6-glucuronide action. *J Am Soc Anesthesiologists* 2000; **92(5):** 1473.

130 Indelicato R, Portenoy RK. Opiod rotation in the management of refractory cancer pain [The art of oncology: when the tumor is not the target]. *J Clin Oncol* 2002; **20:** 348–52.

Chapter 19

Opioid dosing strategies

Paul Glare & Mellar Davis

Introduction

The World Health Organization (WHO) three-step approach to managing cancer pain bases drug choice upon pain severity[1]. Such an approach has been generally accepted as valid[1]. The choice of opioids, whether 'weak' or 'potent', is usually determined by geographic availability, although morphine is preferred by most palliative specialists as the potent opioid of choice. Low doses of morphine are frequently substituted for weak opioids in countries where morphine is readily available without prescription barriers. One of the major drawbacks to the WHO recommendations is that the guidelines do not include dosing strategies for temporal changes in pain severity.

The Agency for Health Care Policy and Research (AHCPR)[2] has provided further recommendations based upon the World Health Organization three-step approach. These recommendations include the following principles:

- medications should be based upon individual needs with the simplest dosing schedule and least invasive route chosen first;
- analgesic choices need to be guided by cost;
- for moderate to severe pain opioid dose titration is preferred;
- around the clock pre-emptive use of opioids should be prescribed for chronic pain and also rescue doses for breakthrough pain;
- alternative routes should be selected if oral administration is impossible—optional routes include transdermal, rectal, parenteral (subcutaneous and intravenous) and spinal (epidural and intrathecal);
- adjuvants should be used to improve analgesia or reduce opioid side effects or both— opioids are to be added to non-steroidal anti-inflammatory drugs or other adjuvants if pain persists on therapeutic doses of the adjuvant or if pain level increases;
- drug rotation (opioid switch) is appropriate if the first analgesic is ineffective or produces intolerable side effects, although the amount of opioid dose or the timing of it may be ill suited to the pain pattern, resulting in an ineffective pain control despite appropriate drug choice according to the AHCPR; dosing strategies needs to be optimized in this type of situation.

The recently published recommendations of the European Association for Palliative Care (EAPC) expert panel recommended morphine as the opioid of first choice[1]. This recommendation is not 'evidence based', but on the fact that none of the alternative opioids are significantly superior to morphine. Morphine has been used extensively and physicians are familiar with morphine—it is available, versatile and is relatively inexpensive. These factors override morphine's negative characteristics such as its poor oral bioavailability, large differences in individual response and tolerance, and neuroactive metabolite. Large variations in morphine kinetics and dynamics between individuals are due to the type of pain and pain severity, and individual pharmacogenetics that makes it difficult to predict doses for a single individual. Optimal dose correlates poorly with body surface area, weight and gender[1]. Analgesic demands in the individual patient may differ widely due to levels of endogenous opioids (enkephalin, endorphin and dynorphin) and release of substance P, excitatory amino acids, cholecystokinin, gamma amino butryic acid and serotonin levels. The activation of N-methyl-d-aspartate receptors and alpha-2 adrenergic receptors will secondarily influence opioid dose responses. Some patients will have a 'steep' dose response such that small opioid increments produce large differences in pain relief, while others may be 'shallow' responders, where dose titration produces small increments in pain relief [3–5].

Titration

For those patients who need titration to pain relief, immediate release morphine is preferred. It usually has an onset to action of 30 min. The EAPC expert panel recommends starting with a morphine dose of 10 mg every 4 h by mouth if the patient is on a step II or 'weak' opioid, and using 5 mg every 4 h if opioid naïve[1]. The EAPC recommendations suggest a rescue dose that is the same dose as the 4-h morphine dose and that it is to be taken at any time during the 4-h period of time. Alternatively, sustained release morphine sulfate (15 mg every 12 h) could be started for the opioid naïve with a provision of 5 mg of immediate release every 4 h as needed[6,7]. If patients still require frequent rescue doses for non-incident breakthrough pain then the around-the-clock (ATC) dosing is inadequate[6,8]. The choice of rescue doses during titration varies in the literature. The EAPC recommends 100% of the 4-hourly dose, while others have recommended either 25–50% of a 4-hourly dose taken once in the 4-h period or 2–5% of the total around the clock opioid dose to be taken once every 4 h as needed[6,9]. There have been no randomized controlled trials to establish the appropriate rescue morphine dose relative to the ATC morphine dose and there is no evidence which confirms that there is a relationship between rescue and ATC doses[1]. For example, if there is incomplete pain control on 30 mg of sustained release oral morphine every 12 h and six breakthrough doses of 10 mg have been taken within 24 h, then the adjusted dose should be 120 mg times 1.5 (a 50% increase in dose due to incomplete control of pain). The adjusted sustained release morphine dose would be 90 mg every 12 h. However, for convenience due to the commercially available dose size of sustained release morphine tablets doses would be adjusted to 100 mg every 12 h in order to reduce the number of daily tablets and a rescue dose of 30 mg may be given every 4 h. The choice of the rescue and around the clock dose is based upon the nearest increment as an approximation. Dosing differently than what would be rational, based upon tablets or elixir strength, produces more stress and potential opioid dosing errors[6]. Dose adjustments should be once daily due to the time it takes morphine to arrive at steady state, which is approximately 20–24 h. Sustained release morphine doses should not be changed more than every 48 h due to the fact that this type of morphine requires 48 h to reach steady state levels[1]. Rescue doses are added as needed, and the around the clock and breakthrough doses adjusted accordingly.

Intravenous or subcutaneous morphine is started at a dose of 1 mg/h in the healthy opioid naïve or a 0.5-mg dose in the frail, opioid naïve elderly or those with renal insufficiency[10,11]. Subcutaneous infusions should use a 25–26-gauge needle placed subclavicular, or in the abdominal wall or deltoid region. It should not be placed in an area of skin that has received radiation. The needle should be inspected daily and changed weekly. Infusion bags are changed every 2–3 days. Subcutaneous infusions will have the same opioid kinetics and conversion ratios as intravenous opioids, but are less technically involved and generally less painful. Inflammatory reactions occur in approximately 9–13% of patients with subcutaneous therapy[12]. Other opioids can be substituted for subcutaneous morphine such as fentanyl or hydromorphine. Approximately 20–25 mcg of fentanyl or 0.2 mg of hydropmorphone is equivalent to 1 mg of morphine/h. Bolus doses for rescue should be provided hourly or every 2 h. Temporarily more frequent dosing may be necessary for acute or crescendo pain until the pain comes under control[1,6]. The EAPC suggests that the parenteral doses can be given as frequently as every 15 min during titration. This recommendation is not evidence based, but consistent with the time to onset of action of parenteral morphine and clinical experience according to the EAPC. The breakthrough dose may need to be adjusted based upon the individual's response and the duration of that response. If pain relief is 50% or less then the dose is doubled. If pain relief is greater than 50%, but less than 100%, then doses may be increased by 50%[6]. At steady state, rescue doses are added to the ATC dose if the rescue dose is for non-incident breakthrough pain.

Intravenous doses are adjusted in a similar fashion. The time to steady state morphine and hydromorphone levels by the parenteral route is the same as oral (20–24 h), whereas for parenteral fentanyl it is 5 h.

Doubling the nighttime dose may avoid wakening the patient in the early morning for a scheduled dose; however, sustained release morphine given at night appears to be a better strategy[13].

The kinetics of morphine are such that titrating frequent small doses to pain response is both effective and safe and can be followed by maintenance[14]. The central nervous system (CNS) dwell time for morphine is prolonged as compared to fentanyl, which may influence opioid titration strategies depending upon the opioid used and certainly will influence intervals between rescue dosing at steady state[14].

Opioid dose titration for severe or catastrophic pain

A different strategy will be necessary for the treatment of acute pain than that used to treat chronic pain[14]. Patients may present with severe pain and require rapid dose titration in order to control pain quickly. In this situation, the use of a continuous infusion will be inadequate and delay pain control. Steady state levels of morphine can be reached quickly by rapid dose titration of small doses. Dosing strategies should use a loading dose of small frequent morphine doses (titration) at less than drug half-life intervals or, alternatively, a planned incremental dose escalation at normal intervals[6]. The normal strategy of using continuous morphine infusions with provision for rescue dosing will delay reaching effective doses in acute severe pain. Determining the response and morphine dose by titration will also facilitate finding the appropriate maintenance dose[15–18].

Nine trials that dealt with dose titration for severe pain in cancer were obtained through a Medline research process (Pubmed, Ovid Med, and Cochrane Reviews)[15–23]. Eight trials were prospective and two were randomized. Four trials used intravenous morphine, two trials used patient-controlled parenteral analgesia (PCA) and three trials involved oral titration strategies. Patient population, the definitions of severe pain and pain scales differed among the trials. The time of assessment that would influence determination of onset to analgesia also differed among the trials. Intravenous dosing involved:

- 10–20 mg of morphine given every 15–30 min;
- 1.5 mg intravenous every 10 min;
- 2 mg intravenous given every 2 min.

The PCA strategies were either morphine at a 1 mg dose or fentanyl at a 50-mg dose, which was available at 5-min lockout intervals. Oral morphine was given at a dose of:

- 10 mg every 4 h with the possible escalation of the dose by 33–50% every 24 h;
- a randomization between immediate or sustained release morphine with planned increments to 60, 90, 120, 180, 270 and 360 mg daily dose increments;
- 5 mg of morphine every 2–4 h with planned dose escalation every 2–4 h at 10, 15, 20, 30, 40, 60, 80, 120, 160 and 200 mg of morphine depending upon response.

Pain responses were seen within 10 min with parenteral morphine doses every 2 min. Response time was less than 1 h for 1.5 mg of parenteral morphine every 10 min and less than 2 h for parenteral morphine 10–20 mg given every 30 min. The PCA strategies produced responses within 5–24 h. Oral routes of administration at 2-h intervals produced analgesia within 6 h and where 4-h oral dosing intervals reduced pain to acceptable levels by 26–48 h[7,15–22]. Respiratory depression was not seen with any of these strategies and there were very few patient dropouts due to toxicity. Not surprisingly, the onset to analgesia was quicker with parenteral dose titration by non-PCA methods since patients would activate the device upon resurgence of pain and the PCA strategy was demand only. Evidence for guidelines cannot be drawn from studies due to the heterogeneity of the studied population, differences in dosing strategies and assessment tools.

The parenteral morphine dose at which pain relief occurs allows for the determination of maintenance doses[18]. Our protocol involves using morphine doses of 1 mg/min for 10 min or to the onset of analgesia as a clinically effective strategy. Patients failing to respond within the first 10 min are given a 5 min respite and the regimen is then repeated (1 mg/min for 10 min) with a second 5 min respite. This may be repeated once more for a maximum of 30 mg over 45 min before a reassessment of pain is needed. Subcutaneous loading doses of morphine at 2 mg every 5 min may be used as an alternative strategy[10]. Either fentanyl 20 mcg or hydromorphone 0.2 mg i.v., or fentanyl 40 mcg and hydromorphone 0.4 mg given subcutaneously may be substituted for morphine[10]. Once the loading dose is established it can be assumed to be an every 4 h dose, and can be converted to oral dosing by multiplying by 3 or the loading dose can be divided by 3–4, and given on an hourly basis as a continuous infusion[18]. If the patient is not opioid naïve prior to titration, the pretitrated opioid doses will need to be added to the maintenance dose[24]. In general, the parenteral route of administration is necessary[1]. Intramuscular injections should not be used. Intravenous infusions should be considered for:

- patient with an existing indwelling line;
- patients with generalized edema;
- patients experiencing soreness or have had a sterile abscess at subcutaneous infusion site;
- patients with coagulopathy;
- those with poor peripheral circulation[1].

Opioid dosing with diurnal variations in pain

Circadian changes in pain patterns have been well documented and will require asymmetrical dosing schemes for pain control, rather than uniformally increasing the ATC dose. Flat dosing schemes will be inadequate in the setting of significant variations in chronic pain severity. Pain severity may increase in the afternoon or early morning. If nocturnal pain is most problematic, sustained release morphine is given at night and immediate release morphine is given during the day. Alternatively, a larger sustained release morphine dose may be used at night and a smaller one used during the day[10]. If pain is worse during the day, then sustained release morphine may be increased in the morning, and either lower doses of sustained release morphine or immediate release morphine may be made available as needed at night.

Opioid dosing strategies with reduced pain

If pain is relieved by radiation, surgery or by the addition of an adjuvant analgesic, opioid doses may be reduced 50% every 1–3 days until the resurgence of pain or until discontinuation of the opioid without the recurrence of pain. The rescue opioid dose should during the time the ATC dose is reduced and should be available if pain should reappear. In general, the ATC and the rescue dose should not be simultaneously reduced[10].

Respiratory depression and opioid dosing

In rare circumstances, patients may unexpectedly develop opioid-induced respiratory depression. Sedation will precede decreased respirations and minute ventilation volume. Miosis is usually prominent. The clinical situations in which this respiratory depression occurs include:

- opioid dose titration while the patient is receiving a single large fraction of radiation therapy—the radiation results in a rapid reduction of pain within 1–2 days;
- cancer induced spinal cord compression with rapid transection resulting in an absence of pain;
- progressive renal or hepatic failure with delayed opioid clearance;
- the addition of an interacting co-medication, which reduces opioid clearance;
- hypotension and sepsis;
- pneumonia, pulmonary embolus and cardiomyopathy[6,23].

Physicians should be aware that not all mental status changes on opioids are due to the opioid, and that the indiscriminate use of naloxone is inappropriate and can be harmful. Mental changes while patients are on opioids can be due to sedating medications other than opioids, metabolic complications, such as hypercalcemia and hyponatremia, brain metastases, sepsis, depression and delirium. If, at assessment, opioid respiratory depression is likely then naloxone (0.4 mg/ml diluted with 10 cm^3 of water and given at 40 mcg every 3 min) is given either intravenously or subcutaneously until arousability occurs and the respiratory rate is >10[6,25]. If a sustained release opioid or methadone caused the respiratory depression, then continuous infusion using the effective dose at titration should be given hourly until the respiratory depression resolves[9,25].

Types of breakthrough pain: dosing strategies

Transient flares of pain are well recognized with cancer. The incidence ranges from 39% of patients with advanced cancer to 86–93% of cancer patients in hospice[9,26–30]. The reported incidence of breakthrough pain varies between countries, and is not related to age, gender, tumor type, site or therapy[31]. Transient flares upon baseline chronic pain are somatic in 39%, visceral in 22% and neuropathic in 36%.[9,26] Breakthrough pain is associated with a lower likelihood of overall pain control[9,29].

Transient flares of pain are either end-of-dose failure, breakthrough pain or incident pain[32,33]. The first end-of-dose failure and breakthrough pain are associated with suboptimal ATC dosing[8]. Incident pain occurs in half or more of patients experiencing transient flares of pain, and causes more functional impairment, mood and anxiety disorders than non-incident breakthrough pain and end of dose failure[8,9]. Incident pain can be divided into volitional or non-volitional pain. Distinctly different dosing strategies are needed in order to successfully manage incident pain. Opioid doses that are high enough to control incident pain will frequently be too much during quiescence times if added to the ATC dose, leading to the likelihood of opioid toxicity[8]. There are no randomized, controlled trials that evaluate opioid dosing strategies for incident pain[8]. Treatment patterns for transient flares of pain in general include:

- supplemental opioid as previously mentioned;
- optimizing analgesic dose and schedule to pain pattern independent of the ATC dose;
- adjuvant analgesics as an option for breakthrough pain;
- non-pharmacological ancillary measures, such as neurolytic blocks, orthotics, radiation and surgery;
- treatment of the underlying cancer[28].

However, there are no prospective studies to suggest that antitumor therapy with chemotherapy will influence transient flares of pain[30].

Management of breakthrough and end-of-dose failure pain

Breakthrough and end-of-dose failure pain will usually respond to increases in the ATC dose of opioid[6,8,9,30]. End-of-dose failure, in particular, should be managed by dose increases before changing the frequency of dosing. By increasing the ATC dose, these pain episodes become less intense and less frequent. The fixed dose of opioid is increased by increments of 25–50% and rescue doses added to the scheduled dose if pain is still a problem[6,30]. With end-of-dose failure and breatkthrough pain there is a general relationship between the ATC dose and breakthrough dose of opioid. As scheduled ATC doses are increased, so should rescue doses for breakthrough pain be proportionally increased[6,28]. Recommendations are by clinical experience and wide individual variability can exist[6,30]. Rescue dose recommendations as previously mentioned include: 100% of the every 4-h dose; 25–50% of the 4-hourly dose; 5–10% of the total opioid dose[1,6,30]. If opioid toxicity occurs and breakthrough pain is still not controlled adequately, simultaneous but separate opioid dose adjustments should be done as per incident pain[6]. Functional status (as measured by activities of daily of living) and patient satisfaction may be acceptable guides to determine the dose amount and schedule frequency, rather than absolute analgesia[6].

Incident pain

The cardinal principles of the successful management of incident pain are:

♦ do not increase the ATC dose through adding rescue doses for incident pain unless the baseline pain is not adequately controlled;

♦ independently dose chronic and incident pain according to severity and response;

♦ use short-acting opioids for incident pain to avoid carry-over effect;

♦ realize that rescue doses can greatly exceed the ATC dose which is quite unusual for breakthrough and end of dose failure pain;

♦ that pre-emptive dosing strategies are preferable if pain is volitional[6,10].

Rescue doses for incident pain are doubled if pain is less than 50% relieved. These doses are increased by 50% if more than 50%, but less than 100% of the pain is relieved[10]. A subset of patients will have incident pain that rapidly peaks and subsides within 30 min[9,30,32]. Oral opioids will not work adequately with the rapid onset of incident pain. If the chronic pain is under control and the incident pain remains severe on oral rescue opioid due to timing of the rescue dose, then other options would include: transmucosal fentanyl; parenteral patient controlled analgesia devices; administration of a non-opioid analgesic adjuvant; the use of spinal opioids; the use of non-pharmacological approaches such as neurolytic blocks, orthotics, radiation and surgery[34–36].

Opioid dosing errors

Opioid dosing errors will result in inadequate pain control and/or opioid toxicity. Errors will lead to premature opioid rotation and add to the patient's symptom burden. Errors frequently arise from taking an inadequate pain history and the failure to adequately assess the individual's response.

A common error is as-needed dosing for continuous pain. This strategy may lead to large periods of time in which pain is uncontrolled and episodes of opioid 'mini' withdrawal. As a result, as-needed opioid doses may be increased in lieu of ATC dosing, which then leads to alternating opioid toxicity and withdrawal[37]. Another common error is ATC opioid without rescue. Since most patients will have some transient pain, they will have inadequate pain control if rescue dosing is not made available.

Patients may not receive pre-emptive opioids for incident pain. Some patients will receive sustained release opioids for incident or breakthrough pain leading to inadequate control and a 'carry over' effect. This 'carry over' toxicity from the sustained release 'as needed' opioid leads to opioid toxicity once the transient pain resolves[37].

Physicians may prescribe several opioids at once in low doses, rather than effectively titrating a single opioid. In this case, if patients develop side effects from combined opioid therapy, the offending opioid will not be known, necessitating the discontinuation of all opioids. An exception to single opioid use is the combination of short-acting opioids such as morphine, hydromorphone or oxycodone with transdermal fentanyl due to the expense of transmucosal fentanyl[37].

The route, dose and drug may be simultaneously changed in instances of inadequate pain control, rather than appropriately changing either drug, route or dose. Changing drug and route or dose and route may lead to confusion regarding the maneuver, which leads to pain relief and/or toxicity[37]. An exception would be an 'opioid sparing' strategy, which adds an adjuvant analgesic to the opioid and reduces opioid doses simultaneously in the case of opioid toxicity and inadequately controlled pain[6].

Physicians frequently fail to use adjuvant analgesics. Adjuvants will widen the therapeutic index of opioids, thus reducing the risk of opioid toxicity. It is relatively common to add rescue doses for incident pain into the ATC dose despite control of chronic pain.

Pharmaceutically inappropriate dosing can occur. For instance, the sustained release opioid may be prescribed every 6 h instead of every 8 or 12 h. Alternatively, immediate release morphine may be prescribed every 6–8 h, rather than every 4 h.

Opioid dosing errors will arise from incorrectly estimating equianalgesia with opioid rotation or opioid conversion doses when changing routes of administration. Some opioid equianalgesia tables have inaccurate equivalences, which leads to delayed and potentially severe opioid toxicity[37].

Opioid rotation

A minority of patients develop intolerable adverse side effects with morphine. If pain is relieved and opioid side effects occur, incremental dose reduction will usually reduce opioid toxicity. The major dose-limiting toxicities are neurotoxicity (as manifested by hallucinations, confusion and myoclonus) and gastrointestinal toxicity (exhibited by persistent nausea and vomiting). Indications for opioid rotation are poorly controlled pain and unacceptable side effects. Uncontrolled pain without side effects should be treated by dose escalation, rather than opioid rotation[1,37]. Switching opioids in the majority allows for dose titration without the occurrence of disabling side effects[1]. The incidence of opioid rotation varies from 18 to 40%[1,38–42]. Some patients will require several opioid rotations until their pain is controlled without burdensome side effects[1]. Opioid rotation requires a fundamental understanding of opioid equivalence[39,43]. Calculated equivalence based upon equianalgesia tables are relatively accurate due to the large individual differences in equivalence reported clinically. Opioids differ in intrinsic efficacy and receptor binding spectrum. Equivalents have been reported to differ depending on order of rotation, opioid dose and individual pharmacokinetics. Age, gender and organ function, as well as co-medications, may influence relative opioid potency[4,5,38,39,43–54]. In addition, incomplete equianalgesic cross-tolerance occurs, which can lead to unanticipated greater opioid response than expected with the second opioid. There are also non-cross-tolerance to side effects, which contributes to the opioid therapeutic index of the second opioid[36]. Reasonable doses for rotation are 50–70% of the opioid equivalence if rotation is for side effects and are 100% of equivalence if for pain[6,38,43,55,56]. Switching to methadone requires a unique dosing strategy[55].

No firm guidelines are available which directs the choice of second line opioids. It is not possible to know in advance whether an opioid switch will increase pain control more than it will create adverse effects. Before rotation one should:

- review the clinical situation and pain syndrome;
- be sure that dosing was according to pain pattern;
- review potential adjuvants;
- reduce doses if opioid toxicity is the problem;
- treat opioid-induced confusion with haloperidol, nausea with metoclopramide, and myoclonus with clonazepam, valproic acid or gabapentin;
- treat underlying metabolic disorders which have similarities to opioid toxicity such as hypercalcemia or hypoxemia[10,38].

Patients on morphine may be rotated to other opioids with a broader opioid receptor profile such as oxycodone and levorphanol. Patients may rotate to opioids with a higher intrinsic efficacy as with fentanyl. Rotations may be to opioids with both a broad receptor profile and higher intrinsic efficacy such as methadone[54,55,57–60]. Alternative strategies to opioid rotation are: the aggressive management of opioid side effects; opioid 'sparing' with adjuvants; opioid conversion to another route (rectal, parenteral or spinal); non-pharmacological intervention including nerve blocks, orthotics, radiation and surgery[59].

Conclusions

Effective pain control in advanced cancer requires the use of analgesics based upon pain severity as outlined by the World Health Organization, and dosing strategies as outlined by the EAPC and AHCPR. Refinements in dosing strategies are based upon pattern and the type of breakthrough pain (incident, breakthrough and end of dose failure), and will facilitate the control of pain and minimize opioid toxicity. Opioid dosing errors lead to premature opioid rotations and added symptom burden to patients. Opioid rotation is required when pain and opioid side effects limit further opioid titration. Rational prescribing is often the key to successful pain management.

References

1 Hanks GW, de Conno F, Cherny N, *et al.* Morphine and alternative opioids in cancer pain: the EAPC recommendations. *Br J Cancer* 2001; **84(5)**: 587–93.

2 Anon. Management of cancer pain guideline overview. *J Nat Med Ass* 1994; **86(8)**: 571–3.

3 **Dickenson AH.** Plasticity: implications for opioid and other pharmacological interventions in specific pain sites. *Behav Brain Sci* 1997; **20:** 392–403.

4 **Pasternak GW.** Insights into mu opioid pharmacology. The role of mu opioid receptor subtypes. *Life Sci* 2001; **68:** 2213–19.

5 **Pasternak GW.** Incomplete cross tolerance and multiple mu opioid peptide receptors. *Trends Pharmacol Sci* 2001; **22(2):** 67.

6 **Walsh D.** Pharmacological management of cancer pain. *Semin Oncol* 2000; **27(1):** 45–63.

7 **Klepstad P, Kassa S, Jystad A, et al.** Immediate- or sustained-release morphine for dose finding during start of morphine to cancer patients: a randomized, double-blind trial. *Pain* 2003; **101:** 193–8.

8 **McQuay HJ, Jadad AR.** Incident pain. *Cancer Surv* 1994; **21:** 17–24.

9 **Portenoy RK, Hagen NA.** Breakthrough pain: definition, prevalence and characteristics. *Pain* 1990; **45(1):** 107–8.

10 **Walsh D, Rivera N, Davis MP, et al.** Opioid dosing in cancer pain: 40 strategies for 10 clinical problems: the Cleveland Clinic Foundation Guidelines. *Support Cancer Ther* 2004; **1(3):** 157–64.

11 **Glare P, Walsh D, Groh E, et al.** The efficacy and side effects of continuous infusion intravenous morphine (CIVM) for pain and symptoms due to advanced cancer. *Am J Hosp Palliat Care* 2002; **19(5):** 343–50.

12 **Ripamonti C, Zecca E, De Conno F.** Pharmacological treatment of cancer pain: alternative routes of opioid administration. *Tumori* 1998; **74:** 289–300.

13 **Todd J, Rees E, Gwilliam B, et al.** An assessment of the efficacy and tolerability of a 'double-dose' of normal-release morphine sulphate at bedtime. *Palliat Med* 2002; **16(6):** 507–12.

14 **Upton RN, Semple TJ, Macintyre PE.** Pharmacokinetic optimisation of opioid treatment in acute pain therapy. *Clin Pharmacokinet* 1997; **33(3):** 225–44.

15 **Hagen NA, Elmwood T, Ernst S.** Cancer pain emergencies: a protocol for management. *J Pain Sympt Manag* 1997; **14(1):** 45–50.

16 **Kumar KS, Naseema AM.** Intravenous morphine for emergency treatment of cancer pain. *Palliat Med* 2000; **14:** 183–8.

17 **Harris JT, Kumar S, Rajagopal MR.** Intravenous morphine for rapid control of severe cancer pain. *Palliat Med* 2003; **17:** 248–56.

18 **Mercandate S, Villari P, Ferrara P, et al.** Rapid titration with intravenous morphine for severe cancer pain and immediate oral conversion. *Cancer* 2002; **95(1):** 203–8.

19 **Radbruch L, Loick G, Schilzeck S, et al.** Intravenous titration with morphine for severe cancer pain: report of 28 cases. *Clin J Pain* 1999; **15:** 173–8.

20 **Zech D, Grond SUA, Lynch J, et al.** Transdermal fentanyl and initial dose-finding with patient-controlled analgesia in cancer pain. A pilot study with 20 terminally ill cancer patients. *Pain* 1992; **50:** 293–301.

21 **Klepstad P, Kassa S, Skauge M, et al.** Pain intensity and side effects during titration of morphine to cancer patients using a fixed schedule dose escalation. *Acta Anesthesiol Scand* 2000; **44:** 656–64.

22 **Klepstad P, Kassa S, Jystad A, et al.** Immediate or sustained release morphine for dose finding during start of morphine to cancer patients: a randomized, double-blind trial. *Pain* 2003; **101:** 193–8.

23 **Lichter I.** Accelerated titration of morphine for rapid relief of cancer. *NZ Med J* 1994; **107(990):** 488–90.

24 **Davis MP.** Acute pain in advanced cancer: an opioid dosing strategy and illustration. *Am J Hosp Palliat Care* 2004; **21(1):** 47–50.

25 **Wasiak J, Clavisi O.** Is subcutaneous or intramuscular naloxone as effective as intravenous naloxone in the treatment of life-threatening heroin overdose? *Med J Aust* 2002; **176(10):** 495.

26 Petzke F, Radbruch L, Zech D, et al. Temporal presentation of chronic cancer pain: transitory pains on admission to a multidisciplinary pain clinic. *J Pain Sympt Manag* 1999; **17(6):** 391–401.

27 Fine PG, Busch MA. Characterization of breakthrough pain by hospice patients and their caregivers. *J Pain Sympt Manag* 1998; **16(3):** 179–83.

28 Swanwick M, Haworth N, Lennard RF. The prevalence of episodic pain in cancer: a survey of hospice patients on admission. *Palliat Med* 2001; **15(1):** 9–18.

29 Zeppetella G, O'Doherty CA, Collins S. Prevalence and characteristics of breakthrough pain in cancer patients admitted to a hospice. *J Pain Sympt Manag* 2000; **20(2):** 87–92.

30 Portenoy RK. Treatment of temporal variations in chronic cancer pain. *Semin Oncol* 1997; **24(5 Suppl 16):** S16-7–S16-12.

31 Lyss AP, Portenoy RK. Strategies for limiting the side effects of cancer pain therapy. *Semin Oncol* 1997; **24(5 Suppl 16):** S16-28–S16-34.

32 Coluzzi PH. Cancer pain management: newer perspectives on opioids and episodic pain. *Am J Hosp Palliat Care* 1998; **15(1):** 13–22.

33 Mercadante S, Radbruch L, Caraceni A, et al. Episodic (breakthrough) pain. *Cancer* 2002; **94:** 832–9.

34 Cleary JF. Pharmacokinetic and pharmacodynamic issues in the treatment of breakthrough pain. *Semin Oncol* 1997; **24(5 Suppl 16):** S16-13–S16-19.

35 Coluzzi PH. Oral patient-controlled analgesia. *Semin Oncol* 1997; **24(5 Suppl 16):** S16-35–S16-42.

36 Mercadante SG, Radbruch L, Caraceni A, et al. Episodic (breakthrough) pain. *Cancer* 2002; **94:** 832–9.

37 Kochhar R, LeGrand SB, Walsh D, et al. Opioids in cancer pain: common dosing errors. *Oncology* 2003; **17(4):** 571–5.

38 Fallon M. Opioid rotation: does it have a role? *Palliat Med* 1997; **11:** 177–8.

39 Cherny NJ, Ripamonti C, Pereira J, et al. Strategies to manage the adverse effects of oral morphine: an evidence-based report. *J Clin Oncol* 2001; **19(9):** 2542–54.

40 Cherny NJ, Chang V, Frager G, et al. Opioid pharmacology in the management of cancer pain. *Cancer* 1995; **76:** 1288–93.

41 Mercadante SG. Opioid rotation for cancer pain. *Cancer* 1999; **86:** 1856–66.

42 Enting RH, Oldenmenger WH, van der Rijt CDC, et al. A prospective study evaluating the response of patients with unrelieved cancer pain to parenteral opioids. *Cancer* 2002; **94:** 3049–56.

43 Anderson R, Saiers JH, Abram A, et al. Accuracy in equianalgesic dosing: conversion dilemmas. *J Pain Sympt Manag* 2001; **21(5):** 397–406.

44 Galer BS, Coyle N, Pasternak GW, et al. Individual variability in the response to different opioids: report of five cases. *Pain* 1992; **49(1):** 87–91.

45 Bernard S, Bruera E. Drug interactions in palliative care. *J Clin Oncol* 2000; **18(8):** 1780–99.

46 Davies G, Kingswood C, Street M. Pharmacokinetics of opioids in renal dysfunction. *Clin Pharmacokinet* 1996; **31(6):** 410–22.

47 Duttaroy A, Yoburn BC. The effect of intrinsic efficacy on opioid tolerance. *Anesthesiology* 1995; **82:** 1226–36.

48 Paktor J, Vaught JL. Differential analgesic cross-tolerance to morphine between lipophilic and hydrophilic narcotic agonists. *Life Sci* 1984; **34(1):** 13–21.

49 Drewe J, Ball HA, Beglinger C, et al. Effect of P-glycoprotein modulation on the clinical pharmacokinetics and adverse effects of morphine. *Br J Clin Pharmacol* 2000; **50(3):** 237–46.

50 Thompson SJ, Koszdin K, Bernards CM. Opiate-induced analgesia is increased and prolonged in mice lacking P-glycoprotein. *Anesthesiology* 2000; **93(5):** 1392–9.

51 Tegeder I, Lotsch J, Geisslinger G. Pharmacokinetics of opioids in liver disease. *Clin Pharmacokinet* 1999; **31(1):** 17–40.

52 Liston HL, Markowitz JS, DeVane CL. Drug glucuronidation in clinical psychopharmacology. *J Clin Psychopharmacol* 2001; **21(5)**: 500–15.

53 Davis MP, Homsi J. The importance of cytochrome P450 monooxygenase CYP2D6 in palliative medicine. *Support Care Cancer* 2001; **9:** 442–51.

54 Morgan D, Picker MJ. Contribution of individual differences to discriminative stimulus, antinociceptive and rate-decreasing effects of opioids: importance of the drug's relative intrinsic efficacy at the mu receptor. *Behav Pharmacol* 1996; **7(3)**: 261–84.

55 Ferrante FM. Principles of opioid pharmacotherapy: practical implications of basic mechanisms. *J Pain Sympt Manag* 1996; **11(5)**: 265–73.

56 Indelicato A, Portenoy RK. Opioid rotations in the management of refractory cancer pain. *J Clin Oncol* 2002; **20(1)**: 348–52.

57 Morley JS. Opioids, confusion and opioid rotation. *Palliat Med* 1998; **12:** 463–8.

58 Twycross R. Opioid rotation: does it have a role? *Palliat Med* 1998; **12(1):** 60–1.

59 Portenoy RK. Managing cancer pain poorly responsive to systemic opioid therapy. *Oncology* 1999; **15(5 Suppl 2):** 25–9.

60 Mercadante SG, Casuccio A, Fulfaro F, *et al.* Switching from morphine to methadone to improve analgesia and tolerability in cancer patients: a prospective study. *J Clin Oncol* 2001; **19(11):** 2898–904.

Chapter 20

Patient controlled analgesia

Mellar P. Davis

Introduction

Opioids are frequently prescribed at too low a dose by physicians and given at less than adequate intervals by nursing staff[1]. There are usually two reasons for inadequate dosing by healthcare professionals. The first concerns addiction and the second a misunderstanding of analgesic tolerance, which 'justifies' inadequate dosing. The fear of opioid toxicity particularly respiratory depression, leads nurses to prolong dosing intervals[1–3]. The development of patient controlled analgesia (PCA) has greatly improved the knowledge of appropriate opioid dosing strategies in patients[1]. PCA was first used in obstetrics in the 1960s and became extensively utilized for postoperative pain in the 1980s[2]. Prior to this, pain management was delegated to the nursing staff and opioids were given intramuscular at rigid or fixed rate intervals, or only upon urgent requests[1].

Most modern PCA devices are electronically controlled infusion pumps supervised by programmable microprocessors. These systems are activated by the patient without requiring a third party for dose delivery. Unauthorized alterations in dosing parameters and overdoses are prevented by a number of safety factors[1]. The adaptability of parenteral PCA may involve strategies that are:

- demand only;
- fixed or diural infusion plus demand;
- fixed rate followed by demand (usually for postoperative analgesia)[1].

Oral PCA strategies are actually the standard recommendation by the AACPR and EAPC, and are not further addressed.

The three variables necessary for PCA dosing are drug, increment or bolus dose, and lockout interval, all of which requires pump programming. The scientific basis supporting the optimal bolus doses for commonly used opioids is lacking[4]. Cancer patients will have distinctively different minimal effective concentration (MEC) for pain relief, and are more likely to achieve optimal dose response and MEC by PCA dosing strategies than by rigid fixed dose rates, particularly if pain is changing in severity[5]. The PCA strategy removes the gap between the physician's estimate of the patient's opioid need and actual requirements as dictated by the patient[1]. The clinical experience with PCA is evidence that opioid pharmacodynamics, rather than the pharmacokinetics are of greater importance to optimal pain relief, since there is both a lack of a universal MEC and highly variable individual requirements[4]. The experience with PCA strategies demonstrates that opioid doses can be programmed to be small enough to avoid adverse effects, but large enough for pain relief and at long enough intervals to avoid toxicity, but short enough to avoid uncontrolled pain[2]. Ideally, well-informed patients will dose themselves to their individual optimal MEC.

The principles of PCA are those established for oral sustained released opioids with immediate release opioid rescue for cancer pain. Although PCA is not superior to other treatment strategies, it does allow for individualization, a cardinal rule for effective opioid dosing in cancer[3,6]. The PCA strategy is adaptable to pain patterns and moves the locus of pain control to the patient, which can dramatically improve patient satisfaction with pain management[7]. Since cancer pain is chronic with transient flares of pain, a PCA strategy needs to be programmed for infusion rate, bolus dose and lockout intervals in order to fit the individual.

The opioids of choice for rapid onset to analgesia (5–10 min) and short duration of actions are fentanyl, morphine and hydromorphone. Methadone, due to the duration of action, half-life and risk of subcutaneous toxicity, should not be used with PCA except in unusual circumstances. The subcutaneous route is preferred by most palliative physicians world wide, there may be regional preferences for intravenous infusions. Due to opioid concentrations in small volumes for subcutaneous infusions, preferred opioids are fentanyl and hydromorphone over morphine when high doses are required[3,7]. The usual recommended subcutaneous infusions are 1–2 ml/h. Maximum recommended morphine concentrations for subcutaneous infusions are 50 mg/ml and will be difficult to deliver subcutaneously if morphine requirements exceed 75 mg/h. Alternatives are to switch opioids when dose requirements exceed this dose or convert to intravenous morphine infusion.

Appropriate lockout intervals are related to peak effect, which for most parenteral opioids occurs within 20 min[3]. However, lockout intervals by published reports are shorter when the dosing strategy was demand only and longer when demand was combined with continuous infusion. A recommended starting PCA regimen for continuous infusion and demand has been published by Ma & Lin[3] (Table 20.1).

Dose adjustments are based upon response with the delivered dose, the number of demand doses and the type of transient pain (incident, breakthrough or end of dose failure). Lockout intervals have not been prospectively compared with the various

Table 20.1 Dose regimen in opioid naive[3]

Fentanyl	20 μ/h	20 μ/h/15 min
Hydromorphone	0.2 mg/h	0.1 mg/15 min
Morphine	1.0 mg/h	0.5 mg/20 min
Oxymorphone	0.1 mg/h	0.1 mg/20 min

Table 20.2 Example of PCA dosing strategy[11]

I	Load of morphine 2–5 mg every 10–20 min until analgesia
II	Maintenance dose is calculated by summing the cumulative morphine divided by the time to analgesia
III	Demand only maintenance phase: provide 50–75% of the loading dose as the rescue with a lockout interval of 10–30 min
IV	Continuous plus demand dosing: infuse 75% of hourly opioid by continuous and 25% as demand with an hour lock-out interval.

opioids. The duration of central nervous system (CNS) dwell time with morphine is much longer than fentanyl and, although CNS dwell time does not predict pain relief, it may, in fact, be an important factor in determining the dosing interval[8,9].

Published morphine equivalents/h range from 6 to 36 mg (0.5–3 mg with a lockout interval of 5–60 min) for cancer. Bolus morphine doses greater than 1 mg have been associated with more side effects. Continuous morphine doses have ranged from 1 to 4 mg. The elderly and very sick should start with morphine at lower doses (0.5 mg). Those who are not opioid naïve usually require greater than 1 mg doses[2]. Recommendations are not based upon high-quality randomized controlled trials[2]. An example of one strategy is provided in Table 20.2.

Indications for bolus only PCA in advanced cancer are:

- incident pain particularly acute onset and no chronic pain;
- diural variations in pain patterns;
- dose finding with renal failure;
- personality characteristics that require 'as needed' dosing for acceptance;
- methadone (due to its prolonged half-life);
- patient fears of opioid side effects;
- parenteral conversion from oral for reasons of side effects;
- dysphagia;
- dose titration[6].

A review of the literature does not provide enough evidence to confirm these indications.

Problems with PCA and counter indications

Respiratory depression with PCA occurs rarely. The safety with PCA relies upon the fact that sedation limits the patient ability to activate the PCA device prior to respiratory arrest in those experiencing toxicity from their opioid[2]. However, respiratory depression has been reported with:

- dehydration associated with evolving pre-renal azotemia;
- sleep apnea;

- upper respiratory tract obstruction;
- operator or prescribing error[2].

PCA precipitated respiratory failure has been documented with upper respiratory tract obstruction in advanced cancer. Minor side effects with PCA, such as drowsiness, dry mouth, constipation, vomiting, urinary retention and pruritus, are related to the opioid rather than to the PCA technique[2].

PCA requires a degree of understanding, compliance and education, which is greater than usually required for traditional parenteral dosing regimens[10]. Over-reliance upon PCA may delay the appropriate addition of adjuvant analgesics or non-pharmacological measures. PCA devices limit mobility to a certain extent and are expensive. The pumps mechanics or electronics can malfunction and a 24-h call system needs to be in place for home care. The PCA strategy is touted to be more effective in the management of uncontrolled severe pain, but review of the literature reveals that the time to analgesia is actually longer than by traditional physician-directed rapid titration and maintenance strategies[11]. There are no controlled trials that have found that PCA strategies improve patient performance status to a greater extent that other traditional dosing methods[11]. Comparisons between the various PCA methods in advanced cancer are rare.

Other problems with PCA include failure to assess new pain during patient directed controlled dosing and dose titration, and the lack of follow-up. In one study, only 27% of patient days on PCA had appropriately documented pain severity by numerical rating[12]. Patients can become dissatisfied with PCA, despite good pain relief, due to reduced nursing attention[6]. Lead time to preparation may produce gaps in dosing unless pro-active planning for pump refills is done. Patients may be anxious (button pusher) and recorded demand doses may reflect anxiety, rather than the lack of pain control. Physicians may count the number of PCA activations as a measure of uncontrolled pain, rather than the response of a nervous patient. Problems can include mechanical pump failures in the demand or lockout mechanism, cracks in drug vials, bags or syringes, and faulty one-way valves and alarms[6].

Patients with a history of alcoholism or polysubstance abuse should not be treated with PCA, particularly at home[6]. Cognitive failure precludes the use of PCA. A passive personality or fear and anxiety with technology may render PCA strategies less effect-ive and less desirable. A plan that includes the transfer of care to a community that is unable to support PCA technology or to a physician untrained in PCA is a contraindication to initiating PCA for pain control.

Morphine is compatible with multiple medications as is fentanyl, hydromorphone and methadone, which can be included in the PCA (Table 20.3). Combining medica-tions with opioids in a continuous infusion and titration by PCA demand will also increase the dose of the co-medication and potentially lead to adverse drug effects[13]. There are distinct differences in PCA strategies due to differences in pain between cancer and postoperative patients, which will influence the method of delivery and appropriate outcomes (Table 20.4).

Table 20.3 Co-medications comparable with morphine, fentanyl, hydromorphone, methadone

Atropine	Lorazepam
Dexamethasone	Methotrimeprazine
Diazepam	Metoclopramide
Diphenhydramine	Midazolam
Haloperidol	Phenobarbital
Hydroxyzine	Scopolamine
Ketorolac	

Table 20.4 Factors that differ between cancer and postoperative patients that will influence PCA

I	Differences in the trajectory of disease, which makes it unlikely that PCA reduces hospitalization as an outcome measure for cancer patients.
II	Changing pain patterns and pain intensity in cancer patients as compared with the usual diminishing pain pattern with postoperative patient.
III	Delirium, cognitive failure and limited manual dexterity is more common with cancer patients.
IV	Functional status of cancer patients will be relatively unchanged with PCA. Activities of daily living and performance status in cancer are due to multiple symptoms, which are usually absent in surgical patients.

Patient controlled analgesia in cancer patients: a systematic review

Introduction

Studies and issues

The use of PCA in cancer pain has been investigated in only a few studies, which usually involved small numbers of patients. Opioid doses and schedules vary widely, and outcome measures are not consistently applied from study to study. Benefits over traditional parenteral dosing strategies are not easily discernable in published studies. There has been no uniform response assessment. As a result there is not enough evidence to develop a valid evidence-based guideline for PCA use in cancer pain[11]. There are 13 PCA trials in cancer pain, which can be gleaned from the published literature through a Medline search (Ovidmed, Pubmed and Cochrane Reviews).

The initial PCA studies in cancer were reported in 1986. Baumann and colleagues reported a two phase trial[14]. The initial phase consisted of morphine 1 mg with a 6-min lockout interval as titration. If there was no response, then a 50% increase in the bolus dose was allowed and the demand only continued. Patients received demand only dosed for titration to pain relief. The second phase involved conversion from parenteral PCA morphine to oral morphine using a ratio of 2 (oral) to 1 (parenteral). Pain severity was measured by verbal rating scale (VRS, 1–5). Sedation was also graded by VRS every 2 h by the nurse. A relative dose indicator (RDI) was obtained by subtracting the pain VRS from the sedation VRS. Patients who were previously receiving opioids were allowed in this trial. All patients responded to the demand phase using the 1-mg bolus and 6-min lockout interval. During the PCA phase of the trial the RDI ranged between +1 and −1. Dosing rates varied widely among individuals ranging from 10.63 + 6.25 mg/h to 0.96 + 1.01 mg/h, a 10-fold difference. Three of eight patients were converted to oral with a final morphine conversion ratio of 1 parenteral to 2.5 oral. Sedation was minimal and respiratory depression not observed. Five did not finish the trial due to death, the need for a cordotomy, oral morphine intolerance, a faulty intravenous site and early discharge.

A second trial was published the same year by Citron and colleagues[13,15]. This was an open labeled trial involving eight male patients with a mean age of 58 (range 54–62). Some were on potent opioids prior to study. All had normal liver and renal function. The PCA strategy was demand only. Pain, subjective sedation and objection sedation were graded by VRS (1–5). The mean morphine dose was 4.2 mg (range 1–5) with a mean lockout interval of 30 min (range 15–90 min). The mean cumulative number of demand doses during the first 24 h was 11.2 (range 0–25). Dosing was required more frequently in the first four h. One patient who before starting the PCA required 10 mg of parenteral morphine every 4 h did not require morphine in the first four h of the study for unknown reasons. The mean pain score was 1.5 on the PCA demand strategy. Sedation was mild and ranged from 1.6 to 2.8 (VRS 1–5). Total morphine requirements ranged from 0 to 87 mg in the first 24 h. No respiratory depression occurred. All patients expressed satisfaction with pain control while on PCA.

A trial by Kerr and colleagues involved cancer patients on opioids with pain not controlled on their potent dose or who were experiencing opioid-related side effects or unable to swallow[16]. A CADD-PCA infusion pump (Pharmacia CADD-PCA, Pharmacia Inc Montreal Quebec Canada) was utilized. The PCA strategy involved continuous infusion plus demand. Patients on parenteral opioids prior to study were placed on a continuous infusion dose based upon the pre-study 24-h total opioid dose. Patients on oral opioids were converted to parenteral using a standard conversion table. Rescue doses were set at 30–100% of the hourly dose, and the lockout interval was kept between 30 and 60 min. Infusion rates were increased if the patient's demand doses were more than 6 within 24 h. A VRS (1–5) was used to gauge pain control. Telephone follow-up was part of this study since most patients were treated at home. Eighteen patients were included on study: 15 for breakthrough pain, six for nausea and vomiting, four for drowsiness, two for inconvenient dosing schedule and one for dysphagia. Several patients had multiple indications for PCA according to the author. The outpatient infusions were maintained for a mean of 54 days (maximum 225 days). Patient's ages ranged from 34 to 64 years. Morphine and hydromorphone were the two most frequently used opioids. Initial doses of hydromorphone (11 patients) ranged between 1 and 22 mg/h with final doses ranging from 1 to 60 mg/h. For morphine (seven patients) initial doses were 2–30 mg/h and final doses ranged from 12.5 to 80 mg/h. Sedation, nausea and vomiting were not a major problem. Four experienced pump failure during the infusion. Improved pain control was noted by all, although eight later developed suboptimal pain control.

This long-term trial with PCA involved higher doses than the two earlier trials, which probably indicates a group of patients with more advanced cancer. Individual differences in dose requirements ranged between 6- and 60-fold. Side effects were minimal for this group of patients, but most had significant prior opioid exposure during which tolerance to side effects was more likely to occur. Mechanical pump failure occurred in four (20%). Seizures occurred in one patient when hydromorphone doses were titrated from 60 to 75 mg/h.

Swanson and colleagues reported one of the largest experiences of PCA for cancer pain[13]. Patients were previously on oral, rectal or parenteral opioids. One-hundred-seventeen patients with a mean age of 61.2 years (range 28–90 years) participated in this study. A CADD-PCA pump (Pharmacia Del-Tech, St Paul, MN) was used and a continuous infusion plus demand dosing strategy was implemented. Conversion from opioid to parenteral opioid used a standard conversion table. Bolus doses were 25% of the hourly dose. Baseline infusions were increased by 10–20% every 60 min until pain was controlled. Once the patient reached stable pain control, the minimal lockout interval was kept to 60–120 min. A VRS (0–5) was used to rate pain. Most received subcutaneous infusions with their PCA. The mean duration of treatment was 3 weeks. Nearly half the patients had pain due to bone metastases, while 22% experienced visceral pain. Ninety-five responded as defined by a reduction in pain from 4 to 1 by VRS and all responded within 12 h. All but two remained on the CADD-PCA until death. The mean baseline subcutaneous morphine dose was 6.5 mg (1–33) and bolus 4 mg (0.5–15). For those receiving intravenous morphine the mean baseline morphine dose was 24 mg/h (2–180). The bolus dose was 4 mg/h (range 2–12). The mean hourly subcutaneous hydromorphone dose was 3 mg (range 0.3–21) and the mean bolus dose was 1 mg/h (0.5–1.5). One patient developed a subcutaneous abscess at the site of infusion, and six were converted from subcutaneous to intravenous infusion due to the high dose requirements. One patient sustained a respiratory arrest within 24 h of starting PCA due to an upper respiratory tract obstruction from recurrent oral cancer. Pump failure occurred in three. Dexamethasone was added in 20%, metoclopramide in 7% and haloperidol in 9% of infusions for inflammation at subcutaneous sites and opioid-induced side effects, respectively. The subjective impression was that the co-medications limited nausea and agitation.

Wagner and colleagues reported their experience using a CADD-PCA (Pharmacia Inc, Del-Tech, St Paul, MN) for patients on oral opioids with poor pain relief or unacceptable adverse effects[17]. Patients experiencing pain arising from below the diaphragm were to have failed epidural opioids before the parenteral PCA was allowed. Patients received a continuous infusion dose based upon prestudy opioid requirements and were provided a demand dose. Patients were monitored every 2 h. A VRS (0–3) was used for pain relief. Once pain was controlled, the PCA infusion was delivered through an implanted central venous catheter. Continuous doses were adjusted based upon demand doses calculated per 24 h. Four patients entered this study. The age ranged from 30 to 80 years. Initial infusion rates prior to study were 3–4 mg morphine/h. Initial infusions by the CADD-PCA were 1–5 mg/h and the final continuous infusion was 0.8–60 mg/h. Only two received demand doses. In those two, demand doses were 3 mg i.v. with a lockout interval of 60 min and 2 mg subcutaneous with a lockout interval of 30 min. Responses were generally rated as good. One had the central catheter removed.

A study of continuous morphine infusions with demand PCA for bone marrow transplant related mucositis was performed by Hill and associates. This study randomized patients between conventional PCA using an Abbott model 4100 PCA pump or a pharmacokinetic modulated PCA pump (PK-PCA)[18]. Initial morphine doses by conventional PCA were 1–2 mg with a lockout interval of 10 min. The PK-PCA was determined individually for each patient on the PCA-PK arm of the study and infusions were based upon their respective MEC. Patients on PK-PCA could increase the infusion rate through the CADD-PCA. A visual analog scale (VAS, 0–100 mm) was used for both pain and side effects. Thirty-five bone marrow transplant patients were randomized between PCA (20) and PK-PCA (15). The PK-PCA predicted morphine requirements for pain control in the first 7 days, but diverged from predicted doses thereafter. The PK-PCA group had a 30% improvement in pain control when compared with the PCA group. Side effects were similar between the groups, although sedation was greater for the PK-PCA group in the first 7 days. Morphine requirements were 2.7 times higher in the PK-PCA group in the first 6 days. The PK-PCA group required twice the morphine within the first 14 days. The mean duration of therapy did not differ between the groups. The severity of mucositis did not differ between groups.

Respiratory depression was not seen in either group.

The PK-PCA strategy predetermines MEC morphine serum levels for individual patients and reduces pain by 30% compared to conventional PCA, but is associated with increased sedation and requires 2.7 times the amount of oral morphine than conventional PCA.

Zech and colleagues performed a two-phase trial using demand PCA fentanyl as an initial strategy until pain control was achieved followed by conversion to transdermal fentanyl[19]. The initial 24-h period PCA dosing used a CADD-PCA pump (Pharmacia Del-Tech, Inc, St Paul, MN). The demand only strategy was fentanyl 50 mcg with a lockout interval of 5 min. Transdermal fentanyl was started on the second day based upon first day requirements. Morphine was used for breakthrough while on transdermal fentanyl. A VAS was used for pain response and side effects. Patients entered on study had severe pain on non-opioids, and weak or potent opioids. Severe pain was defined as to VAS of 80–100. Patients had to have adequate hepatic and renal function. Patients were not included if they were receiving radiation or chemotherapy, suffering from severe obstruction lung disease or actively dying.

Twenty patients with a mean age of 56 years (range 40–88 years) participated in this trial. Fourteen had somatic and/or visceral pain and eight neuropathic pain (two had mixed pain). Sixteen were on oral morphine prior to study with doses ranging between 30 and 200 mg per day for an average of 20 days. Three additional patients were on tramadol and one patient was on high dose subcutaneous morphine prior to study. The mean fentanyl dose on the first day was 1.5 mg (average 30 demand doses). The average bolus dose was 1.25 doses/h. The average VAS decreased to 34 by 24 hours which was 68 prior to PCA. Respiratory depression was not observed. Opioid side effects were increased compared with prestudy. Most patients were on opioids prior to PCA fentanyl and some of the side effects were perhaps carried over from prestudy opioid use. Pain control in this study was achieved in 24 h, though this may be related to the timing of assessment.

In a retrospective review by Devulder, 13 of 92 patients treated for cancer pain over 18 months required PCA morphine as a dosing strategy[20]. A Pharmacia Del-Tech, CADD-PCA pump was used. Both continuous and demand morphine of 1/10th the total daily dose was used with a lockout interval of 30 min. Conversion from oral to subcutaneous morphine was done by using a 2 : 1 ratio. If doses did not adequately reduce pain, a 25% increase in the dose was allowed. Some of these patients were subsequently converted to intrathecal PCA due to the lack of response to parenteral opioid titration after several successive increments in doses. Response to the subcutaneous PCA was not provided in the article, and the rationale for using PCA and patient demographics were not available in the manuscript. The author states that too many rescue boluses were indicative of inadequate doses, which reduced patient satisfaction with PCA.

A second study was published as an abstract by Citron and colleagues in 1993. It compared conventional continuous infusion morphine with PCA in patients on potent opioids with uncontrolled pain or unable to take oral medications[21]. Prior to randomizations, patients received bolus doses of morphine every 15 min for the first 4 h until pain relief was achieved and then were randomized to PCA versus continuous morphine. PCA was by a CADD-PCA pump (Abbott-Life Care 4100). Patients were stratified for neuropathic pain and multiple parameters were followed. Pain was measured by the Memorial Pain Assessment Scale. Pain intensity and pain relief were recorded. A Krantz Health Opinion Survey Behavior subscale, which measures, patient preference and control over ones health, and a Brief Profile of Mood States (BPOMS) for psychological dysfunction, was used for patient characteristics, which may influence response and patient acceptance.

Seventy-nine patients with a mean age of 60 years were admitted to study. Thirty eight were randomized to PCA. In the first 5 days the amount of morphine used was less, but pain intensity was higher in the group receiving PCA morphine by demand. Pain relief was similar between groups. Patients on PCA had less psychological distress and less sedation. The lowest distress was seen in the PCA group who also had adequate pain control. The authors felt that the PCA strategy was superior to continuous infusion morphine due to:

- reduced morphine doses;
- equivalent pain relief;
- less psychological distress.

This study, however, was not a study of pain control, but of pain maintenance using different opioid dosing strategies. The demand only approach to dosing with continuous pain seems at odds with usual recommendations.

Vanier and colleagues performed a randomized double-blind cross-over trial comparing continuous subcutaneous hydromorphone with continuous subcutaneous hydromorphone plus PCA[22]. Eight patients were included in this cross-over trial. Patients were excluded if receiving chemotherapy or radiation, and could not have respiratory compromise. A colored VAS scale was used with the Present Pain Index of the McGill Pain Questionnaire. A VRS was used for side effects.

Prior to study, hydromorphone infusion was titrated to pain control. A CADD-PCA pump (Pharmacia, Quebec, Canada) was utilized. Two pumps per patient were required in this study: one for PCA therapy and one placebo during the continuous infusion (non-PCA) part of the study. All patients received continuous infusion hydromorphone through the second pump. The basal rate was 50–60% of the hourly continuous dose and the bolus was 40–50% of the continuous dose in the PCA arm of the trial. Lockout intervals were 60 min. Cross-over occurred on day 3 of the study.

The mean hourly dose was 1.6 mg with continuous only versus 0.8 mg for PCA. The 36-h hydromorphone dose was 56.3 + 30.1 for continuous infusion and 36.5 + 24.5 for the PCA strategy. Overall, there was a 30% reduction in hydromorphone consumption with the PCA. Rescue doses were greater on PCA as one would anticipate due to reduced continuous infusion doses with the PCA. The pain intensity did not differ between the continuous and the PCA morphine; however, there were large individual differences in pain intensity. No significant respiratory depression or sedation occurred. Three patients felt uncomfortable using the PCA for fear of making a dosing error and two did not activate the PCA device. Four patients preferred the traditional continuous dosing over the PCA. Two patients preferred the PCA[21].

Zech and colleagues expanded their pilot study as previously reviewed to include 70 patients extending the experience with the original 20 patients on their pilot study[22]. Intravenous fentanyl was used to control pain by demand PCA in the first 24 h. Patients were then converted to transdermal fentanyl during the second phase of the study. The mean i.v. fentanyl dose in the first 24 h was the same as in the pilot. Reduction in pain was also similar to the pilot study, which occurred within the first 24 h. Three patients experienced respiratory depression during the demand PCA dose titration. Constipation, nausea and vomiting were not different from prestudy opioid and were actually reduced with the PCA fentanyl.

A consecutive cohort of preterminal cancer patients with severe pain on oral opioids was studied by Meuret and colleagues[23]. A Del-Tech CADD-PCA pump was used for this PCA study. Morphine was given by subcutaneous infusion using a 27-gauge needle. The median daily morphine dose was 93 mg (range 12–464) and the median bolus dose was 5 mg (range 4–10). The lockout interval ranged from 10 to 30 min.

One-hundred-and-forty-three patients were on the study; however, only 120 of the 143 (84%) used self-administered doses by the PCA. The mean study period was 27 days. Morphine requirements increased by a mean of 2.3 mg/day. The mean number of self-administered bolus doses were 1.4/day and the maximum was 61. The median percentage of daily morphine given by demand per day was 5% of the total daily dose with a maximum of 40% delivered by PCA demand. Pain control was excellent in 66%, satisfactory in 30% and insufficient in 4%. Guideline for judging pain response was not provided. Side effects included constipation (42), fatigue (24), nausea (21) and local inflammation at subcutaneous sites (13). Many of the side effects were a carry-over from the prestudy opioid, but this was not addressed by the author.

A randomized cross-over double-blind study of morphine continuous infusion plus PCA was compared epidural and subcutaneous opioid administration[24]. Kalso and colleagues converted other opioids to morphine at equianalgesic doses. After a 2-day washout period, patients were given both subcutaneous and epidural catheters. Physicians who assessed the response of patients in the study were blinded as to the route of administration. Physicians who were responsible for morphine administration were aware of the route. Converting between subcutaneous and epidural infusions was accomplished by using a ratio of 5 : 1 (subcutaneous to epidural). Either 10–20 mg of morphine for subcutaneous PCA or 2–4 mg of morphine for the epidural PCA was initiated. The lockout interval was 60 min for both. A CADD-PCA pump (Pharmacia, Sweden) was used for both subcutaneous and epidural PCA. Patient diaries for pain response were completed four times daily. A VAS (0–100 mm) for both rest and movement related pain were recorded. Pharmacokinetics were done.

Ten patients with an age range of 22–75 years were studied. Nine of the 10 had neuropathic pain. The median prestudy parenteral morphine equivalents were 225 mg (range 120–600). The median calculated 24-h dose determined by dose requirements during the last 4 h of the study was 372 mg for subcutaneous morphine and 106 mg for epidural morphine. Both subcutaneous and epidural morphine were equally effective. The VAS tended to be lower in the subcutaneous group. Nightmares were greater with oral morphine prior to study than subcutaneous or epidural morphine on study. Adverse effects diminished with conversion to subcutaneous or epidural PCA. Five preferred subcutaneous and four preferred epidural PCA. Adverse effects did not differ between epidural and subcutaneous PCA.

This study demonstrates that subcutaneous PCA morphine is as effective for neuropathic pain as epidural morphine. The PCA demand strategy also appears to be effective in incident pain. There were no particular advantages to epidural PCA in this study.

Radbruch and colleagues performed an open-labeled trial involving patients with uncontrolled pain on weak opioids[25]. A PCA demand morphine strategy was utilized. Patients were not admitted to the study if on chemotherapy or radiation. The demand only PCA was morphine 1 mg bolus as needed, with a lockout interval of 5 min for the first 24 h. Conversion to sustained release morphine was done on the second day of the study. The PCA demand dosing continued for breakthrough pain, while on sustained release morphine using 1/12th of the total daily oral dose as rescue and a 20–30-min lockout interval. The PCA was discontinued when less than two rescue doses were required in a 24-h period of time. Patients diaries were completed four times daily using a numerical scale (0–100) for pain severity. Effective analgesia was defined as the numerical score of less than 30. A VRS was used for adverse effects, an 11-step numerical scale was used for mood and a VRS five-step scale for sleep.

Twenty-eight patients participated, 26 were evaluable. The mean morphine dose in the first 24 h was 32 mg (range 4–78, parenteral). On the day of PCA termination the mean morphine dose was 139 mg (range 20–370, oral). The mean conversion ratio was 1–3.8 (parenteral to oral). A subset of patients who were closely followed had a mean time to effective pain control of 5 h (range 1.5–10). Opioid-related side effects included nausea, constipation, vomiting, sedation, dyspnea, pruritus and dry mouth, but were mild and responded to adjuvants. Two patients with lung cancer developed symptoms of bowel obstruction, while on the PCA. Sleep improved, but mood was unchanged by the PCA. Patient satisfaction was 80%.

This study is a PCA titration study. The mean onset to analgesia was 5–6 h in a subset of closely observed patients, which is longer than by traditional titration. The rationale for PCA over and against continuous oral morphine or parenteral morphine was not discussed.

In this systematic review 490 patients were treated in 12 prospective and one retrospective trial using PCA strategies. One study of 20 patient pilot was an extended study of 70 patients. Most patients were receiving potent oral opioids, and had poorly controlled pain or side effects. The mean age ranged from 56 to 61 years, but with a wide range among participants. Six studies were demand only. Seven studies had 20 patients or less. Three were randomized, one compared standard PCA with pharmacokinetic PCA, one with continuous morphine, and one epidural with subcutaneous PCA morphine. Morphine was used as the most frequent opioid with hydromorphone and fentanyl given to a smaller number of patients. The techniques and strategies varied and involved:

- morphine 1 mg on demand with a 6-min lockout interval;
- 4 mg of morphine with a lockout interval of 30 to 60 min;
- continuous morphine plus a demand of 50–100% of the hourly dose and a lockout interval of 30 to 60 min;

- continuous morphine plus 25% of the hourly dose as demand with a lockout interval of 60 to 120 min;
- 3–4 mg of continuous morphine with a demand of 1–5 mg hourly;
- 1–2 mg of morphine with a lockout interval of 10 min;
- fentanyl with a demand of 50 mcg and a lockout interval of 5 min;
- 1/10th of the total daily morphine dose as demand with a lockout interval of 30 min;
- morphine with an infusion of 50 to 60% of the total dose as continuous dose;
- 40–50% of the total daily dose as a demand with a lockout interval of 1 h;
- continuous morphine plus demand at 5 mg every 10–30 min;
- continuous morphine plus 10–20 mg with a lockout interval of 30 min;
- a demand of 1 mg morphine with a lockout interval of 5 min followed by oral sustained release morphine and ongoing PCA demand as rescue at 20–30 min.

This large variety of dosing strategies precludes establishing guidelines and meta-analysis.

Response assessment in five studies involved VRS, five used a VAS, one used an NRS and one a Memorial Pain Assessment Score, and two were not published. Individual opioid dosing requirements varied as much as 20-fold or greater between individuals. Responses occurred in most patients. Patient satisfaction was addressed in a few studies and appears to be high overall. Patient preference was divided, and some patients were uncomfortable with the PCA device and strategy. Respiratory arrest occurred in patients with airway compromise. Two patients with lung cancer developed a bowel obstruction after initiation of PCA. Side effects were related to the opioid, but improved with conversion from oral to parenteral opioid. Pump failure was recorded in a few.

Reasons for opioid conversion to PCA dosing include opioid-related side effects, uncontrolled pain and dose finding. Time to analgesia by PCA was longer (6 and 24 h) than traditional dose titration. The advantages to PCA opioid dosing strategies (with or without a continuous infusion) over traditional continuous infusion plus rescue dosing is not well defined within the published literature. In the one randomized control trial by Citron, there was a reduction in morphine dose requirement and equivalent pain relief with less psychological distress. In the cross-over trial by Vainier, there was a reduction in opioid doses with PCA, but increased rescue doses and equal pain relief without improved patient satisfaction.

Conclusions

The advantages of opioid PCA dosing strategies are theoretically based upon the recommended cardinal principles of oral opioid dosing strategy for cancer pain. Multiple schedules involving both demand only and continuous infusion plus demand have been reported. Comparison between trials is impossible. Pain is improved for most patients using PCA. Comparisons to traditional parenteral dosing strategies have not been done in large groups of patients, but the advantages appear to be relatively small. Larger trials and randomized comparisons will be necessary to fully elucidate the advantages or lack of benefit to PCA opioid dosing strategies.

References

1 Lehmann KH. Patient-controlled analgesia with opioids. In: C. Stein (Eds) *Opioid in Pain Control: basic and clinical aspects.* Cambridge: Cambridge University Press, 1999, pp. 270–94.

2 Smythe M. Patient-controlled analgesia: a review. *Pharmacotherapy* 1992; **12**(2): 132–43.

3 Ma CS, Lin D. Patient controlled analgesia: drug options, infusion schedules, and other considerations. *Hosp Formul* 1991; **26**(3): 198–201.

4 Mather LE. Pharmacokinetics and patient-controlled analgesia. *Acta Anaesthesiol Belg* 1992; **43**(1): 5–20.

5 Woodhouse A, Mather LE. The minimum effective concentration of opioids: a revisitation with patient controlled analgesia fentanyl. *Reg Anesth Pain Med* 2000; **25**(3): 259–67.

6 Ripamonti C, Bruera E. Current status of patient controlled analgesia in cancer patients. *Oncology* 1997; **11**(3): 373–80.

7 Patt RB. PCA: prescribing analgesia for home management of severe pain. *Geriatrics* 1992; **47**(3): 69–72.

8 Walsh D. Pharmacological management of cancer pain. *Semin Oncol* 2000; **27**(1): 45–63.

9 Upton RN, Semple TJ, Macintyre PE. Pharmacokinetic optimisation of opioid treatment in acute pain therapy. *Clin Pharmacokinet* 1997; **33**(3): 225–44.

10 Lindley C. Overview of current development in patient-controlled analgesia. *Support Care Cancer* 1994; **2**(5): 319–26.

11 Lutomski DM, Neimeyer S, Payne C, *et al.* Quality assurance in the prescribing of patient-controlled analgesia and long-acting opioids. *Am J Hlth Syst Pharm* 2003; **60**(14): 1476–9.

12 Swanson G, Smith J, Bulich R, *et al.* Patient-controlled analgesia for chronic cancer pain in the ambulatory setting: a report of 117 patients. *J Clin Oncol* 1989; **7**: 1903–8.

13 Baumann TJ, Batenhorst RL, Graves DA, *et al.* Patient-controlled analgesia in the terminally ill cancer patient. *Drug Intell Clin Pharm* 1986; **20**: 297–301.

14 Citron ML, Johnston-Early A, Boyer M, *et al.* Patient-controlled analgesia for severe cancer pain. *Arch Intern Med* 1986; **146**: 734–6.

15 Kerr IG, Sone M, De Angelis C, *et al.* Continuous narcotic infusion with patient-controlled analgesia for chronic cancer pain in outpatients. *Annl Intern Med* 1988; **108**: 554–7.

16 Wagner JC, Souders GD, Coffman LK, *et al.* Management of chronic cancer pain using a computerized ambulatory patient-controlled analgesia pump. *Hosp Pharm* 1989; **24**: 639–44.

17 Hill HF, Mackie AM, Coda BA, *et al.* Patient-controlled analgesic administration. A comparison of steady-state morphine infusions with bolus doses. *Cancer* 1991; **67**: 873–82.

18 Zech DFJ, Grond SUA, Lynch J, *et al.* Transdermal fentanyl and initial dose-finding with patient-controlled analgesia in cancer pain. A pilot study with 20 terminally ill cancer patients. *Pain* 1992; **50**(3): 293–301.

19 Devulder J. PCA and cancer pain. *Acta Anesthesiol Belg* 1992; **43**(1): 53–6.

20 Citron M, Conaway M, Zhukovsky D, *et al.* Efficacy of patient-controlled analgesia (PCA) vs. continuous intravenous morphine (CIVM) for the treatment of severe cancer pain. *Proc Am Soc Clinical Oncol* 1993; **12**: 433.

21 Vanier MC, Labrecque G, Lepage-Savary D, *et al.* Comparison of hydromorphone continuous subcutaneous infusion and basal rate subcutaneous infusion plus PCA in cancer pain: a pilot study. *Pain* 1993; **53:** 27–32.

22 Zech DFJ, Lehmann LA. Transdermal fentanyl in combination with initial intravenous dose titration by patient-controlled analgesia. *Anti-Cancer Drugs* 1995; **6(Supp13):** 44–9.

23 Meuret G, Jocham G. Patient-controlled analgesia (PCA) in the domiciliary care of tumour patients. *Cancer Treat Rev* 1992; **22(Suppl A):** 137–40.

24 Kalso E, Heiskanen T, Rantio M, *et al.* Epidural and subcutaneous morphine in the management of cancer pain: a double-blind cross-over study. *Pain* 1996; **67:** 443–9.

25 Radbruch L, Loick G, Schulzeck S, *et al.* Intravenous titration with morphine for severe cancer pain: report of 28 cases. *Clin J Pain* 1999; **15:** 173–8.

Chapter 21

Spinal opioids in cancer pain

Mellar P. Davis

Introduction

The initial use of spinal opioid infusions for cancer pain was reported in 1979[1]. Intraspinal drug administration routes are either intrathecal or epidural. Some consider spinal drug infusions as the fourth step in the World Health Organization analgesic ladder[1,2]. Spinal opioid strategies are based upon the theory that the action of opioids is regionally confined to the dorsal horn. This action is thought to be a means of improving analgesia and reducing toxicity, which improves the therapeutic index of opioids. The advantages to spinal opioids compared with spinal anesthetics for pain control is the lack of motor and sensory deficits with spinal opioids, which are dose limiting to spinal anesthetics. In addition, at least with hydrophilic opioids, there is a prolonged period of analgesia per dose due to its regional confinement compared with systemic opioids. A single morphine dose given intrathecally will extend the duration of analgesia to 16 h compared with only 3–6 h for systemically administered morphine. Also, smaller doses of spinal opioids are required to produce the same degree of analgesia produced by systemic morphine[3]. Recommendations by an expert panel from the European Association of Palliative Care are that spinal opioids should be considered for those patients with intolerable side effects from opioids despite optimal systemic dosing, the optimal use of adjuvants and opioid rotation[4]. Other reviews of spinal opioid therapy confirm these recommendations[5]. The addition of bupivicaine and clonidine can improve movement related and neuropathic pain where the exclusive use of spinal opioids fails[4]. The lack of pain response to oral opioids or systemic opioids predicts a poor response to the use of spinal opioids alone[6–8]. It is estimated that 2–8% of patients who have been treated aggressively and optimally with systemic opioids, adjuvants, by opioid conversion and rotation will finally require spinal analgesia for pain control[9]. Spinal opioids, however, should not be used indiscriminately, since there are additional significant risks to this invasive strategy[10].

Neuroanatomy and pharmacology

Opioid receptors are located on peripheral afferent fibers and pre and postsynaptic dorsal horn neurons. All three major opioid receptors, which include mu, delta and kappa opioid receptors (MOR, DOR and KOR) are found in high concentrations within the superficial laminae of the dorsal horn[11]. Opioid receptor activation hyperpolarizes primary afferent fibers and prevents depolarization of postsynaptic fibers. This is done by:

+ stimulating inward rectifying potassium channels;
+ blocking the influx of calcium through voltage gate calcium channels, thereby preventing release of substance P and calcitonin gene-related peptide (CGRP)[11].

In addition opioids inhibit adenylyl cyclase, which prevents cyclic AMP production, a major mediator of pronociceptive[12]. Opioid receptors must couple to certain intracellular G-proteins in order to relieve pain. Subclasses of the three major receptors exist, which are derived from a single gene as a result of post-transcriptional splicing differences of receptor mRNA. These variations in receptor mRNA processing account in part of differences in opioid responses between individuals and opioid analgesic non-cross-tolerance. Distinct populations of opioid receptors can be found in different parts of the central nervous system, which contribute to differences in opioid receptor action[11]. MOR receptors are found in greater abundance within the dorsal horn followed by DOR and KOR.

Opioids also bind to receptors and activate superspinal descending neuromodulating pathways found in the periaqueductal gray (PAG) and rostroventromedial medulla (RVM). Microinjections of morphine within the PAG and RVM reduce pain by increasing PAG and RVM neurotransmission. This results in a blunting of painful afferent neurotransmission through the dorsal horn[13].

Opioid intrinsic efficacy relates to the degree of receptor activation generated by an agonist receptor interaction. This biological effect can be quantified by increases in potassium influx and also quantified by the binding of a radio-labeled (^{35}S, GTPgamma-S) to G proteins (G alpha), which is the initial response that occurs with receptor activation. Intrinsic efficacy can be theoretically viewed as the number of receptors needed to be occupied by opioids in order to produce maximum analgesia. Efficacy directly correlates with the opioid 'receptor reserve'[12]. Intrinisic efficacy is governed by the stimulus (pain), receptor configuration (genetics) particularly G-protein interaction, opioid binding affinity and opioid receptor phosphorylation[12,14]. Spinal opioids do not improve opioid intrinsic efficacy since spinal opioids will not influence many of the factors that determine intrinsic efficacy. Neither the conformation of the receptor nor G protein binding is influenced by opioid concentration. Therefore, if pain is refractory to opioids, spinal opioids alone are unlikely to improve the pain response.

Although there is a poor relationship between opioid receptor binding and opioid physicochemical properties, it is the latter characteristic, which predicts opioid spinal pharmacology along with a second major factor, the anatomy of the spine[12,14].

The epidural space is an area circumscribed by the spinal canal, but outside the dural sac. This space contains fat, which provides both a lubricating and padding function[15,16]. The epidural space is largely a potential space since much of the dural sac fills the spinal canal. Large areas of the epidural sac come into direct contact with the bone and ligaments of the spinal canal. The dura is not actually attached to the spinal canal, but is in close proximity to it. The epidural fat is not uniformly distributed, but layered in a series of circumferential compartments between which the dura approximates the spinal canal wall[15,16]. Epidural catheters can freely enter the epidural space. The posterior compartment, where epidural catheters are most frequently placed, is steeply arched by a paired ligamenta flavum. This triangular space bordered by the ligamenta flavum and dura is filled with fat, which alters the distribution of lipophilic opioids. The lateral epidural space, which is medial to the intraventricular foramen and communicates with the intra-abdominal space is subject to increased intra-abdominal pressures transmitted to the epidural space through the foramina. Increased abdominal pressures will increase spinal anesthetic responses[15,16]. Solutions injected into the posterior epidural space freely, but unevenly distribute throughout the space unless flow is limited by epidural tumor. Small volumes of fluid (i.e. 4 ml) are usually asymmetrically distributed[15–18]. Solutions injected into the epidural space spread through numerous small channels, rather than an advancing wave. Solutions spread non-uniformly, but reliably approximate the nerves in the intervertebral foramina. Both the dorsal root ganglia and the sheath containing the roots are directly bathed by epidural solutions[16–18]. Epidural fluid follows along nerve roots and beyond the dorsal ganglion. The large surface area of the nerve sheath and small volume of CSF surrounding the root within the nerve sheath is a favorable site for spinal anesthetic and analgesics, rather than the spinal cord. This may be a critical reason why catheters location in close proximity to the site of pain is necessary for successful spinal therapy[19].

A blood–brain barrier exists, which regulates the ingress of biologically active molecules into the brain and central nervous system. Brain capillaries are not fenestrated and contain tight junctions with high electrical resistances. Cellular extensions from astrocytes (called foot processes) maintain the blood brain barrier[12,14]. Infusions of drug must pass through a series of alternating lipid and aqueous interfaces, consisting of cell membranes and aqueous cellular cystol. The rate limiting spinal membrane to opioid distribution is the arachnoid and not dura. The lipophilic nature of an opioid dictates its ability to transverse the blood–brain barrier. This is reflected in the drug's partition coefficient. This coefficient, which measures the distribution of a drug between aqueous and lipid (octanol) solvents is expressed as a ratio. Higher numbers indicate greater lipid solubility[12,14]. The higher the partition coefficients, particularly if greater than 100 (log 2 partition coefficient), the more difficult it is for an opioid to transverse the blood–brain barrier to receptor sites. As lipid solubility increases, the drug becomes sequestered in fat (epidural fat) and myelin. Highly lipophilic drugs are prevented from entering the hydrophilic environment of the dorsal horn due to thermodynamically unfavorable factors. Spinal lipophilic opioids, such as fentanyl, methadone, sufentanil, meperidine and alfentanil, are sequestered in myelin and epidural fat before reaching receptors in the dorsal horn. They are then rapidly and systematically absorbed through capillaries. As a result, opioid potency will largely reflect a 'bell-shaped' curve when plotted against partition coefficients[12,14]. Spinal lipophilic opioids lack the relative regional benefits of spinal hydrophilic opioids and will have a relative reduction in potency as compared with hydrophilic opioids. For example, epidural morphine is 5–10 times more potent that parenteral morphine and intrathecal morphine is 5–10 times more potent that epidural. However, epidural fentanyl is only twice as potent as parenteral fentanyl[3,20]. Rapid systemic re-absorption of lipophilic opioids causes rapid analgesia relative to hydrophilic opioids and early side effects such as nausea when compared with morphine due to rapid distribution[1].

Opioid responsiveness and spinal infusion strategies

The pain response to spinal opioids is highly variable. Most patients experience a 50–60% reduction in pain, but many require supplemental systemic analgesics or intraspinal adjuvants such as bupivicaine and clonidine in order to have pain relief to achieve these percentages of pain relief [3,21]. Failure rates with spinal opioids alone are as high as 30%[22]. Certain pains are poorly responsive to spinal opioids and are colic, neuropathic pain, incident pain and pain from cutaneous ulcers[23,24]. Diffuse visceral pain and poorly localized bone pain (particularly involving the lower extremity or pelvis) seem to be most responsive to spinal opioids. Pains that are responsive to systemic opioids are also more likely to respond to spinal opioids[3,23]. Although conversion to spinal opioids does not improve pain relief, it does significantly reduce side effects thereby extending the opioid therapeutic index[10,25]. Dorsal horn opioid receptors are the main target of spinal opioids, however, MOR and DOR are found in the descending bulbospinal pathways, the forebrain, cingulate cortex, limbic lobe and the thalamic nuclei[26]. The degree to which each pathway plays a role in the overall benefits of spinal opioids is not known. The optimal response to an opioid may require opioids to bind to bulbar, spinal and peripheral receptors.

Intrathecal morphine can reduce pain within 15–60 min and will have a duration of action as long as 30 h[27]. There are no consensus guidelines for conversion from systemic to spinal opioids[23]. However, intrathecal morphine doses by clinical experience are approximately 1/10th of epidural does that in turn are 1/10th of parenteral morphine doses[1,8,28,29]. On the other hand, Kalso and colleagues found that a ratio of 3 : 1 was optimal in their experience with conversion from subcutaneous to epidural hydrophilic opioids in a small number of patients[30]. The onset to analgesia with epidural morphine is slower than for the lipophilic opioids. Lipophilic opioids, however, require continuous infusion due to the rapid redistribution, whereas hydrophilic opioids can be bolused for sustained analgesia due to being regionally confined. Systemic absorption of fentanyl with redistribution to fentanyl is much greater than that of morphine and, as a result, there is a greater degree of somnolence with fentanyl[31]. Delayed respiratory depression occurs with both morphine and fentanyl; however, fentanyl has delayed respiratory depression due to systemic redistribution to brainstem, while morphine has delayed respiratory depression from its rostral migration through the CSF to the brainstem[32].

Continuous epidural or intrathecal opioid infusion has a particular advantage in the home setting due to the ease of administration[33,34]. A patient-controlled analgesia (PCA) strategy with intrathecal or epidural opioids by demand only or demand plus continuous infusion is a popular strategy for pain management after surgical procedures, and may be adapted to be used at home[22].

The placement of the spinal catheter should be near the painful spinal segment for greatest anticipated benefit and for the lowest dose. However, many individuals have multiple painful vertebral sites, which make it difficult to choose the best site for catheter placement[7,23]. The most rostral painful site may be a reasonable choice for catheter placement. Patients treated with intrathecal opioids who develop significant epidural tumor extension with spinal canal compression will start to require higher opioid doses than before tumor extension. Patients with epidural tumor will experience radicular pain with intrathecal injection[35]. Prior to committing to spinal therapy (particularly intrathecal) prior to permanent catheter placement and prior to a test dose of morphine for pain response should be done in order to judge the benefits of spinal opioids.

Intrathecal opioids are preferred over epidural dosing in the long run survival is anticipated to be months. Intrathecal therapy has a lower rate of catheter complications in the long run. Intrathecal catheters function longer and lower opioid doses are required for pain control[7,8,23,36,37]. Due to lower drug volumes for intrathecal therapy there will be fewer pump refills over time and a longer time between refills as compared with epidural therapy, which reduces the risk of catheter infections[23]. The choice between an external or implantable pump will be dependent upon prognosis, patient experience, patient preference and cost. The break-even time economically between epidural and intrathecal modes of delivery is approximately 3 months[8]. Other investigators have found the break-even point at 4–6 months[38]. Percutaneous externalized tunneled catheters are most appropriate for those with days to weeks to survive[23]. An alternative for others is a tunneled intrathecal catheter attached to a subcutaneous port, which is accessed percutaneously[39].

Intracerebroventricular opioids

Intracerebroventricular (ICV) opioids are an alternative for patients with intractable pain. In a review of studies involving a total of 268 patients receiving ICV opioids, excellent pain relief was achieved in 75% of patients receiving intracerebroventricular opioids compared with 58% of patients receiving intrathecal and 72% of patients receiving epidural opioids[40,41]. These trials of various routes of administration were not direct comparisons and are certainly subject to individual bias. However, ICV opioid infusions should be considered in patients with severe pain with an obstructed spinal canal and/or intractable face, neck or upper thoracic pain, which is unresponsive to systemic opioids[42].

Spinal opioids and refractory pain dosing strategies

Responses to spinal morphine do not correlate with either cerebrospinal fluid (CSF) or plasma morphine concentrations[43]. Progressive pain with spinal opioids may be due to tumor at a site remote from the catheter placement[44]. Technical problems with catheters and pumps are another cause of failure when technical failure has been ruled out in patients who are not responding to spinal opioids, response can occur either by increasing the spinal opioid dose or by spinal opioid rotation. Initial management of these patients should be an increase by 30–50% of the existing opioid dose titrated every few days until pain relief is achieved or toxicity occurs. Additional precautions should taken to monitor for opioid hyperalgesia syndrome when escalating spinal opioids. This syndrome is characterized by severe neuropathic hypersensitivity in the lower extremity and autonomic abnormalities. Opioid-induced hyperalgesia may be associated with segmental myoclonus and cutaneous piloerection[45]. The opioid hyperalgesic syndrome is a risk with intrathecal doses of morphine that are greater than 20 mg/day. Spinal opioid rotation or a switch from epidural to spinal opioids has been reported to reestablish pain control with opioid induced hyperalgesia[39,46–49].

Pain that is refractory to spinal opioids may respond to dilute concentrations of a local anesthetic like bupivacaine or to an alpha-2 adrenoreceptor agonist like clonidine[39,50]. Bupivicaine is the local anesthetic most commonly used with refractory pain. Forty to ninety per cent of patients with cancer pain that is refractory to epidural or intrathecal morphine alone will respond to the addition of 0.1–0.5% bupivacaine infused at 4–10 ml/h[23,37,47,51–53]. Patients with neuropathic pain or incident pain are more likely to require the addition of bupivacaine[39]. The total bupivacaine dose, rather than its concentration is a more important factor in predicting pain response[52]. Large intrathecal bupivacaine doses (ranging between 60 and 300 mg) are required with deafferentation pain, brachial and lumbar plexopathy, or pain arising from a large ulcerative mucocutaneous tumor[54]. The usual ratio for intrathecal morphine to bupivacaine ratio is 1 : 10 (morphine to bupivicaine) and for epidural the ratio is 1 : 1. The conversion from epidural morphine plus bupivacaine to intrathecal morphine plus bupivacaine will improve pain response in those not responding to the epidural combination[53]. Another advantage to the addition of bupivacaine is a reduction in overall infusion volume. Bupivacaine has antimicrobial properties and may reduce infections. Continuous bupivacaine infusion, rather than bolus dosing is necessary to prevent side effects, since bolus bupivacaine will cause paralysis and hemodynamic instability[52]. Bupivacaine unfortunately produces gait abnormalities and paralysis despite continuous infusion with high doses. This side effect may make it difficult to determine the cause of a neurological deficit as to whether it is a bupivacaine complication or the progression of tumor and spinal cord compression[23,52,53,55,56]. It is unusual to see bupivicaine-induced paralysis if doses are maintained at or below 30–60 mg/day[7,23,35].

Analgesia with morphine will also improve with the addition of spinal clonidine whether given by the epidural or intrathecal route[56–58]. Alpha$_{2C}$ adrenoreceptors are found within the superficial laminae of the dorsal horn close to the opioid receptors, which are bound and activated by clonidine. Clonidine blocks pre- and postsynaptic sensory neurons independent of opioid receptors and this blocking action is no reversed by naloxone[57,59]. Non-overlapping toxicities exist between clonidine and morphine, which provide an additional rationale for this combination[57,60]. Clonidine further improves morphine analgesia and secondarily reduces bupivacaine toxicity when triple drug combination is used for refractory pain. Clonidine will reduce opioid requirements, and as a result indirectly prevents opioid hyperalgesia and myoclonus[23,61,62]. Clonidine infusions are usually started at 30 mcg/h (range 10–40), with an average daily dose of 720 mcg[1]. Intrathecal and epidural clonidine are rapidly systemically absorbed. Common clonidine side effects include hypotension and bradycardia[57,62,63]. Clonidine alone is usually ineffective in reducing neuropathic pain long term. Like morphine, clonidine is best infused close to the critically painful spinal segment[44].

Spinal analgesia and opioid tolerance

Long-term intrathecal morphine increases CSF levels of excitatory amino acids, which are associated with pain and morphine tolerance[64]. Clinically, however, tolerance is not usually a problem in cancer patients and dose adjustments are due to progressive disease for the majority of patients[27]. It is important to rule out technical failure (which can mimic opioid tolerance) when extraordinary morphine dose escalation is required in a patient whose pain was previously controlled before attributing the pain to opioid tolerance. Analgesia tolerance does occur in animal studies with spinal opioids, to a greater extent with continuous infusion compared with bolus dosing[29]. In certain patients, series dose escalations as great as 5% per day without detectable tumor progression have been reported, indicating some degree of analgesic tolerance[28]. Others have demonstrated a much smaller daily dose increment and analgesia tolerance[26]. Management of opioid tolerance like refractory pain can be done by dose escalation, opioid rotation or the addition of bupivacaine or clonidine[50]. Conversion from epidural to intrathecal morphine or spinal opioid rotation may re-establish analgesia[46,48].

Toxicity

The toxicities associated with spinal opioids are divided into those related to opioid, and those related to the procedure, such as catheter complications and pump failure (Tables 21.1, 21.2, 21.3 and 21.4). The incidence of catheter complications is directly related to the frequency of catheter manipulation and the number of refills required.

Table 21.1 Adverse effects of spinal opioids

Constipation
Urinary retention
Nausea
Vomiting
Over sedation
Myoclonus
Nightmares
Pruritus
Sweating
Hyperalgesia syndrome
Hypogonadotrophin hypogonadism
Loss of libido
Impotence
Dry mouth
Worsening lower extremity edema
Analgesic tolerance
Respiratory depression
Perioral paresthesia

Table 21.2 Surgery complications

Skin breakdown
Wound infection
Bleeding
Hematoma
Epidural abscess
Meningitis
CSF leak
Postdural puncture headache

Complications increase with time when epidural catheters are used, but are inversely related to time with intrathecal catheters. If prolonged infusions are necessary then the intrathecal route is preferred. However, exteriorized tunneled intrathecal catheters, which were initially thought to be a great risk for infections, can be safely maintained for 7 days or longer in those patients who are actively dying, and for whom it would be inappropriate to place on implantable systems[65–70].

Table 21.3 Catheter complications

Dislodgement or withdrawal
Intralumen occlusion
Catheter kink and obstruction
Catheter leak
Disconnection between the pump and implanted catheter
Scarring at catheter tip (epidural)
Tip granuloma (intrathecal)
Tunnel infection

Table 21.4 Pump failure

Program dysfunction
Irregular flow rate
Battery failure
Pump torsion
Programing error
Failure of the alarm system

Conclusions

Spinal opioids are necessary to control cancer pain in less than 10% of patients. Morphine is the drug of choice due to its relatively favorable regional confinement and the extensive clinical experience with morphine. The choice of routes, i.e. epidural or intrathecal, and adjuvants will depend upon patient prognosis and demographics, and pain severity and characteristics.

References

1 **Kedlaya D, Reynolds L, Waldman S.** Epidural and intrathecal analgesia for cancer pain. *Best Pract Res Clin Anaesthesiol* 2002; **16(4):** 651–65.

2 **Ripamonti C, Zecca E, De Conno F.** Pharmacological treatment of cancer pain: alternative routes of opioid administration. *Tumori* 1998; **84(3):** 289–300.

3 **Lindley C.** Overview of current development in patient-controlled analgesia. *Support Care Cancer* 1994; **2(5):** 319–26.

4 **Hanks GW, Conno F, Cherny N, et al.** Morphine and alternative opioids in cancer pain: the EAPC recommendations. *Br J Cancer* 2001; **84(5):** 587–93.

5 **Krames ES.** Practical issues when using neuraxial infusion. *Oncology* 1999; **13(5 Suppl. 2):** 37–44.

6 **Arner S, Arner B.** Differential effects of epidural morphine in the treatment of cancer-related pain. *Acta Anaesthesiol Scand* 1985; **29(1):** 32–6.

7 **Mercandante S.** Problems of long-term spinal opioid treatment in advanced cancer patients. *Pain* 1999; **79:** 1–13.

8 **Krames ES.** Intrathecal infusional therapies for intractable pain: patient management guidelines. *J Pain Sympt Manag* 1993; **8(1):** 36–46.

9 **Hogan Q, Haddox JD, Abram S,** *et al.* Epidural opiates and local anesthetics for the management of cancer pain. *Pain* 1991; **46(3):** 271–9.

10 **Zech DF, Grond S, Lynch J,** *et al.* Validation of World Health Organization Guidelines for cancer pain relief: a 10-year prospective study. *Pain* 1995; **63(1):** 65–76.

11 **Cesselin F, Benoliel J, Bourgoin S,** *et al.* Spinal mechanisms of opioid analgesia. In: Stein C. (Ed.) *Opioids in Pain Control Basic and Clinical Aspects.* Cambridge: Cambridge University Press, 1999, pp. 70–95.

12 **Bernards CM.** Clinical implications of physiochemical properties of opioids. In: Stein C. (Ed.) *Opioids in Pain Control Basic and Clinical Aspects.* Cambridge: Cambridge University Press, 1999, pp. 166–186.

13 **Heinricher MM, Morgan MM.** Supraspinal mechanisms of opioid analgesia. In: Stein C. (Ed.) *Opioids in Pain Control Basic and Clinical Aspects.* Cambridge: Cambridge University Press, 1999, pp. 46–69.

14 **Bernards CM.** Understanding the physiology and pharmacology of epidural and intrathecal opioids. *Best Pract Res Clin Anaesthesiol* 2002; **16(4):** 489–505.

15 **Hogan QH.** Epidural anatomy: new observations. *Can J Anaesth* 1998; **45(5):** 40–4.

16 **Hogan Q, Toth J.** Anatomy of soft tissues of the spinal cord. *Region Anesth Pain Med* 1999; **24(4):** 303–10.

17 **Hogan Q.** Distribution of solution in the epidural space: examination by cryomicrotome section. *Region Anesth Pain Med* 2002; **27(2):** 150–6.

18 **Hogan Q.** Anatomy of spinal anesthesia: some old and new findings. *Region Anesth Pain Med* 1998; **23(4):** 340–3.

19 **Liu SS, Bernards CM.** Exploring the epidural trail. *Region Anesth Pain Med* 2002; **27(2):** 122–4.

20 **McQuay HJ, Sullivan AF, Smallman K,** *et al.* Intrathecal opioids, potency and lipophilicity. *Pain* 1989; **36(1):** 111–15.

21 **Krames ES, Gershow J, Glassberg A,** *et al.* Continuous infusion of spinally administered narcotics for the relief of pain due to malignant disorders. *Cancer* 1985; **56(3):** 696–702.

22 **Chrubasik J, Chrubasik S, Martin E.** Patient-controlled spinal opiate analgesia in terminal cancer. Has the time really arrived? *Drugs* 1992; **43(6):** 709–804.

23 **Mercandante S.** Controversies over spinal treatment in advanced cancer patients. *Support Care Cancer* 1998; **6:** 495–502.

24 **Becker R, Jakob D, Uhle EI,** *et al.* The significance of intrathecal opioid therapy for the treatment of neuropathic cancer pain conditions. *Stereotact Funct Neurosurg* 2000; **75(1):** 16–26.

25 **Samuelsson J, Hedner T.** Pain characterization in cancer patients and the analgetic response to epidural morphine. *Pain* 1991; **46:** 3–8.

26 **Jensen TS.** Opioids in the brain: supraspinal mechanisms in pain control. *Acta Anaesthesiol Scand* 1997; **41:** 123–32.

27 **Gilmer-Hill HS, Boggan JE, Smith KA,** *et al.* Intrathecal morphine delivered via subcutaneous pump for intractable cancer pain a review of the literature. *Surg Neurol* 1999; **51:** 12–15.

28 **Samuelsson H, Malmberg F, Eriksson M,** *et al.* Outcomes of epidural morphine treatment in cancer pain: nine years of clinical experience. *J Pain Sympt Manag* 1995; **10(2):** 105–12.

29 **Gourlay GK, Plummer JL, Cherry DA,** *et al.* Comparison of intermittent bolus with continuous infusion of epidural morphine in the treatment of severe cancer pain. *Pain* 1991; **47(2):** 135–40.

30 **Kalso E, Heiskanen T, Rantio M,** *et al.* Epidural and subcutaneous morphine in the management of cancer pain: a double-blind cross-over study. *Pain* 1996; **67(2–3):** 443–9.

31 Chrubasik J, Chrubasik S, Glass P. Equipotent dose regimens required when comparing epidural opioids. *Can J Anaesth* 1993; **40(8)**: 799–801.

32 Chrubasik J, Martin E, Chrubasik S, *et al*. Epidural opioid selection. *Anesth Analg* 1993; **76(3)**: 674–5.

33 Devulder J, Ghys L, Dhondt W, *et al*. Spinal analgesia in terminal care: risk versus benefit. *J Pain Sympt Manag* 1994; **9(2)**: 75–81.

34 Ohlsson L, Rydberg T, Eden T, *et al*. Cancer pain relief by continuous administration of epidural morphine in a hospital setting and at home. *Pain* 1992; **48(3)**: 349–53.

35 Appelgren L, Nordborg C, Sjoberg M, *et al*. Spinal epidural metastasis: implications for spinal analgesia to treat 'refractory' cancer pain. *J Pain Sympt Manag* 1997; **13(1)**: 25–42.

36 Abram SE. Continuous spinal anesthesia for cancer and chronic pain. *Region Anesth* 1993; **18(Suppl 6)**: 406–13.

37 Van Dongen RT, Crul BJ, De Bock M. Long-term intrathecal infusion of morphine and morphine/bupivacaine mixtures in the treatment of cancer pain: a retrospective analysis of 51 cases. *Pain* 1993; **55(1)**: 119–23.

38 Miguel R. Interventional treatment of cancer pain: the fourth step in the World Health Organization Analgesic Ladder? *Cancer Control* 2000; **7(2)**: 149–56.

39 Patt RB, Chiang JS, Dai CT. Intraspinal opioid therapy for intractable cancer pain. *Int Anesthesiol Clin* 1998; **36(3)**: 105–16.

40 Ballantyne JC, Carr DB, Berkey CD, *et al*. Comparative efficacy of epidural, subarachnoid and intracerebroventricular opioids in patients with pain due to cancer. *Region Anesth* 1996; **21(6)**: 543–56.

41 Anon. Comparative efficacy of epidural, subarachnoid and intracerebroventricular opioids in patients with pain due to cancer. *Database Abstr Rev Effectiveness* 2002; **4**: 1–6.

42 Weigl K, Mundinger F, Chrubasik J. Continuous intraventricular morphine- or peptide-infusion for intractable cancer pain. *Acta Neurochir Suppl* 1987; **39**: 163–5.

43 Samuelsson H, Hedner T, Venn R, *et al*. CSF and plasma concentrations of morphine and morphine glucuronides in cancer patients receiving epidural morphine. *Pain* 1993; **52(2)**: 179–85.

44 Ackerman LL, Follett KA, Rosenquist RW. Long-term outcomes during treatment of chronic pain with intrathecal clonidine or clonidine/opioid combinations. *J Pain Sympt Manag* 2003; **26(1)**: 668–77.

45 Portenoy RK, Savage SR. Clinical realities and economic considerations: special therapeutic issues in intrathecal therapy—tolerance and addition. *J Pain Sympt Manag* 1997; **14(3)**: S27–35.

46 De Leon-Casasola OA, Lema MJ. Epidural bupivacaine/sufentanil therapy for postoperative pain control in patients tolerant to opioid and unresponsive to epidural bupivacaine/morphine. *Anesthesiology* 1994; **80(2)**: 303–9.

47 Hogan Q, Haddox JD, Abram S, *et al*. Epidural opiates and local anesthetics for the management of cancer pain. *Pain* 1991; **46(3)**: 271–9.

48 Pfeifer BL, Sernaker HL, Ter Horst UM, *et al*. Cross-tolerance between systematic and epidural morphine in cancer patients. *Pain* 1989; **39(2)**: 181–7.

49 Boersma FP, Noordiun H, Vanden Bussche G. Epidural sufentanil for cancer pain control in outpatients. *Region Anesth* 1989; **14(6)**: 293–7.

50 Van Dongen RT, Crul BJ, van Egmond J. Intrathecal coadministration of bupivacaine diminishes morphine dose progression during long-term intrathecal infusion in cancer patients. *Clin J Pain* 1999; **15(3)**: 166–72.

51 Du Pen SL, Kharasch ED, Williams A, *et al*. Chronic epidural bupivacaine-opioid infusion in intractable cancer pain. *Pain* 1992; **49**: 293–300.

52 Sjoberg M, Nitescu P, Appelgren L, et al. Long-term intrathecal morphine and bupivacaine in patients with refractory cancer pain. Results from a morphine: bupivacaine dose regimen of 0.5 : 4.75 mg/ml. Anesthesiology 1994; 80(2): 287–97.

53 Nitescu P, Appelgren L, Linder LE, et al. Epidural versus intrathecal morphine-bupivacaine: assessment of consecutive treatments in advanced cancer pain. J Pain Sympt Manag 1990; 5(1): 18–26.

54 Sjoberg M, Appelgren L, Einarsson S, et al. Long-term intrathecal morphine and bupivacaine in 'refractory' cancer pain. I. Results from the first series of 52 patients. Acta Anaesthesiol Scand 1991; 35(1): 30–43.

55 Sjogren P, Banning A. Pain, sedation and reaction time during long-term treatment of cancer patients with oral and epidural opioids. Pain 1989; 39: 5–11.

56 Mercandate S. Neuraxial techniques for cancer pain: an option about unresolved therapeutic dilemmas. Region Anesth Pain Med 1999; 24(1): 74–83.

57 Eisenach JC, Du Pen S, Du Bois M, et al. Epidural clonidine analgesia for intractable cancer pain. Pain 1995; 61: 391–9.

58 Klimscha W, Chiari A, Krafft P, et al. Hemodynamic and analgesic effects of clonidine added repetitively to continuous epidural and spinal blocks. Anesth Analg 1995; 80(2): 322–7.

59 Fairbanks CA, Stone LS, Kitto KF, et al. a_{2C}-Adrenergic receptors mediate spinal analgesia and adrenergic—opioid synergy. J Pharmacol Exp Therapeut 2001; 300(1): 282–90.

60 Tallarida RJ, Stone DJ, McCary JD, et al. Response surface analysis of synergism between morphine and clonidine. J Pharmacol Exp Therapeut 1998; 289(1): 8–13.

61 Tumber PS, Fitzgibbon DR. The control of severe cancer pain by continuous intrathecal infusion and patient controlled intrathecal analgesia with morphine, bupivacaine and clonidine. Pain 1998; 78: 217–20.

62 Eisenach JC, Rauck RL, Buzzanell C, et al. Epidural clonidine analgesia for intractable cancer pain: Phase I. Anesthesiology 1989; 71(5): 647–52.

63 Boswell G, Bekersky I, Mekki Q, et al. Plasma concentrations and disposition of clonidine following a constant 14-day epidural infusion in cancer patients. Clin Ther 1997; 19(5): 1024–30.

64 Wong CS, Chang YC, Yeh CC, et al. Loss of intrathecal morphine analgesia in terminal cancer patients is associated with high levels of excitatory amino acids in the CSF. Can J Anaesth 2002; 49(6): 561–5.

65 Nitescu P, Appelgren L, Hultman E, et al. Long-term, open catheterization of the spinal subarachnoid space for continuous infusion of narcotic and bupivacaine in patients with 'refractory' cancer pain. A technique of catheterization and its problems and complications. Clin J Pain 1991; 7(2): 143–61.

66 Nitescu P, Sjoberg M, Appelgren L, et al. Complications of intrathecal opioids and bupivacaine in the treatment of 'refractory' cancer pain. Clin J Pain 1995; 11(1): 45–62.

67 Smitt PS, Tsafka A, Teng-van de Zande F, et al. Outcome and complications of epidural analgesia in patients with chronic cancer pain. Cancer 1998; 83: 2015–22.

68 Abs R, Verhelst J, Maeyaert J, et al. Endocrine consequences of long-term intrathecal administration of opioids. J Clin Endocrinol Metab 2000; 85(6): 2215–22.

69 Aldrete JA, Couto da Silva JM. Leg edema from intrathecal opiate infusions. Eur J Pain 2000; 4(4): 361–5.

70 Gestin Y, Vaino A, Pegurier AM. Long-term intrathecal infusion of morphine in the home care of patients with advanced cancer. Acta Anaesthesiol Scand 1997; 41(1 Pt1): 12–17.

Chapter 22

Opioid-resistant pain

Mellar P. Davis

Introduction

Opioid responsive pain is determined by patient type, drug type, dose and pain characteristics[1]. Several different terms have been used to describe pain that is poorly responsive to opioids; opioid resistant pain, opioid unresponsiveness, opioid insensitive pain, paradoxical or opioid facilitated pain[2]. There are difficulties in determining just when opioid responsiveness ends, since differences in opioid dose requirements are significant between individuals, and what dose titration will relieve pain (rendering an opioid 'refractory' pain responsive)[1]. Under-dosing, poorly prescribed or ineffective dosing strategies, and dosing errors lead to continued severe pain in some patients despite the use of potent opioids. Patients' response to opioids will improve with more skillful prescribing, which considers pain severity and pattern. Certain pains are relatively opioid unresponsive including headache, colic, tenesmus, neuropathic pain, incident pain, cutaneous and idiopathic pain[2–5]. Patients with central neuropathic pain are less responsive to opioids than those with peripheral neuropathic pain[6]. Psychological factors such as anxiety, depression and delirium, will shift opioid dose responses to the 'right'. A history of drug abuse and methadone maintenance is associated with the need for higher opioid doses and opioid refractoriness[2, 7,8]. Advancing cancer increases the incidence of severe pain and, as a result, the need for higher opioid doses that, in turn, increases the risk for dose-limiting toxicity[2,9]. Opioid responsiveness may be limited by the onset of dose-limiting side effects before an adequate level of analgesia is reached[1]. Fortunately, tolerance to side effects such as respiratory depression or nausea develops rapidly with chronic dosing and analgesic tolerance develops slowly[2,9]. Most patients are well served with morphine without the need for opioid rotation, but some will require an opioid switch before their plan becomes responsive.

Pseudo-opioid resistant pain is persistent pain, despite adequate prescribing, and is usually caused by the failure of the family or patient to follow the prescribed regimen. Pseudo-opioid resistance follows from inadequate communication, failure to accept opioids as part of pain management, economic factors (particularly if expensive opioids are used in patients with limited income), and complicated or impossible dosing strategies, which lead to a lack of compliance[10]. A favorable outcome requires many factors on the part of patient and family. These include attention, vigilance, persistence, energy, body control, knowledge acquisition, reasoning, executive function, the ability to prioritize and the integration of the prescribed course of therapy into the patient's daily schedule[10]. At least 30% of patients will not consistently take their medications in the frequency or dose as prescribed[11,12]. Side effects, fear, anxiety and denial often lead to premature discontinuation of opioids. A passive coping style and learned helplessness also contribute to a lack of compliance[10]. Therefore, the patient's compliance to the prescribed course must be verified before labeling the underlying pain as being resistant to opioids.

Opioid tolerance, physical dependence, withdrawal and paradoxical pain

Opioid tolerance is a time-related reduction in response to the same opioid dose. Analgesia diminishes despite continuing stable opioid doses with the caveat that the underlying disease remains unchanged (lack of progression)[1]. Opioid tolerance can occur over days to weeks, and is particular to the individual and type of pain. Opioid schedule and route may also determine analgesic tolerance. Continuous systemic or continuous spinal opioids more readily induce tolerance[13].

Opioid physical dependence can be experienced as an abstinence syndrome from the abrupt withdrawal of potent opioids or with the use of an opioid antagonist. Opioid withdrawal or the introduction of naloxone produces generalized pain, allodynia, hyperalgesia, abdominal cramps, joint and muscle aches. Opioid physical dependence (like tolerance) is clearly due to neuroplastic changes resulting from opioid receptor activation[14].

Sustained opioid administration, which is intended to abolish pain, has been reported to instead produce neuropathic paradoxical pain with dose titration[1,13]. This opioid 'facilitated' pain is an extreme form of opioid tolerance. Spontaneous pain and allodynia with opioid facilitated pain is unrelated to opioid pharmacokinetics or opioid metabolites[1,13]. In summary, opioid dependence, tolerance and facilitated pain are degrees of same neural adaptations from chronic opioid exposure, which result in neuropathic pain and hypersensitivity.

Pathophysiology of opioid refractory pain

The genius of Wall & Melzak's insight into nociceptive processing culminated in the gate theory, which basically states that pain transmitted through the spinal cord from peripheral nociceptors is subject to modulation within the dorsal horn by intrinsic dorsal horn neurons, and downward emanating inhibitory and facilitatory pathways through the supraspinal circuitry[15–18]. Both the facilitation and inhibition of the noxious sensory processing of pain are independently controlled. The pain experience is not set by either the degree of peripheral stimulus intensity or the time of stimulus. A quantum of stimulus does not produce a quantum of pain[18]. Clinically, for instance, not all metastases are painful and pain intensity does not directly correlate with the degree of tissue destruction nor is it quantitatively related to radiographic changes. Opioid requirements may vary among individuals by 100-fold or more, and are unrelated to opioid metabolism. Persistent pathological pain or a persistent peripheral sensory barrage produce central neuroplasticity, which can become self-generating (autonomous). Central pain is self-generating without continuous peripheral sensory input. Persistent peripheral pain will produce neuroplastic changes at several levels within the central nervous system.

Peripheral events

Nerve injury can increase the activity of calcium channels (N-type), decrease MOR density on dorsal root ganglion primary afferents (at least temporarily) and decrease gamma amino butyric acid (GABA) release from the dorsal horn interneurons. Both opioid receptors and GABA neurons are important inhibitors to the depolarization of wide dynamic range (WDR) neurons. WDR neurons are found in lamina IV and V of the dorsal horn[18]. Glutamate release is augmented from injured unmyelinated C-fibers and poorly myelinated A delta fibers and crosses the synaptic junction to bind to N-methyl-D-aspartate (NMDA) receptors. This process enhances the depolarization of sensory afferents and WDR neurons[19]. The loss of MOR and GABA receptors with nerve injury tends to be temporary, but facilitates transiently the noxious sensory input into higher centers[13]. In summary, nerve injury amplifies sensory input and reduces opioid effectiveness[9,18].

Sensory input converges on surrounding afferents (afferents within the same spinal segment dorsal horn laminae) and depolarizes these bystander (metameric) afferents, resulting in secondary hypersensitivity and referred pain[20]. Convergence, spontaneous sensory barrage and reduced sensory thresholds from nerve injury or inflammation continuously depolarize WDR neurons, which accentuates noxious sensory neurotransmission to brainstem, cerebral cortex, prefrontal and cingulate gyrus.

Cellular mechanisms to opioid tolerance

The initial neuronal response to opioids is to reduce adenylyl cyclase activity and reduced cyclic AMP levels, and increase inward rectifying potassium channels, inhibit voltage gate calcium channels, hyperpolarize ascending sensory neurons, and reduce glutamate, substance P and calcitonin gene-related peptide (CGRP) release into synaptic junctions. Bound opioid receptor causes a cascade of events mediated by different G-proteins, which act as a second messenger for opioid responses. Opioid receptor are phosphorylated by G protein-related kinases and other kinases, which desensitize opioid receptors and dampens opioid responses. Adenylyl cyclase activity recovers with chronic opioids and upon opioid withdrawal a rebound response (superactivation)[14].

NMDA receptors and receptor antagonists

NMDA receptors are found in close proximity to opioid receptors in the dorsal horn, and interact with the MOR and DOR[13]. Peripheral nerve injury and activated opioid receptors stimulate NMDA receptors through protein kinase C and phosphorylation of NMDA receptor. Phosphorylation removes magnesium from blocking the receptor's center core which activates the receptor once bound by glutamate. NMDA receptors generate nitric oxide and prostaglandins through nitric oxide synthase and cyclo-oxygenase, respectively[26]. NMDA receptors increase intracellular calcium mobilization, which in turn activates protein kinase C and deactivates opioid receptors through opioid receptor phosphorylation[9]. Inhibiting NMDA receptors and/or blocking nitric oxide synthase reduces opioid tolerance and hypersensitivity from nerve injury[9,26–31]. Certain opioids inhibit NMDA receptors; methadone, meperidine, levorphanol and dextromethorphan[32–35]. Memantine and amantadine are modest NMDA receptor antagonists. Corticosteroids reduce neuropathic pain and are 'opioid sparing' as a co-analgesic, in part through the production of kynurenic acid, an NMDA receptor antagonist and through the inhibition of nitric oxide synthase expression. Corticosteroids will also inhibit calcitonin gene-related peptide, and substance P expression and release[9,36] Non-steroidal anti-inflammatory drugs (NSAIDs) reduce dorsal horn prostaglandins and indirectly dampen NMDA receptor activity. This may require inhibition of both cyclo-oxygenase 1 and 2[9,37–43].

Another cellular adaptation is the recovery of adenylyl cyclase responsiveness, which results in the 'over shoot' production of cyclic AMP upon opioid withdrawal. Superactivation of adenylyl cyclase is a hallmark of opioid physical tolerance[14]. All three major opioid receptors (MOR, DOR, KOR) use inhibitory G proteins (Gi-o) to regulate adenylyl cyclase, ion channels and various kinases[14,44,45]. Opioid physical dependence and tolerance does not depend upon opioid receptor numbers or opioid kinetics but upon an array of subcellular signaling processes, which are triggered by particular components of the heterotrimeric G-proteins[9,14,46–51]. A particular type of G protein dictates the cellular events, which lead to opioid tolerance and receptor desensitization. Opposite effects may be elicited by the various subunits of the G protein complex. For instance, Gx/i blocks a group of adenylyl cyclase isoenzymes, whereas G beta gamma activates other groups of adenylyl cyclase isoenzymes[14,48–51]. Opioid receptors can simultaneously or preferentially interact with different G proteins depending on their CNS location. There are potentially 800 different G protein heterotrimeric combinations based upon known G protein components, which can determine opioid responsiveness. A second group of regulating peptides, the GTPase-activating proteins (RGS) govern the duration of G protein receptor coupling and modulate the duration opioid receptor signaling[14,50,51]. Finally, G proteins induce different oncogene transcripts that, with time, modify opioid receptor responses.

Superspinal signal modifications induced by opioids

The substantia gelatinosa (superficial laminae of the dorsal horn) receives the descending tracts from brainstem nuclei. The unique characteristics of these descending neurons are:

* small receptive fields;
* very prolonged responses to signal stimuli which influences duration of dorsal horn nociceptive processing;
* prolonged habituation;
* shifting receptive fields[15–17].

The most important and best understood pathway is the midbrain periaqueductal gray (PAG) and rostral ventromedial medulla (RVM). Both systems link nociceptive networks within the dorsal horn to neuroaxis and brainstem[52]. The RVM sends projections through the spinal cord dorsolateral funiculus to the superficial layers of the dorsal horn as the final common pathway. Morphine and other opioids suppress nociceptive reflexes and pain behavior in experimental animals when microinjected into the PAG or RVM[52]. RVM-mediated analgesic responses are through the release of monoamines. Morphine responses generated by the RVM are blocked by monoaminergic antagonists, acting on the dorsolateral funiculus of the spinal cord. RVM neurons can be divided into 'on' cells or 'off' cells, based upon physiological responses to acute pain (nocifensive reflex). The action of opioids within the PAG and RVM are mediated by the MOR, which differentially alters the firing frequencies of these two classes of cells within the descending tracts. The 'on' cells are stimulated to fire and 'off' cells inhibited just prior to a reflex pain response[52]. The 'on' cells depolarize to generate a reflex response to painful stimuli, but are otherwise inactive. The 'off' cells are chronically active, but abruptly cease firing prior to a pain response[13,52]. Morphine directly inhibits the 'on' cells and indirectly prevents the 'off' cells from pausing in their usual activity. The 'off' cells are directly blocked by GABA-containing neurons, which are, in turn, blocked by opioids[52]. Thus, morphine causes a 'disinhibition' of RVM 'off' cells.

Neuroplastic changes within the supraspinal circuitry occur with chronic opioids. Cholecystokinin (CCK) receptors, in close proximity to opioid receptors, produce a pronociceptive (anti-opioid) response[1]. Cholecystokinin stimulates spinopedal facilitory pathways ('on' cells) arising from the RVM and inhibits morphine-induced depolarization of 'off' cells[13]. Blockade of the CCK type B receptors (CCK_B receptors) will enhance morphine analgesia.[13]

Dynorphin A is a pronociceptive kappa-related opioid neurotransmitter, which initiates a 'feed forward' pronociceptive response through the release of glutamate and aspartate. Secondarily, dynorphin A enhances the release of substance P and calcitonin gene-related peptide from primary afferents. The release of dynorphin A produces

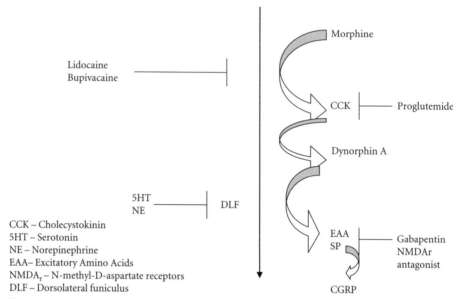

Lidocaine
Bupivacaine

Morphine

CCK —— Proglutemide

Dynorphin A

5HT
NE —— DLF

EAA
SP —— Gabapentin
NMDAr
antagonist

CGRP

CCK – Cholecystokinin
5HT – Serotonin
NE – Norepinephrine
EAA– Excitatory Amino Acids
NMDA$_r$ – N-methyl-D-aspartate receptors
DLF – Dorsolateral funiculus

Fig. 22.1 Neuroplasticity and Opiod Tolerance/Facilatry Pain Supraspinal RVM.

Table 22.1 Opioid tolerance

G-protein uncoupling
G-protein heterotrimeric adaptation
Activation NMDAr through PKC, PIKA
Dynorphin induced release of EAA, SP and CGRP
CCK release
Up regulation of CCK-B receptors
Superactivation of adenylyl cyclase

CCK, cholecystokinin; EAA, excitatory amino acids; NMDA$_r$,
N-methyl-D-asparate receptor; SP, substance P; DLF,
dorsolateral funiculus; 5HT, serotonin; NE, norepinephrine.

allodynia and hyperalgesia. Dynorphin A levels in the spinal fluid are increased with chronic inflammation and nerve injury. This 'feed forward' system is blocked by sectioning the descending dorsolateral funiculus[13].

In summary, prolonged opioid exposure causes both a pronociceptive intracellular and supraspinal response, which leads to opioid tolerance, dependence and, in rare circumstances, paradoxical pain occurs depending upon the degree of neuroplasticity (Fig. 22.1 and Tables 22.1 and 22.2). These changes are counter-regulatory mechanisms, which are responses generated by chronic opioid receptor activation. Intracellular

Table 22.2 Classes of agents that potentially block opioid tolerance[13]

NMDA receptor antagonists
CCK-B receptor antagonists
CGRP antagonists
Calcium channel blockers
NOS inhibitors
PKA inhibitors
PKC inhibitors
Cox inhibitors
Glutamate transport activators
Benzodiazepine antagonists (GABA-B receptor antagonists)

NMDA, N-methyl D-aspartate; CCK-B, cholecystokinin B; CGRP, calcium gene-related protein; NOS, nitric oxide synthase; PKA, protein kinase A; PKC, protein kinase C; Cox, cyclo-oxygenase; GABA, gamma amino butyric acid.

Table 22.3 Pain and patient characteristics predicting opioid responsiveness[3]

Good response	Poor response
Visceral pain	Neuropathic pain
Somatic pain	Mixed pain
Non-incident pain	Incident pain
Absence of somatization	Somatization
Absence of tolerance	Opioid tolerance
Absence of substance abuse	Substance abuse

adaptive changes include increased kinases, altered G-proteins, the activation of NMDA receptors and calcium channels, and transcription of neural oncogenes. In the supraspinal circuitry neurotransmitters, such as CCK and dynorphin A, are released[21–25]. Experimental and clinical experience suggests that interventions that block these adaptive changes improve opioid responsiveness and prevent opioid tolerance (Table 22.3)[13].

Clinical implications and drug choices in the patient with opioid refractory pain or opioid tolerance

Assessment of opioid resistant pain

A prospective study determined the effectiveness of a staging system to predict opioid responsiveness in cancer pain[52]. The Edmondton Staging System divided patients into stage 1 (good risk) and stage 2 (poor risk) based upon pain mechanism, pain characteristics, previous opioid doses, cognitive function, psychological distress, tolerance, and history of alcohol or drug abuse (Table 22.3). This instrument was highly predictive for opioid responsiveness, but inaccurate in predicting pain[3].

A Cancer Pain Prognostic Scale (CPS) by Hwang and colleagues was developed to predict opioid responsiveness during the first 2 weeks of opioid therapy in cancer patients[53]. The CPS instrument used four dimensions to assess pain responsiveness assessed on a weekly basis. The four dimensions were pain characteristics, social situation, symptom distress and overall quality of life. Significant predictors to pain relief differed in the first and second week and none of the variables predicted pain response in the third week after initiating opioids. Independent predictors in the first week were initial pain severity, emotional well being and anxiety. Independent predictors of pain relief during the second week included opioid dose, emotional well-being, nociceptive pain and a history of alcohol abuse[53]. Neuropathic pain was not a predictor. Patients who were initially on lower opioid doses were predicted to respond well to opioids. The authors suggested this was due to the under treatment of pain before entering the study. Higher pain severity predicted better responsiveness for the same reason. Emotional well-being was an important variable for both weeks.

In a study of 7200 hospice patients, opioid doses were inversely related to age and correlated with primary site, but not gender. The mean daily morphine dose (or equivalent) in this study was 140 mg for women and 158 mg for men[54].

In summary, two predictive scales for opioid response have been developed for cancer pain. Both scales better predict opioid responsiveness than resistance. Study variables are more predictable in the short, rather than long term. These variables are multidimensional. Therefore, focusing upon pain characteristics only without taking into account patient characteristics will inaccurately predict opioid responsiveness.

Therapeutic approach to pain poorly responsive to opioids

Several strategies have been used to overcome opioid resistant pain[1,55–57]. Adjuvant analgesics may relieve pain independent of opioids and when added to opioids allow for dose reduction without precipitating pain relapse[56]. Drugs to treat opioid side effects facilitate opioid titration and extend the opioid therapeutic index[56]. Route conversion or opioid switch (rotation) will usually re-establish pain control and resolve side effects[1,56,57].

Adjuvant analgesics

Antidepressants

Tricyclic antidepressants are able to treat both pain-related depression and anxiety, and also facilitate opioid analgesia through the facilitated release of monoamines within the dorsolateral funiculus. Both serotonin and norephinephrine improve the inhibitory response of the RVM. The activity of primary tricylic antidepressants also depend in part upon alpha2 adrenoceptors on the dorsal horn, which are in close proximity to opioid receptors[52]. Responses to pain occur within low doses of tricyclics and within a shorter period of time than anticipated based upon their antidepressant action[57–65]. Amitriptyline also increases morphine levels through inhibition of glucuronidation[64,65]. Selective serotonin reuptake inhibitors are less effective than tricyclic antidepressants in facilitating opioid analgesia.

The anticholinergic activity of tricyclic antidepressants limits their usefulness. Dry eyes, constipation and urinary retention are particularly troublesome[58] Despiramine may be preferred, particularly in the elderly patient, since it is less anticholinergic and sedative[64,65]. The antihistaminic effects of tricyclics cause sedation and hypotension. Arrhythmias can occur in those individuals with a prolonged QTc interval on electrocardiogram or when combined with drugs that can induce arrhythmias.

Sodium channel blocking agents

Resting neurons have sodium channels that are in a 'closed' state. At depolarization, these channels open rapidly and conduct a sodium current across the neural membrane. These channels are then inactivated at the end of depolarization. Anticonvulsants (phenytoin, carbamazepine and oxcarbazepine) and certain antiarrhythmics (lidocaine, flecanide) and tertiary amine local anesthetics (procaine) selectively inhibit sodium channels. These classes of drugs are able to prevent depolarization, suppress repetitive sensory firing and spontaneous action potentials characteristic of neuropathic pain[66].

Anticonvulsants such as gabapentin inhibit glutamate release and block calcium channels[67–69]. Valproic acid increases GABAergic activity and potentiates monoamines[70–72].

Newer anticonvulsants with potential adjuvant analgesic activity are topiramate, (a sodium channel blocker) tiagbine (GABAnergic agonist), vigabatrin (GABAnergic agonist) and lamatrigine (a sodium and calcium channel blocker)[73]. Published experience with these particular agents is limited. Anticonvulsants can be used to treat both central and peripheral neuropathic pain[74–77].

The most common dose-limiting adverse effects with anti-convulsants are sedation and cerebellar dysfunction. Less common adverse effects are peripheral blood dyscrasias and bone marrow suppression. Cardiac arrhythmias can occur with phenytoin and carbamazepine[78]. Comparisons between classical antiseizure medications and newly-released anticonvulsants have not yet been published. However, it does not appear that there is an advantage to a particular anticonvulsant to date. Choices will be dependent upon individual patient's tolerance and drug interactions[79].

Local anesthetics are given orally, by transdermal patch or by spinal infusion. Topical applications of anesthetics are helpful for painful cutaneous ulcers and severe mucositis. Lidocaine patches are useful in treating mononeuropathies without being systemically absorbed and thus with minimum side effects. Mexiteline will work where tricyclic antidepressants or anticonvulsants have failed to relieve pain[80–90].

A recommended treatment algorithm for neuropathic pain divides painful peripheral neuropathies from central neuropathies. For peripheral neuropathies the order of preference is gabapentin, lidocaine patch 5% (if a mononeuropathy), tricyclic antidepressants, opioids and mexilitine[91]. Recommendations for spinal cord injury and central pain are gabapentin, parenteral lidocaine with rotation to mexilitine, tricyclic antidepressants, opioids, and carbamazepine or phenytoin[91]. However, these recommendations are not based upon cancer pain. Many cancer patients have mixed pain and opioids may be used early in the course of illness.

Non-steroidal anti-inflammatory drugs

Recent studies confirm the opioid sparing effect of NSAIDs[92–94]. NSAIDs block the conversion of arachnidonic acid to prostaglandin G2 through cyclo-oxygenase (Cox)[95,96]. Two types of Cox inhibitors exist. The Cox-1 is constitutionally active. Inhibition of this enzyme can lead to gastrointestinal side effects. Cox-2 activity is induced by inflammation, but with Cox-1 is necessary to maintain renal function, and sodium and potassium homeostasis. Analgesia through Cox inhibition was initially thought to be due to its peripheral anti-inflammatory action; however, it is now known that there is a poor correlation between NSAID anti-inflammatory potency and analgesic response[41]. The central analgesic action of NSAIDs probably depends upon Cox-1 and 2 inhibition and the blockade of nitric oxide synthase. NSAIDs inhibit nitric oxide and prostaglandin generated from NMDA receptor activation[97–99]. NSAIDs will also facilitate central serotonergic responses[98,100]. Cox-2 inhibitors relieve pain due to peripheral inflammatory pain syndromes, such as rheumatoid arthritis, osteoarthritis and dental pain, but have not been extensively studied in cancer pain.

NSAIDs reduce opioid analgesic tolerance as a co-analgesic[101–107]. NSAIDs are also documented to have independent analgesic activity, and are reported to relieve somatic, visceral and neuropathic pain.[37,56,97,102,104,106,108–117]. The full benefit of NSAIDs' analgesia takes several days to be realized. Single dose trials will be an inadequate measure of response[92]. In most reported series, opioids have not been optimally titrated before adding NSAIDs so that comparisons with opioid resistant pain may not be valid[92].

NSAID adverse effects may result in end-organ damage, which can be catastrophic at presentation. Renal failure may be irreversible and gastrointestinal bleeding fatal[92]. Paradoxically, cancer patients may have improved appetite and weight gain on NSAIDs through the inhibition of tumor necrosis factor[118,119]. Gastrointestinal damage is both by direct mucosal damage and indirectly through inhibition of Cox-1. Cox-2 inhibitors are not free of gastrointestinal adverse effects and will prevent the healing of gastric ulcers[120]. Elimination of helicobacter pylori infections will reduce the gastrointestinal toxicity of NSAIDs[121–124]. Prophylaxis with double-dose H2 receptor blockers, proton pump inhibitors and misoprostal should be considered if NSAIDs are to be used long term in cancer patients, since they are considered at high risk for peptic ulcer disease[125–128].

Table 22.4 Guidelines for NSAID used in cancer pain

1	Optimize opioid doses before starting NSAIDs
2	An adequate trial is 5 days
3	Start at low doses since toxicity is dose related and analgesia occurs at low doses.
4	Titrate doses to response
5	If used long term, check for *Helicobacter pylori* and use gastrointestinal prophylaxis
6	Be sure the patient is well hydrated
7	Avoid NSAIDs in edematous states, poorly controlled heart failure, hypertension, coagulopathies, hematuria and hemotysis
8	Cox-2 substitution will reduce the risk of bleeding and gastrointestinal toxicity, but may not adequately relieve pain and does not prevent adverse renal effects.
9	Check creatinine after starting NSAIDs (depending upon the duration of therapy and clinical situation).
10	Patients with reduced cognitive function or myoclonus on NSAIDs and opioids should have their creatinine checked often, and doses reduced or NSAID discontinued.

Cox-1 is involved in platelet aggregation such that non-selective Cox inhibitors should be avoided in coagulopathies, thrombocytopenia, dysfunctional platelet syndromes, hematuria and hemoptysis[92].

Both Cox-1 and 2 inhibitors influence renal function. Patients on NSAIDs should be well hydrated in order to reduce the risk of renal failure. Cachexia and reduced albumin levels lead to edema and reduced intravascular volume, predisposing patients on NSAIDs to renal failure and worsening edema[129–133]. Patients with poorly compensated congestive heart failure or poorly controlled hypertension are clinically worsened by NSAIDs. Previously well compensated and easily managed heart failure or hypertension may worsen or become refractory to medical management with NSAID use. Asthma will be precipitated in individuals with nasal polyps by NSAIDs[134,135]. NSAIDs are reported to cause myoclonus and cognitive failure in cancer patients[92,136]. Guidelines for NSAID use in advanced cancer have been reported (Table 22.4)[92].

Corticosteroids

Nitric oxide synthase expression is inhibited by corticosteroids (depending upon the isoenzyme). Type II nitric oxide synthase expression is up-regulated by inflammatory cytokines and blocked by dexamethasone[36,137]. Corticosteroids may be both analgesic and opioid sparing. The former is not as well documented as it is for NSAIDs[56]. Corticosteroids reduce spontaneous discharges from injured nerves. Short-term, high doses of corticosteroids are used for cord compressions. Dexamethasone dose–response relationships are not established. Lower doses reduces the risk of side effects in cancer patients[138,139]. The benefits of corticosteroids decrease with time due, in part, to their side effects: diabetes, cognitive failure, myopathy and cataracts. Initial treatment should be high dose for a rapid response followed by a rapid taper to the lowest effective dose. Corticosteroids will cause hypertension through nitric oxide suppression in the kidney[133].

NMDA receptor antagonists

Ketamine is an NMDA receptor antagonist, which can improve pain in opioid resistant pain syndromes[56, 140]. Hallucinations and other psychotomimetic side effects unfortunately limit ketamine's usefulness. Subhypnotic doses are effective. Both oral and parenteral ketamine are successful by case reports and intrathecal ketamine has been used on occasion[141,142]. Several opioid agonists are NMDA receptor antagonists. These include methadone, meperidine, ketobemidone and the dextrorphan derivatives, dextromethorphan and levorphanol[140,143–147]. In animal studies, synergistic interactions between NMDA receptor antagonists and opioid receptor agonists are limited to MOR receptors[148]. Opioids that block NMDA receptors will relieve pain even if ketamine plus an opioid has failed to do so. Methadone has successfully relieved pain unresponsive to combinations of morphine and ketamine[144]. This is due, in part, to differences in opioid receptors binding and differences in interactions on the NMDA receptor[144]. Difficult pain syndromes such as tenesmus and perineal neuropathic pain unresponsive to morphine, are reported to respond to methadone[149]. Memantine and amantidine are NMDA antagonists, but clinical experience with these agents in advanced cancer pain is meager[145]. Memantine has been demonstrated to reduce opioid physical dependence[150].

Intravenous magnesium (which is assumed to block NMDA receptors) has been reported to reduce neuropathic pain[151].

Calcium channel blockers

Interference with calcium influx reduces opioid tolerance in experimental animals[152–158]. The prevention of calcium influx curtails NMDA receptor activation and opioid receptor phosphorylation. Calcium channel blockers reduces opioid analgesic tolerance. Nimodipine is reported to be opioid sparing in one trial. Nifedipine enhances epidural morphine analgesia[159]. However, not all trials with calcium channel blockers have been positive.

Strategies to treat opioid adverse effects

Opioid side effects are drug-, dose-, route- and patient-dependent. Drug interactions limit the therapeutic index of opioids[56,160]. There are wide individual differences in dose tolerance and unpredictable occurrences of side effects. Tolerance to opioid-induced nausea and vomiting usually develops rapidly over several days. However, some patients have persistent nausea and vomiting requiring a change in opioid and/or antiemetic therapy. Opioids reduce gastric motility, stimulate the area postrema and induce vertigo as a cause of nausea and vomiting[56]. Other causes of nausea and vomiting should be excluded before accepting opioids as the main culprit[161]. Converting opioids to parenteral and/or the use of metoclopramide or haloperidol are appropriate strategies until tolerance to nausea develops. Prochlorperazine, dimenhydrinate, promethazine and transdermal scopolamine may be used particularly if vertigo is present[160]. Opioid rotation may be necessary for persistent nausea and vomiting[160].

Drowsiness occurs with initial opioid titration. Tolerance to drowsiness develops rapidly, usually over several days. Patients with persistent drowsiness should be screened for metabolic disorders, such as hypercalcium or hyponatremia. Sedation is potentiated by other drugs, such as sedatives, or by central nervous system metastases. Progressive drowsiness while on stable opioid doses can be due to organ failure, which delays opioid clearance[161]. If pain is controlled and drowsiness persists, dose reduction, rather than opioid conversion or rotation is the most reasonable approach. Methylphenidate improves opioid sedation in cognitively intact patients[162].

Mild cognitive failure sometimes occurs with the initial use of opioids and with dose titration. Persistent confusion, visual or tactile hallucinations are usually dose limiting. Hallucinations may be due to co-medications, such as sedatives, anticholinergics, tricyclic antidepressants or NSAIDs. Neuroleptics are commonly used for mild cognitive failure or in those actively dying for whom opioid rotation would be inappropriate. If pain is controlled, dose reduction, rather than the addition of a neuroleptic is more appropriate. In the terminally agitated patient, a benzodiazepine is added to the neuroleptic[160]. Opioid rotation or opioid route conversion are alternatives depending upon expected survival[160].

Myoclonus with opioids is relatively common and usually mild. Patients may accept mild myoclonus in exchange for pain control. Oral morphine is associated with a higher risk for myoclonus than parenteral morphine[160]. If pain is controlled, opioid dose reduction may reduce or resolve myoclonus. Reducing or eliminating co-medications, such as neuroleptics or NSAIDs, may also resolve myoclonus. Baclofen, diazepam, clonazepam, midazolam, dantralene sodium, valproic acid and gabapentin have been reported to improve myoclonus[56,160]. Alternatively, opioid rotation will lead to resolution of myoclonus[160].

Opioid-induced pruritus occurs in a minority of patients[160]. This particularly occurs in increasing frequency with spinal morphine. Pruritus also arises also from uremia or cholestasis, and should be considered as the cause of pruritus, particularly if pruritus occurs after stable opioid doses are achieved. Other medications also cause pruritus. Antihistaminics are commonly recommended as treatment, but are rarely effective. Paroxetine has anecdotally been reported to reduce opioid-induced pruritus[163]. Opioid rotation is an option for intractable pruritus[56,164].

Opioid route conversion and opioid rotation

Patients on oral opioids with side effects and poorly controlled pain should be candidates for opioid conversion or rotation. In the presence of intense unstable pain preference should be given to parenteral route conversion[161]. Patients with stable or moderate pain may undergo opioid rotation or conversion to parenteral opioids[161]. These recommendations are based upon expert opinion, rather than prospective trials.

Opioid route conversion reduces opioid dose amounts and extends the opioid therapeutic index[56,165–167]. Route conversion does not make poorly responsive pain more responsive but does reduce opioid side effects.[168] Multiple routes are frequently necessary in terminally ill patients for reasons other than poorly responsive pain.[169–170]

The basis for opioid rotation is 'non-cross-tolerance'. At the present time the mechanisms of 'non-cross-tolerance' are complex and poorly understood. There are no evidence-based guidelines for opioid choices with rotation[167,168]. Equianalgesic tables provide only broad guidelines for selecting dose a type of opioid since there are:

- population differences between from whom equivalents were derived for whom they are applied;
- large individual pharmacokinetic and even larger pharmacodynamic differences in opioid pharmacology[56,170–172].

Opioid conversion tables are frequently based upon single dose studies, which involve non-cancer patients frequently receiving lower doses of opioids than cancer patients[170]. Therefore, equivalences may be expected to be different for cancer patients who are usually on higher doses and require chronic therapy[173,174]. This is particularly true for those patients on methadone. Opioid rotation improves pain and reduces opioid side effects in 75% of patients who are reported to undergo rotation[175]. Pain control occurs at doses significantly lower than predicted based upon equivalence[175]. Therefore, opioid rotation should be started at 50–75% of equivalence, particularly at higher doses[170,171].

Rational choices for second line opioids after morphine involve consideration of differences in:

- the MOR receptor binding (fentanyl and methadone);
- affinity for opioid receptors;
- opioid receptor type compared to morphine (kappa for oxycodone, delta for levorphanol and methadone);
- the capacity to bind to non-opioid receptors involved in analgesia (NMDA receptor antagonist and monoamine reuptake inhibitors such as methadone and levorphanol);
- the ability to influence opioid receptor adaptation and intrinsic efficacy (sufentanil, fentanyl and methadone).

Opioid tolerance inversely relates to opioid intrinsic efficacy, which significantly changes equivalents at higher doses. Intrinsic efficacy accounts for differences in dose response and dose equivalence between opioids, and is the cause, in part, for asymmetrical cross-tolerance between opioids[176–179]. Therefore, choices for rotation can be from a narrow to a broad-spectrum opioid binding profile or from low to high intrinsic efficacy or both.

Palliative sedation

Palliative sedation as a means of pain control is rarely necessary. In an international survey on palliative sedation, it was necessary for pain control in only 1–4% of those who required sedation.

Opioid irrelevant pain

Pain and suffering is modified by social, psychological and spiritual distress[1]. The opioid irrelevant pain syndrome (somatized or idiopathic pain) remains unresponsive to opioids despite titration. CNS side effects are usually experienced without pain relief[1].

Both pain and suffering have an intrinsic existential and spiritual component, which may be attributed by the sufferer to prior transgressions. The Biblical book of Job is a great example. Pain and suffering were signs that repentance was needed in order to gain relief though the answer was not that simple as Job's comforters discovered. Job never received a direct answer to his suffering and pain, but did experience the comfort of God's presence.

The twentieth century took the optimistic view that pain and suffering could be abolished through scientific endeavors[180]. Pain (and suffering) were thought to be neurophysiological and could potentially be eradicated by drugs and surgery. Much of our medical education is based upon this biomedical model[180]. Suffering, to the modern mind, is material in origin and finding the broken part will lead to mending the situation, thereby relieving the suffering[180]. The pervasiveness of the biomedical model accounts for much of the defects in contemporary health care and the dissatisfaction among those patients who truly suffer. Modern medicine cannot find the cause for the suffering nor mend it[180]. These sufferers remain outside the modern medical paradigm. The cause for their existential suffering cannot be found upon physical examination. However, it can be discerned by an attentive mind focused on the patient's narrative. Such attentiveness and discernment can lead to a dialogue that facilitates the sufferer's search for relief through the discovery of meaning. This requires many skills that are beyond the scope of present day medical science.

> Dietrich Bonhoeffer, a Christian theologian who was executed in the Flossenburg concentration camp on April 9, 1945, wrote:
> it once was said 'Pain is a holy angel, who shows treasures to men which otherwise remain forever hidden; through him men have become greater than through all joys of the world.' It must be so and I tell this to myself in my present position over and over again-the pain of longing which often can be felt even physically, must be there, and we shall not need to talk it away. But it needs to be overcome every time, and thus there is an even holier angel than the one of pain, that is the one of joy in God.[181]

References

1 **Hanks GW, Forbes K.** Opioid responsiveness. *Acta Anaesthesiol Scand* 1997; **41(1 Pt 2):** 154–8.

2 **Mercadante S, Portenoy RK.** Opioid poorly-responsive cancer pain. Part 1: clinical considerations. *J Pain Symptom Manage* 2001; **21:** 144–50.

3 **Bruera E, Schoeller R, Wenk R,** *et al.* A prospective multicenter assessment of the Edmonton staging system for cancer pain. *J Pain Symptom Manage* 1995; **10(5):** 348–55.

4 **McQuay HJ, Jadad AR, Carroll D,** *et al.* Opioid sensitivity of chronic pain: a patient-controlled analgesia method. *Anaesthesia* 1992; **47(9):** 757–67.

5 **Hanks GW.** Opioid-responsive and opioid-non-responsive pain in cancer. *Br Med Bull* 1991; **47(3):** 718–31.

6 **Rowbotham MC, Twilling L, Davies PS,** *et al.* Oral opioid therapy for chronic peripheral and central neuropathic pain. *N Engl J Med* 2003; **348(13):** 1223–32.

7 **Liebmann PM, Lehofer M, Moser M,** *et al.* Nervousness and pain sensitivity: II. Changed relation in ex-addicts as a predictor for early relapse. *Psychol Res* 1998; **79(1):** 55–8.

8 **Liebmann PM, Lehofer M, Moser M,** *et al.* Persistent analgesia in former opiate addicts is resistant to blockade of endogenous opioids. *Biol Psychol* 1997; **42(10):** 962–4.

9 **Mercadante S, Portenoy RK.** Opioid poorly-responsive cancer pain. Part 2: basic mechanisms that could shift dose response for analgesia. *J Pain Symptom Manage* 2001; **21(3):** 255–64.

10 **Evers GCM.** Pseudo-opioid-resistant pain. *Support Care Cancer* 1997; **5:** 457–60.

11 **Lewis C, Linet MS, Abeloff MD.** Compliance with cancer therapy by patients and physicians. *Am Med J* 1983; **74(4):** 673–8.

12 **Basch CE, Gold RS, McDermott RJ.** Confounding variables in the measurement of cancer patient compliance. *Cancer Nurs* 1983; **6(4):** 285–93.

13 **Ossipov MH, Lai J, Vanderah TW,** *et al.* Induction of pain facilitation by sustained opioid exposure: relationship to opioid antinociceptive tolerance. *Life Sci* 2003; **73:** 783–800.

14 **Tso PH, Wong YH.** Molecular basis of opioid dependence: role of signal regulation by g-proteins. *Clin Exp Pharmacol Physiol* 2003; **30:** 307–16.

15 **Wall PD.** The role of substantia gelatinosa as a gate control. *Res Publ Ass Nerv Ment Dis* 1980; **58:** 205–31.

16 **Melzack R, Wall PD.** Pain mechanisms: a new theory. *Science* 1965; **150(699):** 971–9.

17 **Dickenson AH.** Gate control theory of pain stands the test of time. *Br J Anaesth* 2002; **88(6):** 755–7.

18 **Dickenson AH, Chapman V, Green GM.** The pharmacology of excitatory and inhibitory amino acid-mediated events in the transmission and modulation of pain in the spinal cord. *Gen Pharm* 1997; **28(5):** 633–8.

19 **Willis WD, Westlund KN.** Neuroanatomy of the pain system and of the pathways that modulate pain. *J Clin Neurol* 1997; **14(1):** 2–31.

20 **Dickenson AH.** Plasticity: implications for opioid and other pharmacological interventions in specific pain states. *Behav Brain Sci* 1997; **20:** 392–403.

21 **Coderre TJ, Katz J.** Peripheral and central hyperexcitability: Differential signs and symptoms in persistent pain. *Behav Brain Sci* 1997; **20:** 404–19.

22 **Mayer DJ, Mao J, Price DD.** The association of neuropathic pain, morphine tolerance and dependence, and the translocation of protein kinase C. *NIDA Res Monogr* 1995; **147:** 269–98.

23 **Mao J, Price DD, Mayer DJ.** Mechanisms of hyperalgesia and morphine tolerance: a current view of their possible interactions. *Pain* 1995; **62(3):** 259–74.

24 **Chen L, Huang LY.** Protein kinase C reduces Mg2+ block of NMDA-receptor channels as a mechanism of modulation. *Nature* 1992; **356(6369):** 521–3.

25 Elliott K, Kest B, Man A, *et al*. N-methyl-D-aspartate (NMDA) receptors, mu and kappa opioid tolerance, and perspectives on new analgesic drug development. *Neuropsychol* 1995; **13(4)**: 347–56.

26 Mao J, Mayer DJ. Spinal cord neuroplasticity following repeated opioid exposure and its relation to pathological pain. *Annl NY Acad Sci* 2001; **933**: 175–84.

27 Hsu MM, Wong CS. The roles of pain facilitatory systems in opioid tolerance. *Acta Anaesth Scan* 2000; **38(3)**: 155–66.

28 Kawamata T, Omote K. Activation of spinal N-methyl-D-aspartate receptors stimulates a nitric oxide/cyclic guanosine 3, 5-monophosphate/glutamate release cascade in nociceptive signaling. *Anesthesia* 1999; **91(5)**: 1415–24.

29 Dickenson AH. NMDA receptor antagonists: interactions with opioids. *Acta Anaesth Scan* 1997; **41(1 Pt 2)**: 112–15.

30 Eisenach J. Update on spinal cord pharmacology in pain. *Acta Anaesth Scan* 1997; **110 (Suppl)**: 124–6.

31 Wiertelak EP, Furness LE, Watkins LR, *et al*. Illness-induced hyperalgesia is mediated by a spinal NMDA-nitric oxide cascade. *Brain Res* 1994; **664(1–2)**: 9–16.

32 Fine PG. Low-dose ketamine in the management of opioid nonresponsive terminal cancer pain. *J Pain Symptom Manage* 1999; **17(4)**: 296–300.

33 Dickenson AH. Neurophysiology of opioid poorly responsive pain. *Cancer Surv* 1994; **21**: 5–16.

34 Church J, Lodge D, Berry SC. Differential effects of dextrorphan and levorphanol on the excitation of rat spinal neurons by amino acids. *Eur J Pharmacol* 1985; **111(2)**: 185–90.

35 Choi DW, Peters S, Viseskul V. Dextrorphan and levorphanol selectively block N-methyl-D-aspartate receptor-mediated neurotoxicity on cortical neurons. *J Pharmacol Exp Therapeut* 1987; **242(2)**: 713–20.

36 Pfeilschifter J, Eberhardt W, Hummel R, *et al*. Therapeutic strategies for the inhibition of inducible nitric oxide synthase-potential for a novel class of anti-inflammatory agents. *Cell Biol Int* 1996; **20(1)**: 51–8.

37 Mercadante S. The use of anti-inflammatory drugs in cancer pain. *Cancer Treat Rev* 2001; **27(1)**: 51–61.

38 Ettinger AB, Portenoy RK. The use of corticosteroids in the treatment of symptoms associated with cancer. *J Pain Symptom Manage* 1988; **3(2)**: 99–103.

39 Pitcher GM, Henry JL. Mediation and modulation by eicosanoids of responses of spinal dorsal horn neurons to glutamate and substance P receptor agonists: results with indomethacin in the rat in vivo. *Neuroscience* 1999; **93(3)**: 1109–21.

40 Pitcher GM, Henry JL. NSAID-induced cyclooxygenase inhibition differentially depresses long-lasting versus brief synaptically-elicited responses of rat spinal dorsal horn neurons *in vivo*. *Pain* 1999; **82(2)**: 173–86.

41 McCormack K. The spinal actions of nonsteroidal anti-inflammatory drugs and the dissociation between their anti-inflammatory and analgesic effects. *Drugs* 1994; **47(Suppl 5)**: 28–45; discussion 46–7.

42 Yamamoto T, Sakashita Y. COX-2 inhibitor prevents the development of hyperalgesia induced by intrathecal NMDA or AMPA. *Neuroreport* 1998; **9(17)**: 3869–73.

43 Willingale HL, Gardiner NJ, McLymont N, *et al*. Prostanoids synthesized by cyclo-oxgenase isoforms in rat spinal cord and their contribution to the development of neuronal hyperexcitability. *Br J Pharmacol* 1997; **122(8)**: 1593–604.

44 Ammer H, Christ TE. Identity of adenylyl cyclase isoform determines the G protein mediating chronic opioid-induced andenylyl cyclase supersensitivity. *J Neurochem* 2002; **83(4)**: 818–27.

45 Tso PH, Wong YH. Deciphering the role of Gi2 in opioid-induced adenylyl cyclase supersensitization. *Neuroreport* 2000; **11(14)**: 3213–17.

46 Borgland SL, Connor M, Osborne PB, *et al*. Opioid agonists have different efficacy profiles for G protein activation, rapid desensitization, and endocytosis of mu-opioid receptors. *J Biol Chem* 2003; **278(21)**: 1876–84.

47 Xu H, Lu YF, Rothman RB. Opioid peptide receptor studies. 16. Chronic morphine alters G-protein function in cells expressing the cloned mu opioid receptor. *Synapse* 2003; **47(1)**: 1–9.

48 Connor M, Christie MD. Opioid receptor signalling mechanisms. *Clin Exp Pharmacol Physiol* 1999; **26(7)**: 493–9.

49 Maher CE, Eisenach JC, Pan HL, *et al*. Chronic intrathecal morphine administration produces homologous mu receptor/G-protein desensitization specifically in spinal cord. *Brain Res* 2001; **895(1–2)**: 1–8.

50 Selley DE, Cao CC, Sexton T, *et al*. Mu opioid receptor-mediated G-protein activation by heroin metabolites: evidence for greater efficacy of 6-monoacetylmorphine compared with morphine. *Biochem Pharmacol* 2001; **62(4)**: 447–55.

51 Law PY, Loh HH. Regulation of opioid receptor activities. *J Pharmacol Exp Therapeut* 1999; **289(2)**: 607–24.

52 Heinricher MM, Morgan MM. Supraspinal mechanisms of opioid analgesia. In: C. Stein (Ed.) *Opioids in Pain Control: basic and clinical aspects*. Cambridge: Cambridge University Press, 1999. p. 46–69.

53 Hwang S, Chang VT, Fairclough DL, *et al*. Development of a cancer pain prognostic scale. *J Pain Symptom Manage* 2002; **24(4)**: 366–78.

54 Hall S, Gallagher RM, Gracely E, *et al*. The terminal cancer patient: effects of age, gender and primary tumor site on opioid dose. *Pain Med* 2003; **4(2)**: 125–34.

55 Portenoy RK. Managing cancer pain poorly responsive to systemic opioid therapy. *Oncology* 1999; **13(5 Suppl 2)**: 25–9.

56 Mercadante S, Portenoy RK. Opioid poorly-responsive cancer pain. Part 3. Clinical strategies to improve opioid responsiveness. *J Pain Symptom Manage* 2001; **21(4)**: 338–54.

57 Guay DR. Adjunctive agents in the management of chronic pain. *Pharmacology* 2001; **21(9)**: 1070–81.

58 McQuay HJ, Tramer M, Nye BA, *et al*. A systematic review of antidepressants in neuropathic pain. *Pain* 1996; **75(1)**: 160–1.

59 McQuay HJ, Carroll D, Glynn CJ. Dose-response for analgesic effect of amitriptyline in chronic pain. *Anaesthesia* 1993; **48(4)**: 281–5.

60 McQuay HJ, Carroll D, Glynn CJ. Low dose amitriptyline in the treatment of chronic pain. *Anaesthesia* 1992; **47(8)**: 646–52.

61 Ventafridda V, Bianchi M, Ripamonti C, *et al*. Studies on the effects of antidepressant drugs on the antinociceptive action of morphine and on plasma morphine in rat and man. *Pain* 1990; **43(2)**: 155–62.

62 Ventafridda V, Ripamonti C, De Conno F, *et al*. Antidepressants increase bioavailability of morphine in cancer patients. *Lancet* 1987; **1(8543)**: 1204.

63 Onghena P, Van Houdenhove B. Antidepressant-induced analgesia in chronic non-malignant pain: a meta-analysis of 39 placebo-controlled studies. *Pain* 1992; **49(2)**: 205–19.

64 Portenoy RK, Rapscak S, Kanner R. Tricyclic antidepressants in chronic pain. *Pain* 1984; **18(2)**: 213–15.

65 Panerai AE, Bianchi M, Sacerdote P, *et al*. Antidepressants in cancer pain. *J Palliat Care* 1991; **7(4)**: 42–4.

66 Ragsdale DS, McPhee JC, Scheuer T, *et al*. Common molecular determinants of local anesthetic, antiarrhythmic, and anticonvulsant block of voltage-gated Na+ channels. *Pharmacology* 1996; **93**: 9270–5.

67 Fink K, Meder W, Dooley DJ, *et al*. Inhibition of neuronal Ca(2+) influx by gabapentin and subsequent reduction of neurotransmitter release from rat neocortical slices. *Br J Pharmacol* 2000; **130(4):** 900–6.

68 Feng Y, Cui M, Willis WD. Gabapentin markedly reduces acetic acid-induced visceral nociception. *Anesthesiology* 2003; **98(3):** 729–33.

69 Finnerup NB, Gottrup H, Jensen TS. Anticonvulsants in central pain. *Expert Opin Pharmacol* 2002; **3(10):** 1411–20.

70 Maneuf YP, McKnight AT. Block by gabapentin of the facilitation of glutamate release from rat trigeminal nucleus following activation of protein kinase C or adenylyl cyclase. *Br J Pharmacol* 2001; **134(2):** 237–40.

71 Shimoyama M, Shimoyama N, Hori Y. Gabapentin affects glutamatergic excitatory neurotransmission in the rat dorsal horn. *Pain* 2000; **85(3):** 405–14.

72 Johannessen CU, Johannessen SI. Valproate: past, present and future. *Cent Nerv Syst Drug Rev* 2003; **9(2):** 199–216.

73 Willmore JL. Choice and use of newer anticonvulsant drugs in older patients. *Drugs Aging* 2000; **6:** 441–52.

74 Tasmuth T, Hartel B, Kalso E. Venlafaxine in neuropathic pain following treatment of breast cancer. *Eur J Pain* 2002; **6(1):** 17–24.

75 Hardy JR, Rees EA, Gwilliam B, *et al*. A phase II study to establish the efficacy and toxicity of sodium valproate in patients with cancer-related neuropathic pain. *J Pain Symptom Manage* 2001; **21(3):** 204–9.

76 Carrazana E, Mikoshiba I. Rationale and evidence for the use of oxycarbazepine in neuropathic pain. *JPSM* 2003; **25(5 Suppl):** S31–5.

77 Backonja MM. Use of anticonvulsants for treatment of neuropathic pain. *Neurology* 2002; **59(Suppl 2):** S14–17.

78 Jensen TS. Anticonvulsants in neuropathic pain: rationale and clinical evidence. *Eur J Pain* 2002; **Suppl A:** 61–8.

79 Sindrup SH, Jensen TS. Efficacy of pharmacological treatments of neuropathic pain: an update and effect related to mechanism of drug action. *Pain* 1999; **83:** 389–400.

80 Strucgartz GR, Zhou Z, Sinnott C, *et al*. Therapeutic concentrations of local anaesthetics unveil the potential role of sodium channels in neuropathic pain. *Nov Found Symp* 2002; **241:** 189–201.

81 Pettersson N, Perbeck L, Hahn RG. Efficacy of subcutaneous and topical local anaesthesia for pain relief after resection of malignant breast tumours. *Eur J Surg* 2001; **167(11):** 825–30.

82 Desai PM, Desai KP. Combined fluphenazine and lidocaine for pain relief in head and neck cancers. *Trop Doct* 2000; **30(2):** 69–70.

83 Robins G, Farr PM. Pain relief with Emla of ulcerating lesions in mycosis fungoides. *Br J Dermatol* 1997; **136(2):** 287.

84 Stegman MB, Stoukides CA. Resolution of tumor pain with EMLA cream: a case report. *Am J Hosp Palliat Care* 1995; **12(1):** 19–21.

85 Stegman MB, Stoukides CA. Resolution of tumor pain with EMLA cream. *Pharmacotherapy* 1996; **16(4):** 694–7.

86 Devers A, Galer BS. Topical lidocaine patch relieves a variety of neuropathic pain conditions: an open-label study. *Clin J Pain* 2000; **16(3):** 205–8.

87 Gammaitoni AR, Alvarez NA, Galer BS. Safety and tolerability of the lidocaine patch 5%, a targeted peripheral analgesic: a review of the literature. *J Clin Pharmacol* 2003; **43(2):** 111–17.

88 **Argoff CE.** New analagesics for neuropathic pain: the lidocaine patch. *Clin J Pain* 2000; **16(2 Suppl)**: S62–6.

89 **Massey GV, Pedigo S, Dunn NL, et al.** Continuous infusion for the relief of refractory malignant pain in a terminally ill pediatric cancer patient. *J Pediat Hemat Oncol* 2002; **24(7)**: 566–8.

90 **Carter GT, Galer BS.** Advances in the management of neuropathic pain. *Phys Med Rehab Clin N Am* 2001; **12(2)**: 447–59.

91 **Galer BS, Dworkin RH.** *A Clinical Guide to Neuropathic Pain.* London: McGraw-Hill Co. 2000.

92 **Jenkins CA, Bruera E.** Nonsteroidal anti-inflammatory drugs as adjuvant analgesics in cancer patients. *Palliat Med* 1999; **13**: 183–96.

93 **Mercadante S, Fulfaro F, Casuccio A.** A randomised controlled study on the use of anti-inflammatory drugs in patients with cancer pain on morphine therapy: effects on dose-escalation and a pharmacoeconomic analysis. *Eur J Cancer* 2002; **38(10)**: 1358–63.

94 **Mercadante S, Arcuri E, Tirelli W, et al.** Analgesic effect of intravenous ketamine in cancer patients on morphine therapy: a randomized, controlled, double-blind, crossover, double-dose study. *J Pain Symptom Manage* 2000; **20(4)**: 246–52.

95 **Dannhardt G, Kiefer W.** Cyclooxygenase inhibitors—current status and future prospects. *Eur J Med Chem* 2001; **36(2)**: 109–26.

96 **Katz N.** Coxibs: evolving role in pain management. *Semin Arthritis Rheum* 2002; **32(3 Suppl 1)**: 15–24.

97 **Bjorkman R, Ullmann A, Hedner J.** Morphine-sparing effect of diclofenac in cancer pain. *Eur J Clin Pharmacol* 1993; **44(1)**: 1–5.

98 **Bjorkman R.** Central antinociceptive effects of non-steroidal anti-inflammatory drugs and paracetamol. Experimental studies in the rat. *Acta Anaesth Scand* 1995; **103**: 1–44.

99 **Bjorkman R, Hallman KM, Hedner J, et al.** Nonsteroidal anti-inflammatory drug modulation of behavioral responses to intrathecal N-methyl-D-asparate, but not to substance P and amino-methyl-isoxzole-propioinic acid in the rat. *J Clin Pharmacol* 1996; **36(12 Suppl)**: 20S–26S.

100 **Cashman JN.** The mechanisms of action of NSAIDs in analgesia. *Drugs* 1996; **52 Suppl 5**: 13–23.

101 **Gordon RL.** Prolonged central intravenous ketorolac continuous infusion in a cancer patient with intractable bone pain. *Annl Pharmacol* 1998; **32(2)**: 193–6.

102 **Joishy SK, Walsh D.** The opioid-sparing effects of intravenous ketorolac as an adjuvant analgesic in cancer pain: application in bone metastases and the opioid bowel syndrome. *J Pain Symptom Manage* 1998; **16(5)**: 334–9.

103 **Mercadante S, Fulfaro F, Casuccio A.** A randomised controlled study on the use of anti-inflammatory drugs in patients with cancer pain on morphine therapy; effects on dose-escalation and a pharmacoeconomic analysis. *Eur J Cancer* 2002; **38(10)**: 1358–63.

104 **Mercadante S, Casuccio A, Agnello A, et al.** Analgesic effects of nonsteroidal anti-inflammatory drugs in cancer pain due to somatic or visceral mechanisms. *J Pain Symptom Manage* 1999; **17(5)**: 351–6.

105 **Myers KG, Trotman IF.** Use of ketorolac by continuous subcutaneous infusion for the control of cancer-related pain. *Postgrad Med J* 1994; **70(823)**: 359–62.

106 **Dellemijn PL, Verbiest HB, van Vliet JJ, et al.** Medical therapy of malignant nerve pain. A randomised double-blind explanatory trial with naproxen versus slow-release morphine. *Eur J Cancer* 1994; **30A(9)**: 1244–50.

107 **Stambaugh JE Jr, Drew J.** The combination of ibuprofen and oxycodone/acetaminophen in the management of chronic cancer pain. *Clin Pharm Therapeut* 1988; **44(6)**: 665–9.

108 **Levick S, Jacobs C, Loukas DF, et al.** Naproxen sodium in treatment of bone pain due to metastatic cancer. *Pain* 1988; **35(3)**: 253–8.

109 Minotti V, Betti M, Ciccarese G, *et al.* A double-blind study comparing two single-dose regimens of ketorolac with diclofenac in pain due to cancer. *Pharmacotherapy* 1998; **18(3):** 504–8.

110 Estape J, Vinolas N, Gonzalez B, *et al.* Ketorolac, a new non-opioid analgesic: a double-blind trail versus pentazocine in cancer pain. *J Int Med Res* 1990; **18(4):** 298–304.

111 Staquet MJ. A double-blind study with placebo control of intramuscular ketorolac tromethamine in the treatment of cancer pain. *J Clin Pharmacol* 1989; **29(11):** 1031–6.

112 Rodriguez MJ, Contreras D, Galvez R, Castro A, *et al.* Double-blind evaluation of short-term analgesic efficacy of orally administered dexketoprofen trometamol and ketorolac in bone cancer pain. *Pain* 2003; **104(1–2):** 103–10.

113 Ripamonti C, Ticozzi C, Zecca E, *et al.* Continuous subcutaneous infusion of ketorolac in cancer neuropathic pain unresponsive to opioid and adjuvant drugs. A case report. *Tumori* 1996; **82(4):** 413–15.

114 Pannuti F, Robustelli della Cuna G, Ventaffrida V, *et al.* A double-blind evaluation of the analgesic efficacy and toxicity of oral ketorolac and diclofenac in cancer pain. The TD/10 recordati Protocol Study Group. *Tumori* 1999; **85(2):** 96–100.

115 Camp Herrero J, Artigas Raventos V, Milla Santos J, *et al.* The efficacy of injectable flurbiprofen in the symptomatic treatment of biliary colic. *Med Clin* 1992; **98(6):** 212–14.

116 Akriviadis EA, Hatzigariel M, Kapnias D, *et al.* Treatment of biliary colic with diclofenac: a randomized, double-blind, placebo-controlled study. *Gastroenterology* 1997; **113(1):** 225–31.

117 Hughes A, Wilcock A, Corcoran R. Ketorolac: continuous subcutaneous infusion for cancer. *J Pain Symptom Manage* 1997; **13(6):** 315–16.

118 McMillan DS, Wigmore SH, Fearon KC, *et al.* A prospective randomized study of megestrol acetate and ibuprofen in gastrointestinal cancer patients with weight loss. *Br J Cancer* 1999; **79(3–4):** 495–500.

119 McMillan DC, O'Gorman P, Fearon KC, *et al.* A pilot study of megestrol acetate and ibuprofen in the treatment of cachexia in gastrointestinal cancer patients. *Br J Cancer* 1997; **76(6):** 788–90.

120 Deviere J. Do selective cyclo-oxygenase inhibitors eliminate the adverse events associated with nonsteroidal anti-inflammatory drug therapy? *Eur J Gastroenterol Hepatol* 2002; **14 (Suppl 1):** S29–33.

121 Laine L, Connors LG, Reicin A, *et al.* Serious lower gastrointestinal clinical events with nonselective NSAID or coxib use. *Gastroenterology* 2003; **124(2):** 288–92.

122 Hawkey CJ. Risk of ulcer bleeding in patients infected with Helicobacter pylori taking non-steroidal anti-inflammatory drugs. *Gut* 2000; **46(3):** 310–11.

123 Hawkey CJ, Wilson I, Naesdal J, *et al.* Influence of sex and Helicobacter pylori on development and healing of gastroduodenal lesions in non-steroidal anti-inflammatory drug users. *Gut* 2002; **51(3):** 344–50.

124 Chan FK, To KF, Wu JC, *et al.* Eradication of *Helicobacter pylori* and risk of peptic ulcers in patients starting long-term treatment with non-steroidal anti-inflammatory drugs: a randomised trial. *Lancet* 2002; **359(9300):** 9–13.

125 Hawkey CJ, Jones JI. Gastrointestinal safety of COX-2 specific inhibitors. *Gastrol Clin N Am* 2001; **30(4):** 921–36.

126 Hawkey CJ, Laine L, Simon T, *et al.* Incidence of gastroduodenal ulcers in patients with rheumatoid arthritis after 12 weeks of rofecoxib, naproxen, or placebo: a multicentre, randomised, double blind study. *Gut* 2003; **52(6):** 820–6.

127 Hawkey CJ, Karrasch JA, Szczepanski L, *et al.* Omeprazole compared with misoprostol for ulcers associated with nonsteroidal anti-inflammatory drugs. Omeprazole versus Misoprostol for NSAID-induced Ulcer Management (OMNIUM) Study Group. *N Engl J Med* 1998; **338(11):** 727–34.

128 Westlund K. Mortality of peptic ulcer patients. *Acta Med Scand* 1963; **174(Suppl 402):** 1–110.

129 Clive DM, Stoff JS. Renal syndromes associated with nonsteroidal anti-inflammatory drugs. *N Engl J Med* 1984; **310(9):** 563–72.

130 Whelton A, Hamilton CW. Nonsteroidal anti-inflammatory drugs: effects on kidney function. *J Clin Pharmacol* 1991; **31(7):** 588–98.

131 Whelton A. Nephrotoxicity of nonsteroidal anti-inflammatory drugs: physiologic foundations and clinical implications. *Am J Med* 1999; **106(5B):** 13S–24S.

132 Whelton A. Renal and related cardiovascular effects of conventional and COX-2-specific NSAIDs and non-NSAID analgesics. *Am J Ther* 2000; **7(2):** 63–74.

133 Whitworth JA, Schyvens CG, Zhang Y, *et al*. The nitric oxide system in glucocorticoid-induced hypertension. *J Hypertens* 2002; **20(6):** 1035–43.

134 Haddow GR, Riley E, Isaacs R, *et al*. Ketorlac, nasal polyposis, and bronchial asthma: a cause for concern. *Anesth Analg* 1993; **76(2):** 420–2.

135 Chen AH, Bennett CR. Ketorlac-induced bronchospasm in an aspirin-intolerant patient. *Anesth Prog* 1994; **41(4):** 102–7.

136 Potter JM, Reid DB, Shaw RJ, *et al*. Myoclonus associated with treatment with high doses of morphine: the role of supplemental drugs. *Br Med J* 1989; **299(6692):** 150–3.

137 Forstermann U, Gath I, Schwarz P, *et al*. Isoforms of nitric oxide synthase. *Biochem Pharmacol* 1995; **50(9):** 1321.

138 Hanks GW. The pharmacological treatment of bone pain. *Cancer Surv* 1988; **7(1):** 87–101.

139 Hanks GW, Trueman T, Twycross RG. Corticosteroids in terminal cancer—a prospective analysis of current practice. *Postgrad Med J* 1983; **59(697):** 702–6.

140 Dickenson AH. Neurophysiology of opioid poorly responsive pain. *Cancer Surv* 1994; **21:** 5–16.

141 Sator-Katzenschlager S, Deusch E, Maier P, *et al*. The long-term antinociceptive effect of intrathecal S(+)-ketamine in a patient with established morphine tolerance. *Anesth Analg* 2001; **93(4):** 1032–4.

142 Kannan TR, Saxena A, Bhatnagar S, *et al*. Oral ketamine as an adjuvant to oral morphine for neuropathic pain in cancer patients. *J Pain Symptom Manage* 2002; **23(1):** 60–5.

143 Mancini I, Lossignol DA, Body JJ. Opioid switch to oral methadone in cancer pain. *Curr Opin Oncol* 2000; **12(4):** 308–13.

144 Sartain JB, Mitchell SJ. Successful use of oral methadone after failure of intravenous morphine and ketamine. *Anaesth Int Care* 2002; **30(4):** 487–9.

145 Sang CN. NMDA-receptor antagonists in neuropathic pain: experimental methods to clinical trials. *J Pain Symptom Manage* 2000; **19(Suppl. 1):** S21–5.

146 Ebert B, Andersen S, Krogsgaard-Larsen P. Ketobemidone, methadone and pethidine are non-competitive N-methyl-D-aspartate (NMDA) antagonists in the rat cortex and spinal cord. *Neurosci Lett* 1995; **187(3):** 165–8.

147 Davis AM, Inturrisi CE. d-Methadone blocks morphine tolerance and N-methyl-D-aspartate-induced hyperalgesia. *J Pharmacol Exp Therapeut* 1999; **289(2):** 1048–53.

148 Baker AK, Hoffmann VL, Meert TF. Dextromethorphan and ketamine potentiate the antinociceptive effects of mu- but not delta- or kappa-opioid agonists in a mouse model of acute pain. *Pharmacol Biol Behav* 2002; **74(1):** 73–86.

149 Mercadante S, Fulfaro F, Dabbene M. Methadone in treatment of tenesmus not responding to morphine escalation. *Support Care Cancer* 2001; **9(2):** 129–30.

150 Bisaga A, Comer SD, Ward AS. The NMDA antagonist memantine attenuates the expression of opioid physical dependence in humans. *Psychopharmacology* 2001; **157(1):** 1–10.

151 Jaitly V. Efficacy of intravenous magnesium in neuropathic pain. *Br J Anaesth* 2003; **91(2):** 302.

152 Omote K, Kawamata M, Satoh O, *et al*. Spinal antinociceptive action of an N-Type voltage-dependent calcium channel blocker and the synergistic interaction with morphine. *Anesth* 1996; **84(3):** 636–43.

153 Dogrul A, Zagli U, Tulunay FC. The role of T-type calcium channels in morphine analgesia, development of antinociceptive tolerance and dependence to morphine, and morphine abstinence syndrome. *Life Sci* 2002; **71(6):** 725–34.

154 Dogrul A, Gardell LR, Ossipov MH, *et al*. Reversal of experimental neuropathic pain by T-type calcium channel blockers. *Pain* 2003; **105(1–2):** 159–68.

155 Yokoyama K, Kurihara T, Makita K, *et al*. Plastic change of N-type Ca channel expression after preconditioning is responsible for prostglandin E2-induced long-lasting allodynia. *Anesth* 2003; **99(6):** 1364–70.

156 Smith FL, Stevens DL. Calcium modulation of morphine analgesia: role of calcium channels and intracellular pool calcium. *J Pharmacol Exp Therapeut* 1995; **272(1):** 290–9.

157 Antkiewicz-Michaluk L, Michaluk J, Romanska I, *et al*. Reduction of morphine dependence and potentiation of analgesia by chronic co-administration of nifedipine. *Psychopharmacology* 1993; **111(4):** 457–64.

158 Martin MI, del Val VL, Colado MI, *et al*. Behavioral and analgesic effects induced by administration of nifedipine and mimodipine. *Pharmacol Biol Behav* 1996; **55(1):** 93–8.

159 Pereira IT, Prado WA, Dos Reis MP. Enhancement of the epidural morphine-induced analgesia by systematic nifedipine. *Pain* 1993; **53(3):** 341–5.

160 Cherny N, Ripamonti C, Pereira J, *et al*. Strategies to manage the adverse effects of oral morphine: an evidence-based report. *J Cancer Oncol* 2001; **9:** 2542–54.

161 Krakowski I, Theobald S, Balp L, *et al*. Summary version of the standards, options and recommendations for the use of analgesia for the treatment of nociceptive pain in adults with cancer (update 2002). *Br J Cancer* 2003; **89(Suppl I):** S67–72.

162 Portenoy RK. Use of methylphenidate as an adjuvant to narcotic analgesics in patients with advanced cancer. *J Pain Symptom Manage* 1989; **4(3)(Suppl. 3):** 2–4.

163 Twycross R, Greaves MW, Handwerker H, *et al*. Itch: scratching more than the surface. *Q J Med* 2003; **96(1):** 7–26.

164 Katcher J, Walsh D. Opioid-reducing itching: morphine sulfate and hydromorphone hydrochloride. *J Pain Symptom Manage* 1999; **17(1):** 70–2.

165 Kalso E, Heiskanen T, Rantio M, *et al*. Epidural and subcutaneous morphine in the management of cancer pain: a double-blind cross-over study. *Pain* 1996; **67(2–3):** 443–9.

166 Osborne R, Joel S, Trew D, *et al*. Morphine and metabolite behavior after different routes of morphine administration: demonstration of the importance of the active metabolite morphine-6-glucuronide. *Clin Pharmacol Ther* 1990; **47(1):** 12–19.

167 Walsh D. Pharmacological management of cancer pain. *Semin Oncol* 2000; **27(1):** 45–63.

168 Mercadante S. Opioid rotation for cancer pain. *Cancer* 1999; **86:** 1856–66.

169 Coyle N, Adelhardt J, Foley KM, *et al*. Character of terminal illness in the advanced caner patient: pain and other symptoms during the last four weeks of life. *J Pain Symptom Manage* 1990; **5(2):** 83–93.

170 Coyle N, Adelhardt J. Cancer patient and subcutaneous infusions. *Am J Nurs* 1996; **96(3):** 61.

171 Indelicato RA, Portenoy RK. Opioid rotation in the management of refractory cancer pain. *J Clin Oncol* 2003; **21(Suppl. 9):** 87–91.

172 Anderson R, Saiers JH, Abram S, *et al*. Accuracy in equianalgesic dosing. Conversion dilemmas. *J Pain Symptom Manage* 2001; **21(5):** 397–406.

173 Ripamonti C, Bianchi M. The use of methadone for cancer pain. *Hemat Oncol Clin N Am* 2002; **16(3):** 543–55.

174 Mercadante S, Casuccio A, Fulfaro F, *et al.* Switching from morphine to methadone to improve analgesia and tolerability in cancer patients: a prospective study. *J Clin Oncol* 2001; **19(11):** 2898–904.

175 De Stoutz ND, Bruera E, Suarez-Almazor M. Opioid rotation for toxicity reduction in terminal cancer patients. *J Pain Symptom Manage* 1995; **10(5):** 378–84.

176 Duttaroy A, Yoburn BC. The effect of intrinsic efficacy on opioid tolerance. *Anesth* 1995; **82(5):** 1226–36

177 Sosnowski M, Yaksh TL. Differential cross-tolerance between intrathecal morphine and sufentanil in the rat. *Anesth* 1990; **73(6):** 1141–7.

178 Dirig DM, Yaksh TL. Differential right shifts in the dose-response curve for intrathecal morphine and sufentanil as a function of stimulus intensity. *Pain* 1995; **62(3):** 321–8.

179 Morgan D, Picker MJ. Contribution of individual differences to discriminative stimulus, antinociceptive and rate-decreasing effects of opioids: importance of the drug's relative intrinsic efficacy at the mu receptor. *Behav Pharmacol* 1996; **7(3):** 261–84.

180 Loeser JD. Pain and suffering. *Clin J Pain* 2000; **16:** S2–S6.

181 Brown JW (Ed.). *The Martyred Christian*, 160 readings from Dietrich Bonhoeffer. New York: Collier Books MacMillan Publishing Co, 1985, p. 170.

Index